CLINICAL CASE STUDY GUIDE TO ACCOMPANY PRINCIPLES AND PRACTICE OF

CARDIOPULMONARY PHYSICAL THERAPY

THIRD EDITION

CLINICAL CASE STUDY GUIDE TO ACCOMPANY PRINCIPLES AND PRACTICE OF
CARDIOPULMONARY PHYSICAL THERAPY

THIRD EDITION

Elizabeth Dean, PhD, PT
University of British Columbia
School of Rehabilitation Sciences
Vancouver, British Columbia

Donna Frownfelter, MA, PT, CCS, RRT
NovaCare, Inc.
Contract Services
Region 7
Northwestern University
Programs in Physical Therapy
Chicago, Illinois
Committed to Excellence
Glenview, Illinois

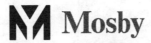

St. Louis   Baltimore   Boston   Carlsbad   Chicago   Naples   New York   Philadelphia   Portland
London   Madrid   Mexico City   Singapore   Sydney   Tokyo   Toronto   Wiesbaden

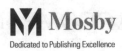

A Times Mirror Company

Publisher: Don Ladig
Editor: Martha Sasser
Developmental Editors: Kellie White, Amy Dubin
Project Manager: Deborah L. Vogel
Production Editor: Mamata Reddy
Designer: Pati Pye
Manufacturing Supervisor: Linda Ierardi

Printed in the United States of America
Composition by Graphic World, Inc.
Editing/project management by Graphic World Publishing Services
Printing/binding by Plus Communications

Mosby–Year Book, Inc.
11830 Westline Industrial Drive
St. Louis, MO 63146

International Standard Book Number 0-8151-2243-8
97 98 99 00 / 9 8 7 6 5 4 3 2

PREFACE

THE EVOLUTION OF THIS BOOK

This book is a companion volume to *Principles and Practice of Cardiopulmonary Physical Therapy*, which is the third edition of *Chest Physical Therapy and Pulmonary Rehabilitation*, edited originally by Donna Frownfelter in 1978 and revised in 1987. Based on an unprecedented number of copies sold and its overall success, this latter book clearly filled a significant void in the textbook market in cardiopulmonary physical therapy. The body of knowledge, that is, physiologic and scientific literature, underlying cardiopulmonary physical therapy, has necessitated significant further revision of this text which is reflected in its revised name, *Principles and Practice of Cardiopulmonary Physical Therapy*, Third Edition, and its conceptual framework, namely oxygen transport. It is clear that efficacious cardiopulmonary physical therapy must be principle-based and prescriptive, and that specific treatment can only be discussed in the context of a specific patient. Therefore this unique companion volume on clinical case studies in cardiopulmonary physical therapy was born.

Because of the increasing specificity of cardiopulmonary physical therapy and the move toward treatment prescription, not every condition could be included in this text. We have therefore selected cases of common primary cardiopulmonary dysfunction, and common, yet often not fully appreciated, cases of secondary cardiopulmonary dysfunction. Consistent with an increasing emphasis on outcomes, defining treatment outcome criteria and selecting optimal outcome measures are emphasized. That optimal treatment prescription should be response-dependent rather than time-dependent is also emphasized.

THE MISSION OF THIS BOOK

Clinical Case Study Guide to Accompany Principles and Practice of Cardiopulmonary Physical Therapy, Third Edition, has been designed to be a learning and teaching tool for students, educators, and physical therapy practitioners.

Students

Students need to establish a solid grounding in the physiology of oxygen transport, the factors that contribute to dysfunction in oxygen transport, and the interventions used to address the various types of deficits in oxygen transport. Students can then practice relating these factors to the selection, prioritization, and application of treatment interventions in actual case scenarios. Proficiency in relating treatment to the underlying pathophysiology requires practice. The progression of the text from basic to advanced cases will enable students to refine their clinical problem solving and decision making skills commensurate with the increasing complexity of the cases.

Educators

Educators can use this book as a source of varied case studies for examination purposes, assignments, and classroom discussion. Each case has been hand-picked to demonstrate a variety of oxygen transport deficits and illustrate the steps in clinical decision making which will be useful to the educator in teaching the principles and practice of cardiopulmonary physical therapy. The progressive complexity of conditions throughout the book parallels the progression of conditions commonly studied in cardiopulmonary physical therapy courses.

Practicing Physical Therapists

Physical therapists without significant background in cardiopulmonary physical therapy will find this book useful in updating themselves in the most recent advances in the specialty and related clinical decision-making skills. Those physical therapists in the specialty will become more proficient at identifying and prioritizing oxygen transport deficits, relating treatments to the underlying deficits, and providing a rationale for treatment selection.

THE INTENDED AUDIENCE

Physical therapy interventions stress the cardiopulmonary system. In this context, every patient can be considered a "cardiopulmonary patient." Regardless of whether they are being treated for soft tissue injuries, or recovering from a stroke, heart attack, or surgery, physical therapy stresses oxygen transport physiologically. The cumulative impact of all these factors in addition to age-related changes in oxygen transport influences treatment outcome. Thus physical therapists in every specialty area benefit from understanding oxygen transport, and the manifestation and impact of deficits in oxygen transport, to treat their patients optimally, that is, with the maximal benefit and least risk. Maximizing the benefit-to-risk ratio of physical therapy practice is particularly important today and in the 21st century because of the demand for evidence-based practice, cost effectiveness, quality care, ethical considerations, and the increased scope of physical therapy practice, e.g., direct access. Further, cardiopulmonary physical therapy has advanced as a unique specialty, thus this book is directed toward physical therapists responsible for basic and advanced levels of practice, and toward physical therapists in other specialties.

THE SPECIFIC GOALS OF THIS TEXT

1. To provide an applied text on clinical problem solving and clinical decision making based on oxygen transport and the remediation of oxygen transport deficits
2. To serve as a study guide for physical therapy students in conjunction with *Principles and Practice of Cardiopulmonary Physical Therapy,* 3rd Edition
3. To provide a source of case studies for the educator for examination purposes, assignments, and class discussion
4. To provide a self-contained text on clinical problem solving and decision making for practicing physical therapists
5. To provide a resource and reference book to physical therapists across all specialties given that physical therapy imposes physiologic stress on oxygen transport and that a vast number of systemic conditions have cardiopulmonary manifestations
6. To provide a broad spectrum of cases involving a variety of oxygen transport deficits for physical therapists preparing for the cardiopulmonary specialty board examinations

THE ORGANIZATION OF THIS BOOK

This book is designed to be used both in conjunction with *Principles and Practice of Cardiopulmonary Physical Therapy,* Third Edition, and on its own. Two introductory chapters, one on the elements of oxygen transport and one on the identification of deficits in oxygen transport, provide the basis for the evidence-based interventions that accompany each case study. The major sections include medical case studies, surgical case studies, special cases, and critical care case studies. The case studies are ordered in a sequential manner such that the complexity of the oxygen transport deficits, hence, level of problem solving, increases throughout the book.

There are four parts to each case study. Each case begins with a concise description of the pathological condition. This is followed by a description of the patient with the specific condition, and a schematic showing the observed and potential deficits in oxygen transport. Finally, in an easy-to-read tabular format, the various cardiopulmonary physical therapy diagnoses appear in order of priority for the patient at that specific stage in the course of recovery, along with the associated signs and symptoms. For each diagnosis, the interventions and their prescriptive parameters are listed, and most importantly, the rationale for the treatment is given.

It is important to note that the cardiopulmonary physical therapy diagnoses and treatment interventions are specific for each individual patient, and not the condition per se.

ACKNOWLEDGMENTS

To Donna Frownfelter for making yet another dream come true. Your dedication to excellence within the specialty and continued support are unparalleled. Thank you for your example.

To Daniel Perlman and Doug Frost for your continued support during the evolution and completion of this project.

To my students and colleagues for your inspiration and inquiry, and for making this volume the best that it can be—my sincere gratitude.

To Kellie White and the Mosby crew for your enthusiasm, support, and excellent editorial capabilities.

My sincere appreciation to you all.

Elizabeth Dean

This case study book represents our view that the cardiopulmonary system needs to be taken into account with all patients. Therapists generally consider the cardiopulmonary system when treating patients with primary cardiopulmonary dysfunction such as asthma or emphysema, yet it is often the limiting factor in the course of rehabilitation of patients with a variety of neuromuscular and musculoskeletal dysfunctions.

Elizabeth and I have always taught our students to take the extra time to evaluate and treat the whole patient, emphasizing the importance of the cardiopulmonary system. This book pulls together our thoughts and specifies the considerations we must make in evaluation and treatment of all patients. I am grateful to my students over many years for your questions and inquiries that have led us to take this mode of teaching to help you find answers. We don't want to give you a "cookbook" method of therapy. We want you to think out the evaluation and treatment plan.

I want to thank Elizabeth from the bottom of my heart for her leadership role in pulling this together. We have been kindred spirits and have discussed and rehashed these considerations on many occasions personally. However, Elizabeth was able to take our thoughts and with physiologic data pull together the cases which would demonstrate our philosophy. The outcome is exciting and one which students and therapists will be able to identify with readily and use immediately.

The response to these cases has been overwhelmingly positive as a teaching tool and an aid to really understanding the role the cardiopulmonary system plays in all patients.

I am thankful to my family, friends, and colleagues who know the toll these endeavors play on personal time and relationships and who have given support and encouragement needed to continue. You are special and appreciated. Thanks. I needed that! I thank God for continued strength and for you all.

I am appreciative to Mosby for their insight and vision that this book was needed as an accompaniment to our text, *Principles and Practice of Cardiopulmonary Physical Therapy,* Third Edition. I also thank them for their leadership and cooperation in this effort.

Donna Frownfelter

CONTENTS

PART I

Clinical Problem Solving in Cardiopulmonary Physical Therapy

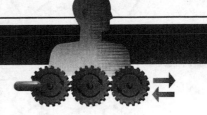

CHAPTER 1

Oxygen Transport: The Basis for Cardiopulmonary Physical Therapy

Cardiopulmonary dysfunction is a medical priority because it contributes to and threatens oxygen transport. In so doing, cardiopulmonary dysfunction can result in reduced function, reduced functional work capacity, and death.

Cardiopulmonary physical therapy is an essential noninvasive medical intervention that prevents, reverses, or mitigates insults to oxygen transport and can avoid, delay, or reduce the need for medical interventions such as supplemental oxygen, intubation, mechanical ventilation, suctioning, bronchoscopy, chest tubes, surgery, and medications. The net effects are reduced morbidity and mortality and improved function and quality of life. A comprehensive understanding of oxygen transport and the factors that determine and influence it is therefore essential to the comprehensive assessment of oxygen transport and its deficits, as well as optimal treatment prescription to effect these outcomes. This chapter describes the fundamental steps in the oxygen transport pathway, their function, and their interdependence.

OXYGEN TRANSPORT

The oxygen transport pathway and its component steps are shown in Figure 1-1. Oxygen transport refers to the delivery of fully oxygenated blood to peripheral tissues, the cellular uptake of oxygen from the blood, the utilization of oxygen in the cells, and the return of partially desaturated blood to the lungs. The oxygen transport pathway consists of multiple steps to effect the delivery, uptake, and utilization of oxygen by tissues. Oxygen transport has become the basis for conceptualizing cardiopulmonary function and diagnosing and managing cardiopulmonary dysfunction (Cone, 1987; Dantzker, 1993; Dantzker, Boresman, and Gutierrez, 1991; Dean, 1994; Dean and Ross, 1992; Ross and Dean, 1989; Samsel and Schumacker, 1991; Weber et al., 1983).

Oxygen transport variables include oxygen delivery ($\dot{D}o_2$), oxygen consumption ($\dot{V}o_2$), and the oxygen extraction ratio (OER). Oxygen demand is the amount of oxygen required by the cells for aerobic metabolism. Usually oxygen demand is reflected by $\dot{V}o_2$; however, in cases of severe cardiopulmonary dysfunction and compromise to oxygen transport, $\dot{V}o_2$ can fall short of the demand for oxygen. Oxygen transport variables, including the components of $\dot{D}o_2$, $\dot{V}o_2$, and the OER, are shown in Figure 1-2. The $\dot{D}o_2$ is determined by arterial oxygen content and cardiac output, oxygen

3

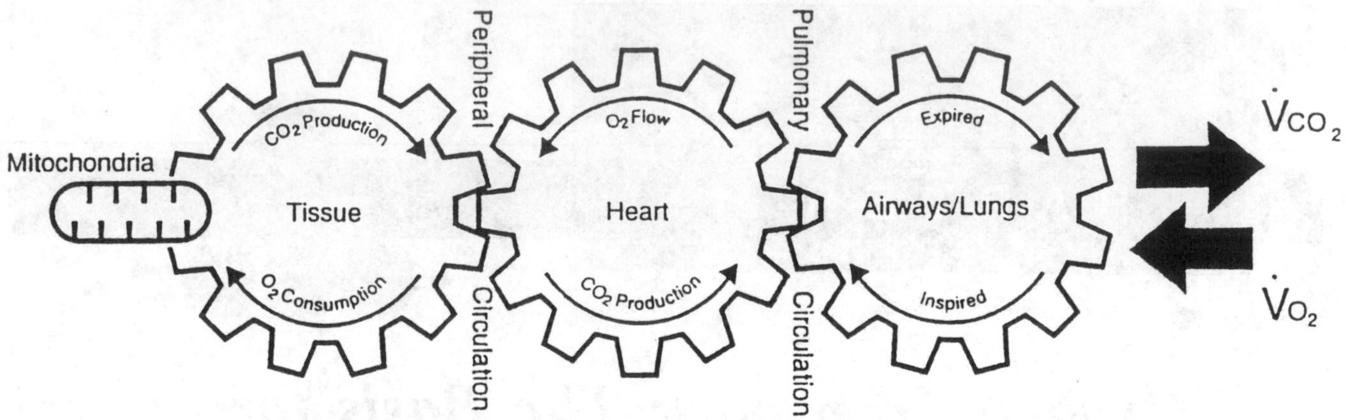

FIGURE 1-1

Scheme of components of ventilatory-cardiovascular-metabolic coupling underlying oxygen transport. (Modified from Wasserman K et al: *Principles of exercise testing and interpretation,* Philadelphia, 1987, Lea & Febiger.)

consumption by the arterial and venous oxygen difference and cardiac output, and the oxygen extraction by the ratio of $\dot{D}o_2$ to $\dot{V}o_2$. Measures and indices of oxygen transport that reflect the function of the component steps of the oxygen transport pathway are shown in the box on pp. 6–7.

THE OXYGEN TRANSPORT PATHWAY

The process of oxygen transport is dependent on several interconnecting steps ranging from oxygen-containing air being inhaled through the nares to oxygen extraction at the cellular level in response to metabolic demand (Figure 1-1). These steps provide the mechanism for ventilatory, cardiovascular, and metabolic coupling. In addition, because blood is the medium responsible for transporting oxygen within the body, its constituents and consistency directly affect this process.

The Quality and Quantity of Blood

Although not considered a discrete step in the oxygen transport pathway, blood is the essential medium for transporting oxygen. To fulfill this function, blood must be delivered in an adequate yet varying amount proportional to metabolic demands and must have the appropriate constituents and consistency. Thus consideration of the characteristics of the circulating blood volume is essential to any discussion of oxygen transport.

Blood volume is compartmentalized within the intravascular compartment such that 70% is contained within the venous compartment, 10% in the systemic arteries, 15% in the pulmonary circulation, and 5% in the capillaries (Sandler, 1986). The large volume of blood contained within the venous circulation permits adjustments to be made as cardiac output demand changes. The veins contrict, for example, when cardiac output needs to be increased. When blood volume is normal and body fluids are appropriately distributed between the intravascular and extravascular compartments, fluid balance is considered normal. When these are disrupted, a fluid balance problem exists. In addition, fluid imbalance affects the concentration of electrolytes, particularly sodium, which is in the highest concentration in the extracellular fluid. Four primary fluid problems that have implications for oxygen transport are water deficit, water excess, sodium deficit, and sodium excess. Other ions that are often affected in fluid and electrolyte imbalance deficits include potassium, chloride, calcium, and magnesium. These electrolyte disturbances also contribute to impaired oxygen transport by affecting the electrical and mechanical behavior of the heart and blood vessels and thus cardiac output and the distribution of oxygenated arterial blood to the periphery.

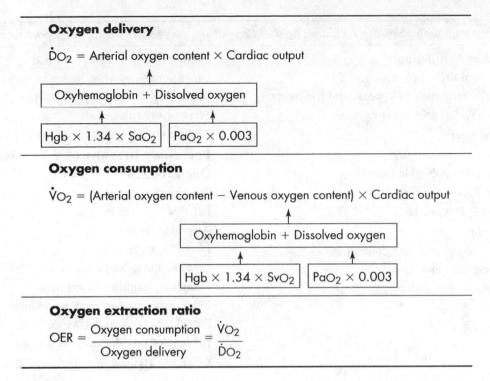

Oxygen delivery

$\dot{D}O_2$ = Arterial oxygen content $\times$ Cardiac output

Oxyhemoglobin + Dissolved oxygen

Hgb $\times$ 1.34 $\times$ SaO_2 PaO_2 $\times$ 0.003

Oxygen consumption

$\dot{V}O_2$ = (Arterial oxygen content − Venous oxygen content) $\times$ Cardiac output

Oxyhemoglobin + Dissolved oxygen

Hgb $\times$ 1.34 $\times$ SvO_2 PaO_2 $\times$ 0.003

Oxygen extraction ratio

$$OER = \frac{\text{Oxygen consumption}}{\text{Oxygen delivery}} = \frac{\dot{V}O_2}{\dot{D}O_2}$$

FIGURE 1-2

Formulas for determining oxygen delivery ($\dot{D}O_2$), oxygen consumption ($\dot{V}O_2$), and oxygen extraction ratio (OER). (Modified from Epstein CD, Henning RJ: Oxygen transport variables in the identification and treatment of tissue hypoxia, *Heart Lung* 22:328-348, 1993.)

Blood is a viscous fluid composed of cells and plasma. Because 99% of the blood is red blood cells, the white blood cells play almost no role in determining the physical characteristics of blood.

Hematocrit refers to the proportion of blood that is cells. The normal hematocrit is 38% for women and 42% for men. Blood is several times as viscous as water; this increases the difficulty with which blood is pumped through the heart and flows through vessels. The greater the number of cells, the greater the friction between the layers of blood, increasing viscosity. Thus the viscosity of the blood increases significantly with increases in hematocrit. An increase in hematocrit such as in polycythemia increases blood viscosity significantly. The concentration and types of protein in the plasma affect viscosity to a lesser extent.

In the adult, red blood cells are produced in the marrow of the membranous bones (e.g., the vertebrae, sternum, ribs, and pelvis). The production of red blood cells from these sites is diminished with age. Tissue oxygenation is the basic regulator of red blood cell production. Hypoxia stimulates red blood cell production through erythropoietin production in bone.

Viscosity of the blood has its greatest effect in the small vessels. Blood flow is considerably reduced in small vessels, resulting in aggregates of red blood cells adhering to the vessel walls. This effect is not offset by the tendency of the blood to become less viscous in small vessels because of the alignment of the blood cells flowing through, which minimizes the frictional forces between layers of flowing blood cells.

The major function of the red blood cells is to transport hemoglobin, which in turn carries oxygen from the lungs to the tissues. Red blood cells also contain a large quantity of carbonic anhydrase, which catalyzes the reaction between carbon dioxide and water. The rapidity of this reaction makes it possible for blood to react with large quantities of carbon dioxide to transport it from the tissues to the lungs for elimination.

Measures and Indices of the Function of the Steps in the Oxygen Transport Pathway

Control of Ventilation

P0.1 (central drive to breathe)

Ventilatory responses to hypoxia and hypercapnia

Pao_2 and Sao_2 responses to exercise

Inspired Gas

Alveolar oxygen pressure

Alveolar carbon dioxide pressure

Alveolar nitrogen pressure

Hematologic Variables

Hemoglobin

Plasma proteins and their concentrations

Red blood cells and count

White blood cells and count

Platelets

Clotting factors

Clotting times

Hematocrit

Pao_2

$Paco_2$ (end tidal CO_2)

$P(A-a)o_2$

Cao_2

$C\dot{v}o_2$

$C(a-v)o_2$ difference

Hco_3

Sao_2

pH

Pao_2/PAo_2

Pao_2/Fio_2

Serum lactate

Pulmonary Variables

Minute ventilation

Tidal volume

Respiratory rate

Dead space volume

Alveolar volume

Alveolar ventilation

Distribution of ventilation

Static and dynamic lung compliance

Airway resistance

Functional residual capacity

Closing volume

Vital capacity

Forced expiratory volumes and flows

Pulmonary Variables—cont'd

Other pulmonary volumes, capacities, and flow rates

Inspiratory and expiratory pressures

Work of breathing

Respiratory muscle strength and endurance

Pulmonary Hemodynamic Variables

Cardiac output

Total perfusion

Distribution of perfusion

Anatomic shunt

Physiologic shunt

Systolic and diastolic pulmonary artery pressures

Pulmonary capillary blood flow

Pulmonary capillary wedge pressure

Pulmonary vascular resistance

Pulmonary vascular resistance index

Systemic Hemodynamic Variables

Heart rate

Electrocardiogram

Systemic blood pressure

Mean arterial blood pressure

Systemic vascular resistance

Systemic vascular resistance index

Central venous pressure

Pulmonary artery pressures

Wedge pressure

Blood volume

Cardiac output

Cardiac index

Stroke volume

Stroke index

Shunt fraction

Ejection fraction

Left ventricular work

Right ventricular work

Fluid balance

Renal output

Creatinine clearance and blood urea nitrogen

Diffusion

$\dot{D}(A-a)o_2$

Diffusing capacity

Diffusing capacity/alveolar volume

Measures and Indices of the Function of the Steps in the Oxygen Transport Pathway—cont'd

Gas Exchange

Oxygen consumption ($\dot{V}o_2$)

Carbon dioxide production ($\dot{V}co_2$)

Respiratory exchange ratio ($\dot{V}co_2/\dot{V}o_2$)

Ventilation and perfusion matching

Pao_2/PAo_2

$P(A-a)o_2$

Oxygen Extraction and Utilization

Oxygen extraction ratio ($\dot{V}o_2/\dot{D}o_2$)

$C(a-v)o_2$ difference

Oxygen Extraction and Utilization—cont'd

$P(a-v)o_2$ difference

Svo_2

Metabolic enzymes at the cellular level

Oxyhemoglobin dissociation

Adequacy of Tissue Perfusion and Oxygen Transport

Tissue oxygenation

Tissue pH

Hemoglobin is contained within red blood cells up to a concentration of 34 gm per 100 ml of cells. Each gram of hemoglobin is capable of combining with 1.34 ml of oxygen (Figure 1-2). Thus in healthy women 19 ml of oxygen can be carried in the blood, given that the whole blood of women contains an average of 14 gm per 100 ml of blood; in healthy men 21 ml of oxygen can be carried in the blood, given that the whole blood of men contains 16 gm per 100 ml of blood.

Clotting factors of the blood are normally in a proportion that does not promote clotting. Factors that promote coagulation (procoagulants) and factors that inhibit coagulation (anticoagulants) circulate in the blood. In the event of a ruptured blood vessel, prothrombin is converted to thrombin, which catalyzes the transformation of fibrinogen to fibrin threads. This fibrin mesh captures platelets, blood cells, and plasma to form a blood clot.

The extreme example of abnormal clotting is disseminated intravascular coagulation, in which both hemorrhage and coagulation occur simultaneously. The acute form of this syndrome occurs in critically ill patients with multiorgan system failure. The chronic form of the syndrome occurs in chronic conditions such as neoplastic disease.

Plasma is the extracellular fluid of the blood and is 7% proteins, namely, albumin, globulin, and fibrinogen. The primary function of the albumin and to a lesser extent globulin and fibrinogen is to create osmotic pressure at the capillary membrane and prevent fluid leaking into the interstitial spaces. The globulins serve as carriers for transporting substances in the blood and serve as antibodies to fight infection and toxicity. Fibrinogen is fundamental to blood clotting. The majority of blood proteins, including hemoglobin, are excellent acid-base buffers and are responsible for 70% of all buffering capability of whole blood.

Blood flow (Q) depends on a pressure gradient (P) and vascular resistance (R); that is, $Q = P/R$. Hence, blood flow equals the pressure gradient divided by resistance. The length of a given blood vessel and the viscosity of the blood are also determinants of blood flow.

The average blood volume is 5000 ml. Approximately 3000 ml of this is plasma and 2000 ml is red blood cells. These values vary according to gender, weight, and other factors. Normally, changes in blood volume reflect deficits and excesses of fluid through imbalances created by losses through the skin and respiratory tract and through urinary, sweat, and fecal losses. Exercise and hot weather are major challenges to fluid balance in health.

The plasma contains large quantities of sodium and chloride ions and small amounts of potassium, calcium, magnesium, phosphate, sulfate, and organic acid ions. In addition, plasma contains a large amount of protein. The large ionic constituents of the plasma are responsible for regulating intracellular and extracellular fluid volumes and the osmotic factors that cause shifts of fluid between the intracellular and extracellular compartments.

Oxyhemoglobin Dissociation

The demand for oxygen at the cellular level changes with moment-to-moment fluctuations in metabolic demand. The properties of oxyhemoglobin dissociation ensure that there is a continuous supply of oxygen at the cellular level. Oxygen combines with the hemoglobin molecules in the pulmonary circulation and then is released in the tissue capillaries in response to a reduced arterial oxygen tension. The S-shaped oxyhemoglobin dissociation curve shifts to the right in response to reduced tissue pH, increased CO_2, increased temperature, and increased diphosphoglycerate (DPG, a constituent of normal blood cells).

The delivery of blood and its ability to effectively transport oxygen is central to all steps in the oxygen transport pathway and must be considered at each step in clinical problem solving and decision making.

STEPS IN THE OXYGEN TRANSPORT PATHWAY
Step 1: Inspired Oxygen and Quality of the Ambient Air

In health, the concentration of inspired oxygen is relatively constant at 21% unless the individual is at altitude. The fraction of inspired oxygen is reduced the higher the elevation.

Atmospheric air consists of 79% nitrogen, 20.97% oxygen, and 0.03% carbon dioxide. Because nitrogen is not absorbed in the lungs, it has a crucial role in maintaining the patency of lung tissue. The constituents of the air have become an increasingly important social, environmental, and health issue because of environmental hazards, pollution, and thinning of the ozone layer resulting in deterioration of air quality, an increase in toxic oxygen free radicals, and a reduction in atmospheric oxygen pressure.

Many factors influence air quality, including geographical area, season, population density, elevation, home environment, work environment, level of ventilation, air conditioning, enclosed buildings, areas with high particulate matter, areas with gaseous vapors and toxic inhaled materials, and smoky versus smoke-free environments. Poor air quality contributes to changes in the filtering ability of the upper respiratory tract, airway sensitivity, and lung damage acutely and over time. Chronic irritation of the lungs from poor air quality can lead to allergies, chronic inflammatory reactions, fibrosis, and alveolar capillary membrane thickening. At the alveolar level, the inspired air is saturated with water vapor. In dry environments, however, the upper respiratory tract may become dehydrated, lose its mucus protective covering, become eroded, and provide a portal of infection even though the air is adequately humidified by the time it reaches the lower airways and alveoli.

Step 2: Airways

The structure of the airways down the respiratory tract changes according to their function. The main airway, the trachea, consists of cartilagenous rings, connective tissue, and small amounts of smooth muscle. This structure is essential to provide a firm and relatively inflexible conduit for air to pass from the nares through the head and neck to the lungs and avoid airway collapse. As the airways become smaller and branch throughout the lung tissue, they consist primarily of smooth muscle. Airway narrowing, which causes obstruction and increased resistance to airflow, is caused by multiple factors, including edema, mucus, foreign objects, calcification, particulate matter, space-occupying lesions, and hyperreactivity of bronchial smooth muscle. The airways are lined with cilia, fine microscopic hairlike projections, which are responsible for wafting debris, cells, and microorganisms away from the lungs into larger airways to be removed and evacuated. The airways are also lined with mucus, which consists of two layers, the upper gel layer and the lower sol layer with which the cilia communicate.

Step 3: Lungs and Chest Wall

Air entry to the lungs depends on the integrity of the respiratory muscles, in particular the diaphragm, the lung parenchyma, and the chest wall. Contraction and descent of the diaphragm inflates the lungs. The distribution of ventilation is primarily determined by the negative intrapleural pressure gradient down the lungs. The negative intrapleural pressure gradient results in the normal uneven distribution of ventilation down the lung (interregional differences). However, there are other factors, such as intraregional differences, that contribute to uneven ventilation within regions of the lung. These intraregional differences reflect regional differences in lung compliance and airway resistance (Ross and Dean, 1992). In patients with partially obstructed airways, reduced lung compliance and increased airway resistance increase the time for alveolar filling. Gas exchange is compromised if there is inadequate time for alveolar filling or emptying, that is, increased time constants (West, 1995). Different time constants across lung units contribute to uneven patterns of ventilation during inspiration. A lung unit with a long time constant is slow to fill and to empty, and it may continue to fill when surrounding units are emptying. A second factor is altered diffusion distance. In diseases in which diffusion distance is increased, ventilation along lung units is uneven.

The lungs and the parietal pleura are richly supplied with thin-walled lymphatic vessels (Guyton, 1991). Lymphatic vessels have some smooth muscle, thus they can actively contract to propel lymph fluid forward. This forward motion is augmented by valves along the lymphatic channels. The rise and fall of the pleural pressure during respiration compresses lymphatic vessels with each breath, which promotes a continuous flow of lymph. During expiration and increased intrapleural pressure, fluid is forced into the lymphatic vessels. The visceral pleura continuously drains fluid from the lungs. This creates a negative pressure in the pleural space, which keeps the lungs expanded. This pressure exceeds the elastic recoil pressure of the lung parenchyma, which tends to collapse the lungs.

The peritoneal cavity of the abdomen consists of a visceral peritoneum containing the viscera and a parietal peritoneum lining the abdominal cavity. Numerous lymphatic channels interconnect the peritoneal cavity and the thoracic duct; some arise from the diaphragm. With cycles of inspiration and expiration, large amounts of lymph are moved from the peritoneal cavity to the thoracic duct. High venous pressures and vascular resistance through the liver can interfere with normal fluid balance in the peritoneal cavity. This leads to the transudation of fluid with a high protein content into the abdominal cavity. This accumulation of fluid is referred to as ascites. Large volumes of fluid can accumulate in the abdominal cavity and significantly compromise cardiopulmonary function secondary to increased intraabdominal pressure on the underside of the diaphragm.

Optimal diaphragmatic excursion requires a balance between thoracic and intraabdominal pressures. Increases in abdominal pressure secondary to factors other than fluid accumulation can impair diaphragmatic descent and chest wall expansion, including gas entrapment, gastrointestinal obstruction, constipation, space-occupying lesions, and paralytic ileus.

Step 4: Diffusion

Diffusion of oxygen from the alveolar sacs to the pulmonary arterial circulation depends on the following factors: the area of the alveolar capillary membrane, diffusing capacity of the alveolar capillary membrane, pulmonary capillary blood volume, and ventilation-perfusion ratio (Ganong, 1993). The transit time of blood at the alveolar capillary membrane is also an important factor determining diffusion. The blood remains in the pulmonary capillaries for 0.75 seconds at rest. The blood is completely saturated within one third of this time. This provides a safety margin during exercise or other conditions in which cardiac output is increased and the pulmonary capillary transit time is reduced. The blood can normally be fully oxygenated even with reduced transit time.

Step 5: Perfusion

The distribution of blood perfusing the lungs is primarily gravity dependent, so the dependent lung fields are perfused to a greater extent than the nondependent lung fields. In the upright lung, the bases are better perfused than the apices. Ventilation and perfusion matching is optimal in the mid zones of the upright lungs (West, 1985). In health, the ventilation-perfusion ratio is a primary determinant of arterial oxygenation. In the upright lung this ratio is 0.8 in the mid zone.

Step 6: Myocardial Function

Optimal myocardial function and cardiac output depend on the syncronized coupling of electrical excitation of the heart and mechanical contraction. The sinoatrial node located in the right atrium is the normal pacemaker for the heart and elicits the normal sinus rhythm with its component P-QRS-T configuration. This wave of electrical excitation spreads throughout the specialized neural conduction system of the atria, interventricular septum, and ventricles and is followed by contraction of the atria and then the ventricles. Contraction of the right and left ventricles ejects blood into the pulmonary and systemic circulations, respectively.

Cardiac output depends on several factors in addition to the integrity of the conduction system and the adequacy of myocardial depolarization (dromotropic effect). The amount of blood returned to the heart (preload) determines the amount ejected (Starling's law of the heart). The distensibility of the ventricles to accommodate this blood volume must be optimal, neither too restrictive nor too compliant. The contractility of the myocardial muscle must be sufficient to eject the blood (inotropic effect). Finally, cardiac output is determined by the aortic pressure needed to overcome peripheral vascular resistance and eject the blood into the systemic circulation (afterload).

The pericardial cavity, like the pleural and peritoneal cavities, is a potential space containing a thin film of fluid. The space normally has a negative pressure. During each expiration, pericardial pressure is increased and fluid is forced out of the space into the mediastinal lymphatic channels. This process is normally facilitated with increased volumes of blood in the heart and each ventricular systole.

Step 7: Peripheral Circulation

Once oxygenated blood is ejected from the heart, the peripheral circulation provides a conduit for supplying this blood to metabolically active tissue. Blood vessels throughout the body are arranged both in series and in parallel. The arteries and capillaries are designed to advance blood to perfuse the tissues with oxygenated blood. Like airways, the vasculature is architected such that the proximal large arteries have a higher proportion of connective tissue and elastic elements than distal medium and small arteries, which have a progressively higher proportion of smooth muscle. This structure enables the large proximal arteries to withstand high pressure when blood is ejected during ventricular systole. Considerable potential energy is stored within the elastic walls of these blood vessels as the heart contracts. During diastole, the forward propulsion of blood is facilitated with the elastic recoil of these large vessels. The thin-walled muscular arterioles serve as the stopcocks of the circulation and regulate blood flow through regional vascular beds and maintain peripheral vascular resistance to regulate systemic blood pressure. Blood flow through these regional vascular beds is determined by neural and humoral stimulation and by local tissue factors. Blood pressure control is primarily regulated by neural stimulation of the peripheral circulation in these vascular beds.

The microcirculation consists of the precapillary arteriole, the capillary, and the venule. Starling's principle governs the balance of hydrostatic and oncotic pressures within the capillary and the surrounding tissue. The balance of these pressures is 0.3 mm Hg; its net effect is a small outward filtration of fluid from the microvasculature into the interstitial space. Any excess fluid or loss of plasma protein is drained into the surrounding lymphatic vessels, which usually have a small negative pressure, as does the interstitium. The integrity of the microcirculation is essential to regulate the diffusion of oxygen across the tissue capillary membrane and to remove carbon dioxide and waste products.

The greater the muscular component of blood vessels, the greater their sensitivity to both exogenous neural stimulation and endogenous stimulation via circulating humoral neurotransmitters, such as catecholamines, and local tissue factors. This sensitivity is essential for the moment-to-moment regulation of the peripheral circulation with respect to tissue perfusion and oxygenation commensurate with tissue metabolic demands and control of total peripheral resistance and systemic blood pressure.

Step 8: Tissue Extraction and Utilization of Oxygen

Perfusion of the tissues with oxygenated blood is the principal goal of the oxygen transport system (Dantzker, 1993). Oxygen is continually being used by all cells in the body; it diffuses out of the circulation and through cell membranes rapidly to meet metabolic needs. Diffusion occurs down a gradient from areas of high to low oxygen pressure. The distance between the capillaries and the cells is variable, and a significant safety factor is required to ensure adequate arterial oxygen tensions. Intracellular Po_2 ranges from 5 to 60 mm Hg, with an average of 23 mm Hg (Guyton, 1991). Given that an oxygen pressure of only 3 mm Hg is needed to support metabolism, 23 mm Hg of oxygen pressure provides an adequate safety margin. These mechanisms ensure an optimal oxygen supply over a wide range of varying oxygen demands in health and in the event of impaired oxygen delivery because of illness. Normally, the rate of oxygen extraction by the cells is regulated by their oxygen demand, that is, the rate at which adenosine diphosphate (ADP) is formed from ATP, and not by the availability of oxygen.

The adequacy of the quality and quantity of the mitochondrial enzymes required to support the Krebs cycle and electron transfer chain, and the availability of myoglobin may be limiting factors in the oxygen transport pathway secondary to nutritional deficits and muscle enzyme deficiencies. Myoglobin is a comparable protein to hemoglobin that is localized within muscle mitochondria. Myoglobin combines reversibly with oxygen to provide an immediate source of oxygen with increased metabolic demands and to facilitate oxygen transfer within the mitochondria.

Normally, the amount of oxygen extracted by the tissues is 23%, the ratio of oxygen consumed to oxygen delivered. This ratio ensures that considerably greater amounts of oxygen can be extracted during periods of increased metabolic demand.

Step 9: Return of Partially Desaturated Blood and Carbon Dioxide to the Lungs

Partially desaturated blood and carbon dioxide are removed from the cells via the venous circulation to the right side of the heart and lungs. Carbon dioxide diffuses across the alveolar capillary membrane and is eliminated from the body via the respiratory system, and the deoxygenated venous blood is reoxygenated. The oxygen transport cycle repeats itself and is sensitively tuned to adjust to changes in the metabolic demand of the various organ systems (e.g., digestion in the gastrointestinal system, cardiac and muscle work during exercise).

Factors that interfere with tissue oxygenation and the capacity of the tissue to use oxygen include abnormal oxygen demands, reduced hemoglobin and myoglobin levels, edema, and poisoning of the cellular enzymes (Kariman and Burns, 1985).

SUMMARY

This chapter describes the oxygen transport system, its component steps, and their interdependence. This framework provides a conceptual basis for the practice of cardiopulmonary physical therapy.

The oxygen transport system is designed to deliver oxygen from the ambient air to every cell in the body to support cellular respiration, the metabolic utilization of oxygen at the cellular level. Blood is the essential medium whose cellular and noncellular components are central to transporting oxygen from the cardiopulmonary unit to the peripheral tissues. The fundamental steps in the oxygen transport pathway were described. These steps included the quality of the ambient air, the airways, lungs, chest wall, pulmonary circulation, lymphatics, heart, peripheral circulation, and the peripheral tissues of the organs of the body. In disease, numerous factors impair and threaten oxygen transport, including underlying pathophysiology, restricted mobility, recumbency, factors related to the patient's care, and factors related to the individual. Thus the physical therapist needs a detailed understanding of these concepts to diagnose these deficits and prescribe efficacious treatments.

References

Cone, J. B. (1987). Oxygen transport from capillary to cell. In Snyder, J. V., Pinsky, M. R. (Eds.). *Oxygen transport in the critically ill.* Chicago: Year Book.

Dantzker, D. R. (1993). Adequacy of tissue oxygenation. *Critical Care Medicine, 21,* S40-S43.

Dantzker, D. R., Boresman, B., & Gutierrez, G. (1991). Oxygen supply and utilization relationships. *American Review of Respiratory Diseases, 143,* 675-679.

Dean, E. (1994). Oxygen transport: A physiologically-based conceptual framework for the practice of cardiopulmonary physiotherapy. *Physiotherapy, 80,* 347-355.

Dean, E., & Ross, J. (1992). Oxygen transport: The basis for contemporary cardiopulmonary physical therapy and its optimization with body positioning and mobilization. *Physical Therapy Practice, 1,* 34-44.

Epstein, C. D., & Henning, R. J. (1993). Oxygen transport variables in the identification and treatment of tissue hypoxia. *Heart & Lung, 22,* 328-348.

Ganong, W. F. (1993). *Review of medical physiology* (16th ed.). Los Altos: Lange Medical Publications.

Guyton, A. C. (1991). *Textbook of medical physiology* (8th ed.). Philadelphia: W. B. Saunders.

Kariman, K., & Burns, S. R. (1985). Regulation of tissue oxygen extraction is disturbed in adult respiratory distress syndrome. *American Review of Respiratory Diseases, 132,* 109-114.

Ross, J., & Dean, E. (1989). Integrating physiological principles into the comprehensive management of cardiopulmonary dysfunction. *Physical Therapy, 69,* 255-259.

Ross, J., & Dean, E. (1992). Body positioning. In Zadai, C. (Ed.). *Clinics in physical therapy: Pulmonary management in physical therapy.* New York: Churchill Livingstone.

Samsel, R. W., & Schumacker, P. T. (1991). Oxygen delivery to tissues. *European Respiratory Journal, 4,* 1258-1267.

Sandler, H. (1986). Cardiovascular effects of inactivity. In Sandler, H., & Vernikos, J. (Eds.). *Inactivity physiological effects.* Orlando: Academic Press.

Wasserman, K., Hansen, J. E., Sue, D. Y., & Whipp, B. J. (1987). *Principles of exercise testing and interpretation.* Philadelphia: Lea & Febiger.

Weber, K. T., Janicki, J. S., Shroff, S. G., & Likoff, M. J. (1983). The cardiopulmonary unit: The body's gas exchange system. *Clinics in Chest Medicine, 4,* 101-110.

West, J. B. (1985). *Ventilation, blood flow and gas exchange* (4th ed.). Oxford: Blackwell Scientific Publication.

West, J. B. (1995). *Respiratory physiology—the essentials* (5th ed.). Baltimore: Williams & Wilkins.

CHAPTER 2

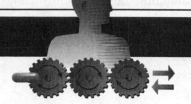

Deficits in Oxygen Transport: The Basis for Diagnosis and Treatment Prescription

Diagnostic skill and optimal treatment prescription in cardiopulmonary physical therapy depend on the therapist's ability to identify specific deficits in the oxygen transport pathway, prioritize their relative clinical significance, and select and apply the most efficacious treatment interventions.

This chapter first identifies four principal categories of factors that contribute to oxygen transport deficits and cardiopulmonary dysfunction: the underlying pathophysiology (acute or chronic), recumbency and restricted mobility, external factors related to the patient's care (e.g., surgery, anesthesia, medications), and internal factors related to the patient (e.g., age, smoking history, obesity). Second, some common deficits in the oxygen transport pathway that impair or threaten oxygen transport are described. Third, a physiologic hierarchy of cardiopulmonary physical therapy interventions is presented. Interventions at the top of the hierarchy are those with the greatest physiologic and scientific basis. Consistent with the thrust toward evidence-based practice, these interventions warrant being exploited first. Depending on the patient's status, interventions in the hierarchy are exploited in descending order. Those interventions with the least physiologic and scientific basis are at the bottom of the hierarchy. These interventions are the treatment of choice when interventions higher on the hierarchy have been exploited and their maximal benefits attained. Multiple treatment interventions from the hierarchy are often prescribed in conjunction with "between-treatment" prescriptions for which the patient or, if appropriate, the nurse can carry out. Fourth, modalities and aids that may further augment oxygen transport and cardiopulmonary function are described. Fifth, evaluation of treatment response is presented.

CATEGORIES OF FACTORS THAT CONTRIBUTE TO OR THREATEN OXYGEN TRANSPORT

Factors that contribute to or threaten oxygen transport are presented in the box on p. 14. The four categories are as follows:
1. Underlying cardiopulmonary pathophysiology
2. Recumbency and restricted mobility
3. External factors related to the patient's care
4. Internal factors related to the individual patient

The contribution of these four factors to cardiopulmonary dysfunction is determined based on the patient's presentation and history.

Factors Contributing to Cardiopulmonary Dysfunction

Cardiopulmonary Pathophysiology

Acute

Chronic

  Primary

  Secondary

Both

Restricted Mobility and Recumbency

Extrinsic Factors

Hospitalization (increased risk of infection, sense of loss of control, anxiety, fear)

Altered feeding and hydration schedules

Surgical procedures (type, position of surgery, duration, type and level of anesthesia, sedation, other drugs, fluid loss, type and number of incisions, type of ventilation, use of the cardiopulmonary bypass machine, blood transfusions, fluid resuscitation)

Dressings and bindings

Casts, splinting devices, traction

Invasive lines, drains, and catheters

Monitoring equipment (invasive and noninvasive)

Medications, including supplemental oxygen and neuromuscular blockade

Medication side effects and interactions

Intubation

Mechanical ventilation (mode, adjuncts, and parameters)

Suctioning

Discomfort and pain (secondary to pathology, wounds, body position)

Intrinsic Factors

Age

Gender

Ethnicity

Religious affiliation

Social support network

Socioeconomic status (lifestyle, nutrition, healthcare)

Education (access to health information)

Congenital and acquired abnormalities

Smoking history and exposure to secondhand smoke

Intrinsic Factors—cont'd

Air quality exposure

Occupational environment

Other environments (indoor, outdoor, rural, urban, industrial)

Ergonomic characteristics of work and home environments

Psychosocial stressors

Coping strategies

Perceived control over health and life

Attitudes and belief systems

Physical restrictions of the chest wall (corsets, restrictive clothing)

Mobility aids, orthoses, and adaptive devices

Occupation (type, hours, environment, commute)

General activity level

Cardiopulmonary conditioning level

General strength

General mobility range of motion of spinal column, rib cage, head and neck, hips, arms, legs

Postural alignment, deformities, limb length discrepancy

Obesity

Underweight

Sleep habits (quality and quantity)

Nutritional deficits

Nutritional status (normal, enteral, or parental feeds)

Absorption deficits

Spinal alignment, static and dynamic posture; thoracic mobility

Chest wall or other deformities

Hydration

Fluid and electrolyte balance

Impaired immunity

Thyroid abnormalities

Diabetes

Electrocardiogram abnormalities

Previous medical and surgical histories

Adapted from Dean E: Physiotherapy skills: positioning and mobilization of the patient. In Webber BA, Pryor JA, editors: *Physiotherapy for respiratory and cardiac problems,* Edinburgh, 1994, Churchill Livingstone.

Recumbency and restricted mobility can be considered to be external factors related to the patient's care. However, they warrant being a separate category because body positioning and mobilization are essential to life, they are primary noninvasive interventions used by physical therapists to directly affect oxygen transport, patients are continually subjected to the effects of gravity and movement stress, and inadvertent positioning and restricted mobility have significant deleterious consequences on oxygen transport and gas exchange.

SPECIFIC DEFICITS IN OXYGEN TRANSPORT

Specific deficits in and threats to steps in the oxygen transport pathway are presented in the box below. The categories of factors that affect oxygen transport can exert their effects at all steps of the pathway (Dantzker, 1983; Weber et al., 1983). Cardiopulmonary assessment and treatment outcome measures are discussed in Chapter 1.

Examples of Deficits in and Threats to Steps in the Oxygen Transport Pathway

Central Control of Breathing

Altered central nervous system (CNS) afferent input and control of breathing

Impaired efferent pathways

Pharmacological depression

Substance abuse depression

Airways

Aspiration related to lack of gastrointestinal motility

Aspiration secondary to esophageal reflux

Obstruction secondary to airway edema, bronchospasm, or mucus

Inhaled foreign bodies

Lungs

Altered breathing pattern secondary to decreased lung compliance

Ineffective breathing pattern related to decreased diaphragmatic function and increased lung volumes, respiratory muscle weakness, respiratory muscle fatigue, CNS dysfunction, guarding, reflex, fatigue, and respiratory inflammatory process

Ineffective airway clearance related to restricted mobility, immobility, sedation, and pulmonary dysfunction secondary to long smoking history, impaired mucociliary transport, absent cilia, dyskinesia of cilia, retained secretions, ineffective cough and mucociliary mechanisms, airway infection, inability to cough efficiently, artificial airway/intubation with endotracheal tube, drug-induced paralysis and sedation

Large airway obstruction secondary to compliant oropharyngeal structures

Chest wall rigidity and decreased compliance

Loss of normal chest wall excursion movements (pump and bucket handle motions) and capacity to move appropriately in all three planes of motion

Chest wall and spinal deformity

Impaired lung fluid balance and acute lung injury

Blood

Bleeding abnormalities, altered body temperature (hypothermia, hyperthermia), fever, inflammation, hypermetabolism secondary to mediator systems

Altered body temperature related to integumentary disruption

Low hematocrit secondary to gastrointestinal (GI) bleeding (more prone to hypoxia)

Anemia

Continued.

Examples of Deficits in and Threats to Steps in the Oxygen Transport Pathway—cont'd

Blood—cont'd

Thrombocytopenia

Disseminated intravascular coagulation

Abnormal clotting factors (balance between clotting and not clotting), sludging of blood

Thromboemboli

Bleeding disorders with liver disease; abnormal clotting factors

Gas Exchange

Alveolar collapse, atelectasis, intrapulmonary shunting or pulmonary edema, shallow breathing and tenacious mucus, body position, consolidation and alveolar collapse, V/Q mismatch, airway constriction, fluid volume excess, pleural effusions, breathing at low lung volumes, abdominal distention and guarding, ineffective airway clearance, pulmonary microvascular thrombi and altered capillary permeability secondary to circulating mediators, closure of small airways secondary to dynamic airway compression, decreased functional residual capacity, intrapulmonary shunting, increased lung surface tension

Diffusion defects

Increased extravascular lung water

Respiratory Muscles

Upper abdominal surgery, weakness, fatigue, neuromuscular disease, ileus related to gastric distention, mechanical dysfunction

Myocardial Perfusion

Coronary artery occlusion

Tachycardia

Potential for cardiac dysrhythmia related to reperfusion

Cardiac dysrhythmia related to myocardial hypoxia

Compression by edema or space-occupying lesions

Heart

Decreased venous return, hence cardiac output, secondary to volume deficit, ascites, myocardial ischemia, hemorrhage, and coagulopathies

Conduction defects

Mechanical defects

Defects in electromechanical coupling

Abnormal distention characteristics

Abnormal afterload

Blood Pressure

Volume deficit/bleeding

Alteration in peripheral tissue perfusion related to acute myocardial infarction, myocardial depression, maldistribution of blood volume, and altered cellular metabolism

Volume excess

Tissue Perfusion

Impaired cardiac output

Impaired tissue perfusion secondary to disseminated microvascular thrombi

Atherosclerosis and thromboembolic events, decreased circulating blood volume, decreased circulating blood volume, decreased vascular integrity, and inflammatory process

Decreased cardiac output related to reduced venous return, impaired right ventricular function, dysrhythmias, increased afterload, and bradycardia

---

Examples of Deficits in and Threats to Steps in the Oxygen Transport Pathway—cont'd

Tissue Perfusion—cont'd

Low oxygen content in the blood

Thromboembolism, vasoconstriction secondary to toxins or sepsis, blood flow alterations, and hypermetabolism secondary to mediator systems

Fluid Volume Excess

Related to excessive intravenous administration

Related to impaired excretion

Apparent hypervolemia secondary to restricted mobility and recumbency, such as occurs from hemodynamic instability

Renal failure

Water intoxication

Therapeutic volume expansion, acute myocardial infarction (MI) and acute renal failure related to renal retention of sodium and water and increased levels of aldosterone, renin, angiotensin II, and catecholamines

Fluid Volume Deficit

Fluid volume deficit related to volume losses during surgery and inadequate oral intake, blood loss, internal injuries such as hematoma, third spacing phenomenon, hormonal imbalance such as increased intestinal motility, vomiting, diarrhea, fluid sequestration in tissues, nasogastric suction and diarrhea, hypovolemia, sepsis, shock, surface capillary leak and fluid loss as in burns and excoriated wounds, fluid shifts

Tissue Oxygenation

Multisystem organ failure with altered peripheral tissue perfusion and gas exchange at the cellular level

---

PHYSIOLOGIC TREATMENT HIERARCHY

A hierarchy of cardiopulmonary physical therapy interventions directed at achieving specific goals related to optimizing oxygen transport is presented in the box on pp. 18-19 (Dean, 1996). The human body functions optimally (including cardiopulmonary function and oxygen transport) when upright and moving. Thus the most physiological and scientifically supported interventions, such as mobilization and exercise, are at the top of the hierarchy, and those that are least physiological or scientifically unsubstantiated are at the bottom of the hierarchy, such as manual techniques and suctioning. With respect to a given treatment goal, the effects of those interventions at the top of the hierarchy are exploited first and those interventions at the bottom of the hierarchy are considered last. Thus interventions such as manual techniques and suctioning are used selectively, that is, if more physiologic interventions do not produce the desired result or if these interventions cannot be applied as necessary to effect the response desired.

Multiple interventions are often indicated to address multiple goals identified in the assessment. The selection of each intervention is based on its indications, determined from the history and assessment and consideration of the contraindications and side effects. Optimal treatment outcome reflects the selection, prioritization, and application of those interventions with the greatest benefit-to-risk ratios.

Mobilization and Exercise

Mobilization and exercise are prescribed differentially to exploit one of three types of effects on oxygen transport:
1. Acute effects
2. Long-term effects
3. Preventive effects

Physiological Treatment Hierarchy for Treatment of Impaired Oxygen Transport

Premise: Position of optimal physiological function is being upright and moving

I. Mobilization and Exercise

Goal: To elicit an exercise stimulus that addresses one of the three effects on the various steps in the oxygen transport pathway, or some combination

    a. Acute effects, e.g., increased alveolar ventilation, mucociliary transport and airway clearance

    b. Long-term effects, i.e., enhanced oxygen transport efficiency at all steps in the pathway

    c. Preventive effects, i.e., to counter negative effects of restricted mobility

II. Body Positioning

Goal: To elicit a gravitational stimulus that simulates being upright and moving as much as possible, that is, active, active assisted, or passive

Goal: To relieve dyspnea

    a. Hemodynamic effects related to fluid shifts

    b. Cardiopulmonary effects on ventilation and its distribution, perfusion, ventilation and perfusion matching, and gas exchange

    c. Body positions to relieve dyspnea and the increased work of breathing

III. Breathing Control Maneuvers

Goal: To augment alveolar ventilation, facilitate mucociliary transport, and stimulate coughing

    a. Coordinated breathing in specific body positions and with activity and exercise

    b. Spontaneous eucapnic hyperventilation

    c. Inspiratory phase coordinated with extension movements, and expiratory phase coordinated with flexion movements

    d. Maximal tidal breaths and movement in three dimensions

    e. Sustained maximal inspiration

    f. Purse lips breathing to end tidal expiration

    g. Autogenic drainage

    h. Incentive spirometry

IV. Coughing Maneuvers

Goal: To facilitate mucociliary clearance with the least effect on dynamic airway compression and adverse cardiovascular effects

    a. Active and spontaneous cough with closed glottis

    b. Assist (self-supported or by other)

    c. Modified coughing interventions with open glottis, such as forced expiratory technique, huff

V. Relaxation and Energy Conservation Interventions

Goal: To minimize the work of breathing, of the heart, and undue oxygen demand overall

    a. Relaxation procedures at rest and during activity

    b. Pacing of activities, exercise, and activities of daily living (ADL)

    c. Energy conservation, that is, balance of activity to rest, performing activities in an energy-efficient manner, improved movement economy during activity

    c. Pain control interventions

    d. Quality and quantity of night's sleep

    e. Quality and quantity of rest periods

VI. Range-of-Motion Exercises (Cardiopulmonary Indications)

Goal: To stimulate alveolar ventilation and alter its distribution

    a. Active

   b. Assisted active

   c. Passive

VII. Postural Drainage Positioning

Goal: To facilitate airway clearance using gravitational effects

   a. Bronchopulmonary segmental drainage positions

   b. Effects on alveolar volume of the nondependent lung, alveolar ventilation, perfusion and ventilation and perfusion matching overall, and chest wall motion and respiratory mechanics

VIII. Manual Techniques

Goal: To facilitate airway clearance in conjunction with specific body positioning

   a. Autogenic drainage

   b. Manual percussion

   c. Shaking and vibration

   d. Deep breathing and coughing

IX. Suctioning

Goal: To facilitate the removal of airway secretions collected centrally

   a. Open suction system

   b. Closed suction system

   c. Tracheal tickle

   d. Instillation with saline

   e. Use of manual inflation bag ("bagging")

Modalities and Aids

Goal: To incorporate the use of those modalities and aids that enhance the preceding interventions

Treadmill, ergometer, chair and bed pedals, treadmill, rowing machine

Weights

Pulleys

Monkey bar

Nebulizers and aerosols

Flutter valve

Bilevel positive airway pressure (BIPAP) and continuous positive airway pressure (CPAP) ventilation

Resistive ventilatory muscle training devices

Incentive spirometer

Cough-stimulating machine

Electrically rotating and moving beds

Silicon inflated mattresses

Walking aids: canes, crutches, walkers, scooters, wheelchairs

Pharmacologic agents

   Oxygen

   Bronchodilators

   Antiinflammatories

   Mucolytics

   Surfactant

   Analgesics

The prescription is based on the underlying etiology of cardiopulmonary dysfunction, that is, an analysis of the four categories of factors contributing to cardiopulmonary dysfunction. The prescriptive parameters include the following:
1. Type of mobilization or exercise
2. Intensity
3. Duration
4. Frequency
5. Course and progression

Body Positioning

Body positioning is prescribed to elicit a gravitational stimulus that physiologically simulates being upright and moving as much as possible. Specifically, gravitational effects associated with the upright position stimulate fluid shifts that preserve the pressure- and volume-regulating mechanisms of the circulating blood volume; the loss of these mechanisms is the primary determinant of bed-rest deconditioning. Additional clinically significant physiological effects of the upright position on oxygen transport include increased neural drive to the respiratory muscles, arousal, alveolar volumes, alveolar ventilation, optimal distributions of alveolar ventilation, perfusion and ventilation and perfusion matching, functional residual capacity, arterial saturation, lymphatic flow, lymphatic drainage, mucociliary transport, secretion clearance, distribution of extravascular lung water, respiratory mechanics, lung compliance, respiratory muscle function, three-dimensional movement of the chest wall, bucket handle and pump handle motion of the chest, cough effectiveness, and work of breathing; and reduced airway resistance, closing volumes, intraabdominal pressure, and work of the heart.

Other body positions, such as side lying, head down, and prone, are prescribed separately to alter lung and chest wall compliance, the distributions of ventilation, perfusion and ventilation and perfusion matching, functional residual capacity, and closing volume and the distribution of pulmonary secretions.

The parameters of the body positioning prescription include the following:
1. Specific body position
2. Duration in each position
3. Frequency of changes
4. Course and progression

The 360-degree rotation schedule is prescribed to simulate the physiological perturbation and "stir-up" effect associated with normal movement and positioning. This rotation schedule is distinct from specific therapeutic positioning prescribed to achieve a specific therapeutic goal. The turning schedule includes as many positions in 360° as possible, including prone, semiprone, side lying, one-half side lying, supine (judiciously), and head of bed up and down variants.

Breathing Control Maneuvers

Breathing control maneuvers are primarily coordinated with movement and body positioning to maximize alveolar ventilation, facilitate mucociliary transport and airway clearance, and stimulate coughing. Inspiration is performed during extension movements and expiration during flexion movements. Maximal inspirations are performed gradually with a 3- to 5-second hold, followed by passive expiration to the end of normal tidal volume. Avoiding breathing below end tidal volume minimizes breathing below functional residual capacity, which predisposes the patient to airway closure.

Pursed lips breathing is a maneuver prescribed for patients with chronic airflow limitation to maintain some splinting of the floppy airways with a post–end-expiratory pressure and promote intrapulmonary gas mixing and gas exchange. It is also prescribed for patients with reversible airway disease, such as asthma, to reduce respiratory flow rates, maintain patency of airways, and minimize dynamic airway compression. Although pursed lips breathing is prescribed, this maneuver is adopted spontaneously by patients in respiratory distress to reduce the work of breathing.

Breathing maneuvers associated with autogenic drainage selectively drain secretions from small to larger airways for evacuation by coughing.

Glossopharyngeal breathing has a role in patients with high spinal cord lesions and patients with progressive neuromuscular weakness. Glossopharyngeal breathing can sustain breathing for several hours or minimally provide respiratory support during short periods off the ventilator.

The prescription of breathing control maneuvers includes the starting position, type of breathing control maneuvers, the depth of breath, the rate, the number of breaths (duration), the frequency of breathing control sessions, and its course and progression. Breathing control is usually coupled with coughing maneuvers.

Coughing Maneuvers

Normal coughing involves a maximal inspiration, increased intrathoracic and intraabdominal pressures, and forceful exhalation and is the single best physiological means of clearing airway secretions. Cough can be voluntary or assisted, the latter being necessary in patients after surgery or with neuromuscular dysfunction (Frownfelter and Massery, 1996; Massery and Frownfelter, 1996). Self-assisted coughing can be achieved using rocking motions, preferably in the upright position or on hands and knees, or a self-administered Heimlich-type maneuver. Maximal inspirations are encouraged during the extension phase of a movement, such as rocking, and a forceful cough is encouraged in the flexion phase of the movement. Assistance can involve the use of a pillow or rolled blanket for support or manual assist, such as applying firm pressure over the anterior chest wall or applying the abdominal thrust during exhalation.

The prescription of coughing maneuvers includes the starting position, assisted or nonassisted, type, intensity of the expiration, number of coughs, frequency of sessions, and course and progression of the prescription.

Relaxation and Energy-Conservation Techniques

Relaxation and energy-conservation techniques are prescribed to reduce oxygen and energy demands on a compromised oxygen transport system. Tension alters breathing mechanics and patterns, causing breathing to become less efficient and more energy costly. Increased tension also increases sensitivity to discomfort and pain, which in turn further interferes with deep breathing and gas exchange. Relaxation can avoid, delay, or reduce the need for potent medications, including narcotics, which are respiratory depressants. These medications also significantly reduce arousal and the patient's ability to participate in treatment. Common relaxation procedures include relaxed controlled breathing, Jacobsen's relaxation procedure, the Benson method, autogenic relaxation, visual imagery, biofeedback, music, and talking reassuringly to the patient. During treatments, relaxation can be promoted by the attentiveness of the therapist to the patient's concerns, speaking in a reassuring and unhurried manner, pacing treatments to minimize pain and suffering, and whenever possible including the patient in decision making and determining how treatment will be carried out to minimize pain.

The patient must learn the relaxation procedure that has the best effect and when to apply it. The prescription parameters of relaxation include the specific relaxation procedure, the duration and frequency of its application, and the course and progression of the relaxation prescription.

The prescription of energy conservation may pertain to activities in general or to conserving energy in a particular activity, such as ambulation.

Stretching and Range-of-Motion Exercises

Stretching of the chest wall, shoulders, and neck is important to cardiopulmonary function to maintain muscle and soft tissue at optimal lengths to optimize chest wall excursion, preserve normal three-dimensional chest wall movement, and preserve normal bucket handle and pump handle motions. Stretching is performed slowly and progressively within the limits of the patient's tolerance. Breathing control is emphasized during stretching. Breath holding, straining, excessive static contraction, and the Valsalva maneuver are discouraged.

The prescription parameters for stretching include the starting position, the specific stretches required, the duration and frequency of their application, and the course and progression of the stretching prescription.

Range-of-motion exercises have important cardiopulmonary effects. Active, passive, or active-assisted range of motion exercises can be prescribed for the upper extremities, trunk, and lower extremities. Sensory input from the joints and muscles and from altered hemodynamics leads to ventilatory stimulation, altered intrapleural pressure, and increased lymphatic flow. Breathing control is emphasized during range-of-motion exercises.

The prescription of range-of-motion exercises includes the specific range-of-motion exercises, the particular movements to be effective, coordination with breathing control, the rate of movement, the number of repetitions, the duration of the session, and the course and progression of the prescription.

Postural Drainage Positioning

In the event that secretions do not sufficiently clear with mobilization and breathing and coughing maneuvers, postural drainage may be added to the treatment regimen. Each bronchopulmonary segment has a particular drainage position. It is important to note that although these positions drain specific bronchopulmonary segments, their effect reflects increased arousal, movement, and positioning effects, including improved alveolar volume of the nondependent lung fields and improved alveolar ventilation and perfusion of the dependent lung fields, in the presence or absence of any effect of pulmonary drainage.

To produce their optimal effects with respect to secretion drainage the specific positions must be used with the specified degree of bed tip. Modified positions are used only with cause—for example, when the patient is too hemodynamically unstable to tolerate the full position safely or is limited by traction or immobilization devices.

The prescription of postural drainage positions includes the specific postural drainage positions, coordination with breathing control and coughing maneuvers, whether manual techniques will be included, specification of the treatment outcomes to establish treatment effect and hence treatment duration, frequency, and the course and progression of the prescription.

Manual Techniques

Manual techniques refer to chest wall percussion, shaking, and vibration and are usually coupled with breathing control and coughing maneuvers. These techniques have not been found conclusively to augment the effects of postural drainage despite being practiced for about 100 years. In addition, these techniques have been reported to be associated with significant side effects. If manual techniques are indicated (when secretion clearance interventions higher in the hierarchy are not sufficiently effective or cannot be applied appropriately, such as in children), they are applied cautiously with appropriate monitoring. Fewer side effects may be associated with single-handed percussion at a frequency of one cycle per second compared with two-handed percussion performed at faster frequencies.

The prescription of manual techniques includes the body positions or postural drainage positions in which they are to be applied, the type of technique or techniques to be performed, treatment outcome criteria to establish treatment effect and duration, frequency, and course and progression of the prescription.

Suctioning

Suctioning is an invasive procedure used to remove pulmonary secretions with the use of a catheter inserted orally, nasally, or tracheally, if the patient has a tracheostomy, and the application of low-pressure wall suction. Suctioning is indicated if the patient has excessive secretions that cannot be adequately mobilized and cleared using other procedures higher on the physiological treatment hierarchy. The procedure is performed in a sterile manner. Instillation of hypertonic saline may facilitate the removal of tenacious secretions. The suction pass time should be within 10 seconds. Mechanically ventilated patients are hyperoxygenated and hyperventilated before and after the procedure to minimize arterial desaturation and airway closure. Closed suction systems are preferable in mechanically ventilated patients because they maintain positive end-expiratory pressure. Hyperinflation can be achieved automatically with the mechanical ventilator. Manual hyperinflation with a manual resuscitation bag must be done cautiously and with close monitoring (e.g., arterial saturation) given the variable tidal volume that may be delivered. An effective cough may be stimulated in some patients from a tracheal tickle, stimulation of the trachea by the catheter without full insertion to the carina.

Based on appropriate indications for suctioning, the prescription of suctioning includes type, size of catheter, use of hyperoxygenation and hyperinflation, means of hyperoxygenating and hyperventilating the patient, use of instillation, depth of suctioning, pass time of the suction catheter (may need to be less than 10 seconds in unstable patients), frequency of passes within a session, and course and progression of the prescription.

USE OF MODALITIES AND AIDS

The interventions in the treatment hierarchy can be augmented with various modalities and devices. Exercise modalities such as the cycle ergometer, chair or table pedals, treadmill, rowing machine, and steps can be incorporated into the exercise prescription. Strength and endurance modalities such as weight training equipment, free weights, and pulleys also can be used. Monkey bars inserted over the bed provide an excellent exercise stimulus for an exercise program, as well as an aid for bed mobility. Walking aids are essential to promote ambulation and exercise stress, such as canes, crutches, and walkers. Lifts are important aids to move patients and change their positions. Lifts are essential for positioning the heavy patient into the upright sitting position with legs dependent. Such aids, however, do not replace the patient's own attempts or assisted attempts at repositioning or mobilizing and are prescribed judiciously.

Specialized airway clearance aids include the cough-stimulating machines and the flutter valve. The incentive spirometer is a device prescribed for patients who are breathing at low lung volumes and may be particularly useful for patients with considerable postsurgical pain.

Pharmacological agents are important aids to augment cardiopulmonary physical therapy, including supplemental oxygen, bronchodilators, coronary vasodilators, antiinflammatories, mucolytics, surfactants, antihypertensive agents, diuretics, and analgesics. The type of medication, dose, possible drug interactions, and time to and duration of peak efficacy are identified to determine the window of peak effect for carrying out treatment. Narcotics are respiratory depressants, have adverse multisystemic effects, and reduce arousal. All these effects significantly interfere with the patient's ability to cooperate with and benefit from cardiopulmonary physical therapy. The team must be aware of the need to maintain the patient in as aroused a state as possible to maximize treatment benefit; alternative medications must be considered that will provide optimal pain control, minimize suffering, and enable the patient to derive maximal benefit from treatment.

Severely ill patients in the critical care unit who are hemodynamically unstable may benefit from advances in bed technology, such as the Circoelectric bed and the Rotobed, which are designed to continuously and slowly move patients in a circular direction or from side to side. Improved mattress technology has improved means of intermittently relieving pressure on the dependent chest wall, bony prominences, and pressure points. By manipulating the mattress pressure, the patient can be moved into different positions more easily.

When using modalities and aids, the patient is monitored closely.

Among the most important aids to maximize the benefits of cumulative treatment are individualized written prescriptions that the patient follows at prescribed times between supervised treatments. Treatment benefit can be forfeited if when unsupervised the patient forgets or fails to perform treatments according to their prescriptive parameters. The written prescription allows the patient to review frequently the relevant interventions and perform selected aspects of treatment correctly. In addition, the therapist can refer to the handout at the beginning of each supervised session to determine if the patient is performing treatments correctly; this is good preparation for discharge. Information that is general as well as specific to treatment is included in the patient's handout.

EVALUATING TREATMENT RESPONSE

Treatment response is based on the use of valid and reliable measures. Relevant cardiopulmonary assessment and treatment outcome measures are presented in Chapter 1. Measures are recorded before and after treatment and often during treatment. These measurements provide a basis for modification or progression of the treatment and an indication of the response to treatment. Measurements reflect the cumulative effect of all interventions that constituted the treatment rather than an individual treatment response, as well as confounding factors such as increased arousal.

SUMMARY

This chapter presented the basis for diagnosis in cardiopulmonary physical therapy, specifically the identification of deficits in the steps of the oxygen transport pathway. Specific diagnosis in turn leads to those interventions that will reverse or mitigate the diagnosis or prevent cardiopulmonary dysfunction. A physiological hierarchy of cardiopulmonary physical therapy interventions was presented. Those interventions at the top of the hierarchy are those with the greatest physiological and scientific evidence; therefore, in keeping with the thrust toward evidence-based practice, these interventions warrant being exploited first. Modalities and aids that may further augment oxygen transport were described.

References

Dantzker, D. R. (1983). The influence of cardiovascular function on gas exchange. *Clinics in Chest Medicine, 4,* 149-159.

Dean, E. (1994). Physiotherapy skills: Positioning and mobilization of the patient. In Webber, B. A., Pryor, J. A. (Eds.). *Physiotherapy for respiratory and cardiac problems.* Edinburgh: Churchill Livingstone.

Dean, E. (1996). Optimizing treatment prescription: Relating treatment to the underlying pathophysiology. In Frownfelter. D., Dean, E. (Eds.). *Principles and practice of cardiopulmonary physical therapy.* St. Louis: Mosby.

Frownfelter, D., & Massery, M. (1996). Facilitating airway clearance by cough. In Frownfelter. D., Dean, E. (Eds.). *Principles and practice of cardiopulmonary physical therapy.* St. Louis: Mosby.

Massery, M., & Frownfelter, D. (1996). Ventilatory strategies. In Frownfelter. D., Dean, E. (Eds.). *Principles and practice of cardiopulmonary physical therapy.* St. Louis: Mosby.

Weber, K. T., Janicki, J. S., Shroff, S. G., & Likoff, M. J. (1983). The cardiopulmonary unit: The body's gas exchange system. *Clinics in Chest Medicine, 4,* 101-110.

PART II

Medical Case Studies

CHAPTER 3

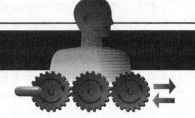

Pneumonia

PATHOPHYSIOLOGY

Pneumonia is an acute inflammation of the lung parenchyma (the portion of the lung distal to the conducting airways) and involves the respiratory bronchioles and alveoli. It may affect a segment, a lobe, or an entire lung. Pneumonia can develop acutely in a healthy person or in a chronically ill patient with another underlying disease. It is characterized by hypertrophy of the mucous membranes of the lung, increased capillary permeability resulting in excess fluid in the interstitial spaces, impaired gas exchange, inflammation of pleurae, respiratory acidosis, and bacteremia. These changes result in an increase in sputum production, cough, dyspnea, chest pain, and fever. Signs of lung consolidation (inspiratory crackles, bronchial breath sounds) can be heard on auscultation of the chest. A chest x-ray is essential in confirming the presence and location of pneumonitis. Pneumonia may be caused by inhalation of infectious agents such as bacteria, viruses, fungi, or protozoa; by aspiration of secretions into the alveolar system, via the bloodstream; or by radiation treatment. Bacterial pneumonia is divided into community-acquired pneumonia (CAP) and hospital-acquired pneumonia. CAP most often infects persons with preexisting disease (e.g., chronic airflow limitation, coronary artery disease) or those with impairments in their immune system. The mortality rate for persons with CAP who are hospitalized ranges from 5% to 15%. About 0.5% to 1% of patients develop pneumonia while they are in the hospital. The mortality rate for these patients is much higher (30% to 50%) because they also suffer from coexisting diseases and there is a high prevalence of gram-negative bacteria, which are resistant to many antibiotics. Thus prevention of pneumonia in hospital is a high priority. Atypical pneumonia is another type of pneumonia caused by bacterial or viral infection in which patients have sore throat, nonproductive cough, headaches, arthritis, myalgias, gastrointestinal symptoms, and viral prodromal symptoms instead of the classic symptoms of acute pneumonia.

Case Study

The patient is a 63-year-old man. He lives with his wife in a two story home. He is the chief executive officer for a major pharmaceutical company and has been under considerable work-related stress over the past few years. He often works 7 days a week. He was admitted with a diagnosis of community-acquired pneumococcal pneumonia. He is approximately 5 feet 5 inches (166 cm) tall and weighs 143 pounds (65 kg); his body mass index is 23.6. He has never smoked. He is acutely and severely ill with the classic signs and symptoms of lobar pneumonia, including a temperature of

103.8°F (39.9°C), heart rate 122 beats per minute, respiratory rate 25 breaths per minute, blood pressure 152/88 mm Hg, dyspnea, tachycardia, pleuritic chest pain over the right chest, hypoxemia, and cough productive of moderate amounts of purulent sputum. His chest x-ray shows infiltrates and signs of consolidation over the right middle and lower lobes. Arterial blood gases (ABGs) on room air are pH 7.48, Pao_2 (arterial partial pressure of oxygen) 78 mm Hg, $Paco_2$ (arterial partial pressure of carbon dioxide) 38 mm Hg, HCO_3 (bicarbonate levels) 28 mEq/L, and Sao_2 (arterial saturation of oxygen) 90%. His past medical and surgical histories are unremarkable except for juvenile-onset diabetes, which becomes labile when he is under stress.

Oxygen Transport Deficits: Observed and Potential

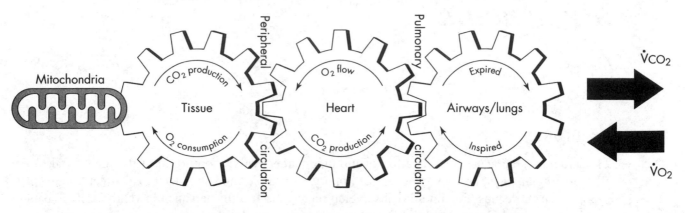

↑ Oxygen extraction

↑ Oxyhemoglobin
dissociation

↑ Heart rate
↑ Cardiac output
↑ Work of the heart

Bronchospasm
↓ Mucociliary transport
Mucus obstruction
↑ Resistance
Closure of dependent
    airways
Inflammatory response
Inflammatory mediators
Exudation
Crackles
Alveolar congestion
Consolidation
↓ Compliance
Alveolar collapse
Atelectasis
Pleural effusion
Pleural irritation
Bronchial breath sounds
Dyspnea
↓ Diffusing capacity
↑ Work of breathing

↑ Blood pressure

Hypoxic vasoconstriction
Shunt
Lymphatic congestion
↓ Lymphatic drainage

Blood: ↑ White blood cell count
febrile

↑	Increase
↓	Decrease

PHYSICAL THERAPY DIAGNOSES AND TREATMENT PRESCRIPTION

Physical Therapy Diagnosis: Altered cardiopulmonary function, oxygen transport and gas exchange: airway obstruction, decreased lung compliance, ventilation-perfusion mismatch, atelectasis, shunt

Signs and Symptoms: Pao_2 (sitting) $< 104.2 - 0.27$ age (± 7) mm Hg; $Sao_2 < 98\%$, increased white blood cell count, increased respiratory rate, increased minute ventilation, increased work of breathing, increased work of the heart, radiographic evidence of atelectasis, and consolidation

INTERVENTIONS	RATIONALE
Serial monitoring of vital signs, dyspnea, white blood cell count, ABGs, and oxygen transport variables	To provide a baseline, ongoing assessment and measure of treatment response To identify factors contributing to hypoxemia and select optimal interventions
Serial monitoring of blood sugar levels	Blood sugar fluctuations alter the patient's response to treatment; treatment may require modification
Monitor respiratory rate, tidal volume, and alveolar volume	To identify cause of increased work of breathing and select optimal interventions
Define outcome criteria: reversal or mitigation of the signs and symptoms	To provide a basis for defining treatment goals and criteria for discontinuing treatment
Place in high or semi-Fowler's position, and in the erect upright position with feet dependent Supplemental oxygen	To optimize alveolar volume, ventilation, forced expiratory volumes and flow rates, functional residual capacity, diaphragmatic excursion, mucociliary transport, mucociliary clearance, lung motion, lymphatic drainage, chest wall symmetry, chest wall excursion, respiratory muscle function, minimize closing volumes, decrease the work of breathing, decrease the work of the heart To reduce central blood volume and effects of cephalad fluid shifts with recumbency
Low-intensity mobilization without undue myocardial work	To prescribe low-intensity mobilization sufficient to exploit its *acute* effects on cardiopulmonary function but within the patient's capacity to meet its oxygen and metabolic demands
Monitor vital signs	To monitor hemodynamic status
Monitor chest pain	To rule out signs of ischemia, ischemic damage, and cardiac compromise
Optimize fluid intake	Ensure IV fluids are flowing and lines are not obstructed during treatment
Avoid active mobilization for at least 40 minutes after eating	To minimize oxygen demand after eating, when blood is shunted to gastrointestinal tract during digestion
Assess for orthostatic hypotension	To prevent orthostatic hypotension and syncope
Monitor serial chest x-rays for signs of and resolution of consolidation and signs of possible pleural effusion	To provide a baseline, ongoing assessment and measure of treatment response
Teach breathing control and coughing maneuvers: inspiration on extension and expiration on flexion, maximal inspiratory hold breaths, passive expiration to normal end-tidal volume, and supported coughing	To promote alveolar ventilation and reduce airway closure, particularly in conjunction with mobilization and body positioning
Teach coughing maneuvers that reduce intrathoracic pressure	To minimize pleuritic pain by teaching the patient to support chest during coughing maneuvers
Coordinated breathing control and supported coughing maneuvers with mobilization, body positioning, and changes in body positioning	To minimize cough-induced chest pain
Mobilization: dangle over bed; stand erect, low-intensity walking (increase in heart rate < 20 beats per minute) Bilateral upper extremity exercises; nonresisted proprioceptive neuromuscular facilitation patterns coordinated with breathing control and coughing maneuvers	To increase alveolar ventilation, tidal volume, vital capacity, ventilation and perfusion matching, expiratory flow rates, mucociliary transport, mucociliary clearance, lymphatic drainage, surfactant production and distribution, chest wall symmetry, chest wall excursion, and respiratory muscle function; and minimize closing volumes in both the affected and unaffected lung fields and thereby optimize gas exchange

Continued.

INTERVENTIONS	RATIONALE
Chest wall mobility exercises coordinated with breathing control and coughing maneuvers (flexion, extension, side flexion, rotation, and diagonal rotation)	
Mobilization: whole body	
Mobilization: upper extremity	
Mobilization: chest wall	
Rhythmic, unresisted exercise coordinated with breathing control and coughing maneuvers	
Intensity—increase in heart rate < 20 beats per minute, increase in blood pressure < 20 mm Hg	
Duration—as indicated; Sao_2 > 90%, within patient's fatigue limits	
Frequency—as indicated; if short duration, frequent sessions indicated	
Course and progression—as indicated by treatment outcomes	
Body positioning: coordinated with breathing control and coughing maneuvers	To maximize alveolar volume, alveolar ventilation, perfusion and ventilation and perfusion matching, functional residual capacity, lung movement, and lymphatic drainage; minimize atelectasis; and stimulate mucociliary transport mucociliary clearance, coughing, and cough effectiveness
Frequent body position changes coordinated with breathing control and coughing maneuvers	
Teach chest wall mobility exercises, such as proprioceptive neuromuscular facilitation	
Type—upper extremity and trunk movements coordinated with breathing control maneuvers, such as maximal inspiration with extension followed by an inspiratory hold, and passive expiration on flexion	
Postural drainage coordinated with breathing control and coughing maneuvers	To promote airway clearance
Right middle lobe	To minimize closure of the dependent airways, emphasis is on passive expiration to normal end-tidal volume
Left side lying, ¾ supine, head of bed down 20°-30°	
Right lower lobe	
Anterior segment—supine, head of bed down 30°-45°	
Lateral segment—left side lying, head of bed down 30°-45°	
Posterior segment—prone, head of bed down 30°-45°	
Superior segment—prone, no tip	
Left lower lobe	
Anterior segment—supine, head of bed down 30°-45°	
Lateral segment—right side lying, head of bed down 30°-45°	
Posterior segment—prone, head of bed down 30°-45°	
Superior segment—prone, no tip	
Postural drainage with selected manual techniques	If indicated, single-handed percussion at a frequency of 1 per second reduces the risk of untoward effects
Frequent position changes at least every 1-2 hours when in bed	Frequent position changes elicit the beneficial effects of physiological "stir-up" necessary for normal cardiopulmonary function, such as altered distribution of ventilation, gas exchange, and pulmonary secretions
Monitor cardiopulmonary responses to treatment	Monitor cardiopulmonary and oxygen transport variables before, during, and after treatment to gauge treatment response and effectiveness and to establish the need to modify treatment prescription parameters
Teach patient to perform mobilization, chest wall mobility exercises, and body positioning coordinated with breathing control and coughing maneuvers between therapist-supervised treatments provided the patient is not likely to have an adverse effect	To prescribe between-treatment interventions that are safe and unlikely to have an adverse effect, so that the cumulative effect of treatments can be enhanced

INTERVENTIONS	RATIONALE
Write out the prescription parameters of the between-treatment interventions (types of intervention and their intensity, duration, and frequency)	Between-treatment interventions enhance the cumulative treatment effects and minimize the negative effects of recumbency and restricted mobility
Check with patient each session regarding the between-treatment interventions to ensure that they are being performed according to the prescription	

Physical Therapy Diagnosis: Ineffective breathing patterns

Signs and Symptoms: Dyspnea, tachypnea, increased respiratory rate, decreased tidal volume, altered chest excursion, diminished breath sounds, cough with purulent, tenacious sputum, abnormal ABGs, increased work of breathing

INTERVENTIONS	RATIONALE
Assess cardiopulmonary status	To provide a baseline, ongoing assessment and measure of treatment response
Monitor respirations for ease, rate, and depth	
Auscultate and percuss chest for decreased breath sounds and dullness	
Assess skin color, constitutional symptoms, chills and fever, and pleuritic chest pain; note sputum and its viscosity, amount, and change in color	
Assess fluid balance	
Define outcome criteria: reversal or mitigation of the signs and symptoms	To provide a basis for defining treatment goals and criteria for discontinuing treatment
Instruct patient in relaxation and positions of comfort	To promote slow deep breaths and an efficient breathing pattern
Mobilize patient to upright position coordinated with breathing control and coughing maneuvers	To exploit the *acute* effects of mobilization on breathing pattern and efficiency
Teach thoracic mobility exercises and coordinate with breathing control and coughing maneuvers	
Place in body positions to maximize alveolar volume and ventilation: upright and moving as frequently as possible within tolerance	Physical manipulation of the patient with body position is the only means of altering the intrapleural pressure gradient and the distribution of ventilation to enhance breathing pattern and normal chest wall movement
Place patient in postural drainage positions	The postural drainage positions augment gas exchange in the dependent lung and alveolar volume of nondependent lung
Monitor cardiopulmonary response to each position	No single position should be maintained indefinitely; even beneficial positions will become deleterious if maintained for longer than 1-2 hr

Physical Therapy Diagnosis: Pain

Signs and Symptoms: Verbal expressions of pain, observation of pain behaviors, guarding of chest, favoring recumbent positions and restricted mobility, breathing at low lung volumes, changes in breathing pattern

INTERVENTIONS	RATIONALE
Assess pain location, severity, frequency, and characteristics, its relationship to condition and activity	To provide a baseline, ongoing assessment and measure of treatment response
Define outcome criteria: reversal or mitigation of the signs and symptoms	To provide a basis for defining treatment goals and criteria for discontinuing treatment
Be responsive to the patient's pain	The therapist's acknowledgement and sensitivity toward patient's discomfort will enhance rapport and cooperation

Continued.

INTERVENTIONS	RATIONALE
Teach patient positions of comfort and relaxation and aids	To minimize pain and chest wall and intraabdominal splinting
Pace treatment and allow for rest periods as indicated within treatment sessions	
Encourage pacing and rest periods of general activity	
Reinforce breathing control and supported coughing maneuvers	To assist resolution of atelectasis, pneumonia, and associated pleural discomfort
Coordinate treatments with medications, (e.g., analgesics and bronchodilators)	To maximize patient's ability to cooperate with treatment and to derive maximal benefit from treatment

Physical Therapy Diagnosis: Altered nutritional state and hydration: malaise, hyperthermia, increased nutritional and fluid requirements, changes in appeal of food, changes in bowel routine

Signs and Symptoms: Too fatigued to eat or drink adequately, inadequate intake of food and fluids, decreased body weight, decreased blood proteins (e.g., albumin), decreased appetite, hypotension, increased heart rate

INTERVENTIONS	RATIONALE
Monitor food and fluid intake	To provide a baseline, ongoing assessment and measure of treatment response
	Interventions are selected commensurate with patient's caloric and energy intake; caloric requirements may double
Monitor intravenous fluid input and urinary output	To assess fluid balance
Note reports of gastrointestinal status	To evaluate gastrointestinal status and intraabdominal effects
Monitor weight	To assess effectiveness of nutritional and fluid regimens and modify mobilization and exercise demands so energy demands can be met by energy supply
Define outcome criteria: reversal or mitigation of the signs and symptoms	To provide a basis for defining treatment goals and criteria for discontinuing treatment
Encourage food and fluid intake	To minimize the effects of nutritional deficits (reduced energy, weakness, increased fatigue, reduced blood protein, reduced iron) and dehydration (reduced plasma volume, impaired ciliary activity, increased tenaciousness and viscosity of secretions, increased airway obstruction, difficulty to mobilize and expectorate secretions)

Physical Therapy Diagnosis: Hyperthermia

Signs and Symptoms: Increased body temperature, increased respiratory rate, diaphoresis, chills, increased white blood cell count

INTERVENTIONS	RATIONALE
Serial monitoring of vital signs, blood work	To provide a baseline and ongoing assessment
Monitor serial white blood cell count	To monitor signs of infections
Monitor fluid intake and output, fluid and electrolyte balance	Hyperthermic, febrile patients lose increased amounts of fluid and may develop electrolyte disturbances
Monitor sputum culture results	Fever is a sign of infection that is likely associated with lung pathology; however, other sources should be ruled out

Physical Therapy Diagnosis: Anxiety caused by cardiopulmonary distress

Signs and Symptoms: Agitation, restlessness, confusion, impaired concentration, hyperventilation, diaphoresis, tachycardia, sleepiness, shakiness, facial tension, distracted behavior, withdrawal, increased heart rate and blood pressure, increased arousal, increased oxygen demand

INTERVENTIONS	RATIONALE
Serial monitoring of oxygenation and associated anxiety levels	To provide a baseline, ongoing assessment and measure of treatment response
Position patient to maximize cardiopulmonary function and gas exchange and minimize respiratory effort	Dyspnea and hyperventilation are signs of cardiopulmonary insufficiency and produce high anxiety in patients, which worsens cardiopulmonary function and gas exchange; body positions are selected to maximize ventilation and perfusion matching and reduce shortness of breath
	To reduce undue demands of anxiety on the compromised oxygen transport system
Define outcome criteria: reversal or mitigation of the signs and symptoms	To provide a basis for defining treatment goals and criteria for discontinuing treatment
Teach relaxation procedures	To reduce anxiety and promote effective rest
Teach pacing within and between treatments	To reduce anxiety
Prepare patient for interventions and what can be expected	To minimize anxiety and maximize cooperation
Provide emotional support	To assist patient in coping with illness

Physical Therapy Diagnosis: Activity and exercise intolerance

Signs and Symptoms: Weakness, fatigue, reduced endurance, inability to perform ADL, dyspnea on exertion; exaggerated increase in heart rate, blood pressure, and perceived exertion

INTERVENTIONS	RATIONALE
Assess premorbid level of independence and ability to perform ADL	To provide a baseline assessment and measure of treatment response
Monitor vital signs, ABGs, and oxygen transport variables	
Monitor blood sugar levels	To monitor blood sugar fluctuations before and after mobilization and exercise and modify prescription as necessary; work with team to regulate insulin requirements
Establish premorbid functional work capacity	To establish the premorbid functional status to define treatment goals
Define outcome criteria: reversal or mitigation of the signs and symptoms	To provide a basis for defining treatment goals and criteria for discontinuing treatment
Prescribe mobilization/exercise commensurate with improvement of acute cardiopulmonary dysfunction	To exploit the *long-term* effects of mobilization/exercise; specifically to increase functional work capacity, enable the patient to perform ADL independently and maintain an optimal level of cardiopulmonary and cardiovascular conditioning, and muscular strength commensurate with the premorbid level of conditioning
Prepare home exercise prescription at discharge	To promote patient-driven care, continuity of care, and health promotion
Plan home program and follow-up in consultation with the patient	

Continued.

Physical Therapy Diagnosis: Threat to cardiopulmonary function and oxygen transport: alveolar hypoventilation, impaired mucociliary transport, ineffective airway clearance, atelectasis, effusion, bronchospasm, inadequate Fio_2 (fraction of inspired oxygen), increased pulmonary vascular resistance, infection

Signs and Symptoms: Abnormal ABGs, blood work, and oxygen transport deficits, cyanosis, chest x-rays indicating atelectasis, effusion, pneumothorax, or hemothorax, secretion accumulation, increased respiratory rate, wheezing, dyspnea, asymmetric chest wall expansion, changes in mental status, fluid overload

INTERVENTIONS	RATIONALE
Serial monitoring of ABGs and oxygen transport variables	To provide indicators of improvement or deterioration in cardiopulmonary function and oxygen transport efficiency
Monitor breath and lung sounds for absent, diminished, or abnormal sounds and chest wall expansion	To detect changes early and modify treatment accordingly
Monitor ABGs, Sao_2, and chest x-rays for lung expansion, width of mediastinum, presence of pleural fluid	
Define outcome criteria: reversal of mitigation of the signs and symptoms	To provide a basis for defining treatment goals and criteria for discontinuing treatment
Facilitate mucociliary transport and airway clearance with mobilization, coordinated with breathing control and coughing maneuvers	To mobilize and remove secretions, optimize oxygenation, and open collapsed alveoli
Facilitate mucociliary transport and airway clearance with body positioning coordinated with breathing control and coughing maneuvers	
Facilitate airway clearance with postural drainage and manual techniques as indicated, such as manual percussion, shaking, and vibration	
Monitor level of arousal and oxygen levels	Indicator of deteriorating ABGs, such as hypoxemia and hypercapnia
Assess for crackles, jugular vein distention, peripheral edema, pulmonary edema, decreased diffusing capacity, ventilation-perfusion mismatch	Signs of impending respiratory failure leading to cardiac failure and pulmonary congestion
Avoid exposing patient to infection	Patients on antibiotics are susceptible to infection

Physical Therapy Diagnosis: Risk of the negative sequelae of recumbency

Signs and Symptoms: Within 6 hr evidence of reduced circulating blood volume, decreased blood pressure on sitting and standing compared with supine, light-headedness, dizziness, syncope, increased hematocrit and blood viscosity, decreased lung compliance, increased work of breathing, altered fluid balance in the lung, impaired pulmonary lymphatic drainage, decreased lung volumes and capacities, decreased forced expiratory flow rates, decreased functional residual capacity, increased closing volume, decreased Pao_2 and Sao_2, and increased work of the heart

INTERVENTIONS	RATIONALE
Monitor fluid balance	To provide a baseline and ongoing assessment
Define outcome criteria: reversal or mitigation of the signs and symptoms	To provide a basis for defining treatment goals and criteria for discontinuing treatment
Sitting upright position, standing, and walking	The upright position is essential to shift fluid volume from central to peripheral circulation and maintain fluid volume and pressure-regulating mechanisms and circulating blood volume
	The upright position maximizes lung volumes and capacities and functional residual capacity
	The upright position maximizes expiratory flow rate and cough effectiveness

INTERVENTIONS	RATIONALE
	The upright position optimizes the length-tension relationship of the respiratory muscles for efficient breathing and neural stimulation of the respiratory muscles and abdominal muscles for effective coughing
	The upright position coupled with mobilization and breathing control and coughing maneuvers maximizes alveolar ventilation, ventilation and perfusion matching, and pulmonary lymphatic drainage

Physical Therapy Diagnosis: Risk of negative sequelae of restricted mobility

Signs and Symptoms: Reduced activity and exercise tolerance, muscle atrophy, reduced muscle strength, reduced endurance, decreased oxygen transport efficiency, increased heart rate, blood pressure, and minute ventilation at submaximal work rates, reduced respiratory muscle strength, circulatory stasis, thromboemboli (e.g., pulmonary emboli), pressure areas, skin redness, skin breakdown, and ulceration

INTERVENTIONS	RATIONALE
Monitor the negative sequelae of restricted mobility	To provide a baseline and ongoing assessment
Define outcome criteria: reversal or mitigation of the signs and symptoms	To provide a basis for defining treatment goals and criteria for discontinuing treatment
Preventive mobilization and exercise prescription commensurate with recovery	Mobilization and exercise optimize circulating blood volume, optimize the oxygen-carrying capacity of the blood, and enhance the efficiency of all steps in the oxygen transport pathway

Physical Therapy Diagnosis: Knowledge deficit

Signs and Symptoms: Lack of information about pneumonia, relapse, complications, and prevention

INTERVENTIONS	RATIONALE
To assess specific knowledge deficits related to pneumonia and cardiopulmonary physical therapy	To provide a baseline and ongoing assessment
Define outcome criteria: reversal or mitigation of the signs and symptoms	To provide a basis for defining treatment goals and criteria for discontinuing treatment
Promote a caring and supportive patient-therapist relationship	To focus on treating the patient with pneumonia rather than the disease
Consider every patient interaction an opportunity for patient education	To promote cooperative and active participation of patient in treatment
Instruct regarding avoidance of respiratory tract infections, nutrition, weight control, hydration and fluid balance, exercise, stress reduction	Promote patient's sense of responsibility for health, health promotion, and prevention
Reinforce medications, their purpose, and the medication schedule	
Teach, demonstrate, and provide feedback on interventions that can be self-administered	Between-treatment interventions are as important as treatments themselves to provide cumulative treatment effect
Teach patient regarding balance of activity and rest	Optimal balance between activity and rest essential to exploit short-term, long-term, and preventive effects of mobilization and exercise
Provide individualized handout of information on mobilization, positioning, and breathing control and coughing maneuvers	To provide comprehensive care and continuity of care at home
At discharge, provide an individualized handout on exercise prescription and lifestyle modification strategies	

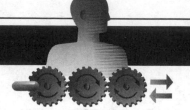

CHAPTER 4

Chronic Airflow Limitation

PATHOPHYSIOLOGY

Chronic airflow limitation (CAL) refers to a variety of conditions, including chronic bronchitis and emphysema. Chronic bronchitis and emphysema are caused by inhalation of irritants from cigarette smoking or air pollution, viral or bacterial infections, alpha-1-antitrypsin deficiency, and the aging process. These conditions are characterized by destruction of parenchyma, impaired mucociliary function, hyperreactivity of the large airways to stimuli, changes in the alveolar walls and air spaces, loss of elastic recoil of the lungs, impaired gas exchange, hypertrophy of mucous glands, and mucus hypersecretion. Excess mucus in the airways often causes bronchospasm and increased airway resistance. The destructive changes in pulmonary function contribute to obstruction to airflow, particularly on expiration, and result in dyspnea on exertion, cough, cyanosis, finger clubbing, shortness of breath, use of accessory muscles to breathe, and increased sputum production. Chronic airflow limitation frequently results in chronically elevated carbon dioxide (CO_2) levels. In turn, the patient's sensitivity to CO_2 is decreased, which increases the patient's hypoxic drive to breathe. Inappropriate oxygen administration can therefore diminish the patient's drive to breathe and contribute to ventilatory failure. Chronically low oxygen levels contribute to polycythemia, increased blood viscosity, and increased work of the heart. Late complications associated with CAL include respiratory muscle weakness, fatigue, right-sided heart failure, respiratory failure, and multiorgan system failure.

Case Study

The patient is a 66-year-old woman. She is a retired school teacher. She lives in the family home with her husband, who is also retired. He is in good health. Her grown son and his family visit frequently. She is about 5 feet 2 inches (160 cm) tall and weighs 143 pounds (65 kg); her body mass index is 31.3. She has developed increased shortness of breath over the past 2 months, including breathlessness during eating, and complains of morning headaches, daytime somnolence, and disturbed sleep. She was admitted with cardiopulmonary insufficiency. She has a 47 pack-year smoking history and has had a prolonged history of chronic bronchitis. Her pulmonary function test results from 6 months ago were forced expiratory volume in one second (FEV_1) 65% of predicted, forced vital capacity (FVC) 89% of predicted, and FEV_1/FVC 73% of predicted. Arterial blood gases (ABGs) on room air were pH 7.36, Pao_2 (arterial oxygen pressure) 65 mm Hg, $Paco_2$ (arterial carbon dioxide pressure) 54 mm Hg, HCO_3

(bicarbonate level) 30 mEq/L, and Sao_2 (arterial saturation of oxygen) 87%. She has small amounts of tenacious secretions that she is unable to clear effectively. Her chest x-ray showed bilateral hyperinflation, depressed hemidiaphragms, and right ventricular hypertrophy. Infiltrates were noted in both bases but more so on the right side. She was started on low-flow oxygen therapy and a course of ampicillin and aminophylline. The nursing staff reported that she objected to lying on her left side because of arthritis.

Oxygen Transport Deficits: Observed and Potential

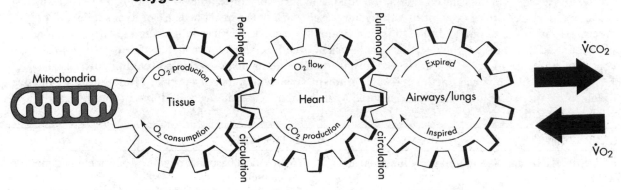

↑ Oxygen extraction

↑ Oxyhemoglobin dissociation

Right ventricular dilatation
↑ Right ventricular work
↑ Heart rate
↑ Blood pressure
↓ Stroke volume
↓ Cardiac output
Axis deviation
Heart displacement
Right heart enlargement

↓ Mucociliary transport
↑ Secretion retention
Mucus obstruction
Distant breath sound
Bronchospasm
↑ Resistance
↑ Dynamic airway closure
↑ Total lung capacity
　with inspiratory reserve
　volume and residual volume
↑ Compliance
↑ Time constants
Atelectasis
Impaired gas mixing
Impaired gas exchange
↑ Work of breathing
Chest wall hyperinflation
↑ AP diameter chest wall
↑ Transverse diameter chest
　wall
Flattened diaphragms
Hypoxic drive to breathe
Hyperinflated chest wall
↓ Mechanical efficiency of
　respiratory muscles
↓ Respiratory muscle strength
↓ Respiratory muscle endurance
Respiratory muscle fatigue
↓ Lung and chest wall motion
↑ Energy cost of breathing
Ciliary dyskinesis
Dyspnea
Prolonged expiration
Prolonged respiratory cycle
　time
↓ Forced expiratory flow rates
↓ Diffusing capacity

Blood: ↑ Red blood cells
　　　Polycythemia
　　　↑ Viscosity
　　　↑ Hematocrit
　　　Thrombus formation
　　　Thromboemboli
　　　Hypoxemia
　　　Hypercapnia
　　　↓ pH

Microemboli

Hypoxic vasoconstriction
↑ Central venous pressure
↑ Pulmonary artery systolic pressure
↑ Pulmonary vascular resistance
Shunt
↓ Lymph flow

↑	Increase
↓	Decrease

PHYSICAL THERAPY DIAGNOSES AND TREATMENT PRESCRIPTION

Physical Therapy Diagnosis: Altered cardiopulmonary function: impaired gas exchange, alveolar hypoventilation, and shunt

Signs and Symptoms: Pao_2 (alveolar partial pressure of oxygen) < 104.2 − 0.27 age (±7) mm Hg; Pao_2 < 75 mm Hg on room air, Sao_2 < 90%, $Paco_2$ > 45 mm Hg, bronchospasm, diminished breath sounds, carbon dioxide retention, cyanosis, altered respiratory mechanics (increased airway resistance); loss of elastic recoil of the lungs and increased compliance; hyperinflation of chest wall, air trapping, impaired gas mixing, decreased chest wall compliance, increased time constants for inspiration; abnormal position of respiratory muscles on their length-tension curves (diaphragm flattened), use of accessory muscles of respiration, increased work of breathing; increased energy cost of breathing, increased work of the heart because of hypoxemia and polycythemia, impaired pulmonary function (volumes and flow rates), decreased diffusing capacity, morning headaches and daytime somnolence, increased work of breathing; gasping, short inspiratory time, prolonged expiratory time; use of accessory muscles of respiration, spontaneous pursed lips breathing, increased $P(A - a)o_2$ (alveolar-arterial partial pressure) gradient, hypoxemia, increased $Paco_2$, radiographic evidence of atelectasis, increased lung compliance caused by loss of elastic recoil, decreased breath sounds; end-expiratory crackles

INTERVENTIONS	RATIONALE
Monitor serial ABGs and Sao_2, pulmonary function, and chest x-rays	To provide a baseline, ongoing assessment and measure of treatment response
Monitor respiratory, hemodynamic, and gas exchange variables before, during, and after treatment	To determine factors contributing to hypoxemia so treatment can be directed at reversing or mitigating their effects
Assess pulmonary function, including lung compliance	
Establish index of the work of breathing and capacity of patient to sustain spontaneous ventilation and an efficient breathing pattern	
Monitor in detail patient's ventilatory and functional capacities	
Define outcome criteria: reversal or mitigation of the signs and symptoms	To provide a basis for defining treatment goals and criteria for discontinuing treatment
Oxygen and ventilatory support (bronchodilators, nebulizers, and aerosols)	To remediate hypoxemia
Mobilization and body positioning coordinated with breathing control and coughing maneuvers	To minimize carbon dioxide retention
Promote passive expiration to normal end-tidal volume	To exploit the effects of gravity to optimize the intrapleural pressure gradient and the distributions of ventilation, perfusion, and ventilation, perfusion matching, intrapulmonary gas mixing and gas exchange
	To minimize breathing below functional residual capacity and minimize closure of dependent airways
Body positioning for relaxation and decreasing dyspnea: sit leaning forward with or without leaning on knees; breathing control maneuvers (pursed lips breathing and prolonged expiration)	To exploit the effects of gravity on pulmonary function; the sitting forward position also displaces the diaphragm upward from pressure of viscera beneath
	To exploit the effects of gravity on cardiac function
	To exploit the effects of gravity on pulmonary function
Body positioning: head of bed down	Some patients benefit from head-down position secondary to enhance viscerodiaphragmatic action and caudal displacement of the diaphragm
	Some patients may experience extreme distress in supine and head of bed down positions
Monitor patient closely when recumbent or head down	These positions reduce functional residual capacity and contribute to airway closure and arterial desaturation
Minimize duration in deleterious body positions (e.g., recumbent positions)	
Administer low-flow oxygen	Pao_2 should increase with fraction of inspired oxygen (Fio_2); low flow is indicated because patients rely on their hypoxic drive to breathe

INTERVENTIONS	RATIONALE
Mobilization and exercise coordinated with breathing control (pursed lips breathing) and coughing maneuvers	To exploit the *acute* effects of mobilization (e.g., optimize alveolar ventilation, and the distributions of ventilation, perfusion, and ventilation and perfusion matching, chest wall motion, lung movement, mucociliary transport airway clearance, lymphatic drainage)
Type—dangle over edge of bed, transfer to chair, chair sit; mobilization in these positions includes upper extremity movements, trunk mobility exercises, and lower extremity movement	
Intensity—$Sao_2 > 85\%$; breathlessness 3-5 (0-10 scale), and heart rate and blood pressure within acceptable levels in relation to rest	As the patient tolerates increases in intensity and duration, the frequency of the mobilization and exercise sessions decreases
Duration—short; 5-20 minutes	
Frequency—frequent; 2 or more times a day	
Course and progression—as indicated	
Body positioning coordinated with breathing control (pursed lips breathing) and coughing maneuvers	To exploit the effects of gravity on optimizing the intrapleural pressure gradient and optimize alveolar volume and the distribution of ventilation and ventilation and perfusion matching
1. Upright sitting	
2. Chest wall mobility exercise positions	
3. Standing and walking	
Avoid excessive time in recumbent positions and deleterious positions	Recumbency increases compression of the diaphragm and its cephalad displacement, thoracic blood volume, and airway closure

Physical Therapy Diagnosis: Impaired gas exchange: airway resistance

Signs and Symptoms: Radiographic evidence of alveolar collapse and atelectasis; airway secretions, alveolar consolidation; pneumonia

INTERVENTIONS	RATIONALE
Monitor serial ABGs and Sao_2	To provide a baseline, ongoing assessment and measure of treatment response
Monitor airway secretions; amount, color, change in color, viscosity	To ensure adequate gas exchange
Define outcome criteria: reversal or mitigation of the signs and symptoms	To provide a basis for defining treatment goals and criteria for discontinuing treatment
Administer low-flow oxygen	Pao_2 should increase with increases in Fio_2; low-flow oxygen administered to avoid eliminating the hypoxic drive to breathe
Secretion clearance interventions: mobilization and exercise coordinated with breathing control and coughing maneuvers (continuous or interval)	To exploit the *acute* effects of mobilization and exercise on reducing airflow resistance (e.g., mobilizing secretions from the peripheral to central airways and increasing airway diameter)
Intensity—low intensity rhythmic	
Duration—short; 10-30 minutes	
Frequency—often; several times daily to 2 times a day	
Course and progression—as indicated	
Body positioning: postural drainage positions for the lower lobes coordinated with breathing control and coughing maneuvers	To mobilize secretions, remove accumulated secretions, reduce work of breathing and work of the heart, optimize alveolar volume, improve ventilation, and decrease shunt
Premedicated as necessary to minimize left hip pain on left side lying	To maximize patient's ability to cooperate with treatment
Body positioning: postural drainage positions with manual techniques (e.g., percussion, shaking, and vibration) coordinated with breathing control and coughing maneuvers	If indicated, single-handed percussion at a frequency of 1 per second may reduce the untoward effects of this intervention

Continued.

Physical Therapy Diagnosis: Decreased ability to perform activities of daily living (ADL), decreased activity and exercise tolerance

Signs and Symptoms: Shortness of breath, dyspnea on exertion, fatigue, weakness, reduced endurance, exaggerated increase in heart rate, blood pressure, rate pressure product, and minute ventilation; decreased Sao_2, increased ventricular work caused by cardiomegaly, impaired night's sleep, supplemental low-flow oxygen reduces respiratory distress and improves ability to perform ADL

INTERVENTIONS	RATIONALE
Establish premorbid ability to perform ADL and exercise tolerance	To provide a baseline, ongoing assessment and measure of treatment response
Define outcome criteria: reversal or mitigation of the signs and symptoms	To provide a basis for defining treatment goals and criteria for discontinuing treatment
Premedicated as necessary to reduce left hip pain and facilitate mobilization	To minimize musculoskeletal discomfort during activity and exercise
Conduct a modified exercise test Type—6-minute walk test	A standardized well-controlled exercise test provides a baseline and the basis for prescribing an exercise program
Prescribe an exercise program Type—walking Intensity—rating of 3-5 on breathlessness scale Duration—15-20 minutes Frequency—3 times a day Course and progression—as indicated	Prescriptive aerobic exercise improves the efficiency of oxygen transport overall (i.e., all steps in the pathway) The *long-term* effects and benefits of a modified aerobic exercise program for patients with chronic airflow limitation include improved efficiency of oxygen transport, desensitization to dyspnea, improved ventilatory muscle strength, improved movement efficiency and economy, improved motivation and sense of well-being, and increased endurance
Supplemental oxygen is increased before, during, and after exercise (throughout recovery)	Supplemental oxygen may be increased to meet the increased metabolic demands of exercise but at low flow rates
Upper extremity and chest wall mobility exercises, including forward flexion, extension, side flexion, rotation, and diagonal rotation	To optimize three-dimensional movement of chest wall, the bucket handle and pump handle motions of the chest wall, and normal thoracoabdominal motion
General strengthening exercises	To maintain optimal strength to perform aerobic exercises and to perform ADL with least physical and metabolic stress
Ensure that patient is appropriately premedicated before exercise	To maximize patient's performance and reduce negative effects of exercise
Ensure that medications are administered appropriately, and are taken within an appropriate time frame to reach maximum potency during activity or exercise	
Ventilatory muscle training with flow rate control	Ventilatory muscle training improves functional capacity
Intensity—maximal resistance load patient can tolerate without desaturating or becoming dyspneic for 5-10 breaths Frequency: 2-3 times a day Course and progression: as indicated	To ensure that the patient is receiving the benefit of a given inspiratory resistive load, flow rate must be controlled
Ergonomic assessment of home and recreational activities	To review the home and recreational activities with respect to biomechanics and energy cost of performing activities in these settings, to make recommendations to minimize energy expenditure (e.g., avoiding wasting energy and pacing while performing the activity and between activities over the course of a day or week), and integrating relaxation procedures

INTERVENTIONS	RATIONALE
Sexual counseling: review time of day patient is at peak energy, review positions of comfort associated with the least shortness of breath, review medication schedule to derive maximum benefit, review techniques to minimize cardiopulmonary distress	To review problems related to sexual performance (e.g., decreased tolerance and shortness of breath) and to reduce these concerns; side effects of medications
Optimize efficiency of energy expenditure	To optimize functional capacity by minimizing undue wasteful energy expenditure
1. Teach relaxation procedures and how to integrate these during activity	
2. Teach pacing of activities (within and between)	
3. Teach energy conservation procedures and alternate means of achieving same functional goals with the least energy expenditure	
4. Teach means of reducing cardiopulmonary strain (e.g., avoid breath holding during activities, avoid straining and the Valsalva maneuver, avoid activities that require heavy resistive work, isometrics, and excessive muscle stabilization)	
5. Teach the benefits of interval versus continuous work output and how to integrate this concept into ADL as well as in an exercise program	
6. Review the use of walking aids and devices	
7. Review the use and prescription of supplemental oxygen	
8. Review the need for intermittent noninvasive mechanical ventilation (e.g., nocturnal CPAP)	
9. Avoid exercise for 45 minutes after meals	
10. Prescribe rest periods (indications, type, quality, duration, frequency)	Ensure that rests and the patient's night sleep are maximally restorative; if not, identify factors interfering with the restorative effects of rest and sleep and make suggestions to help remediate them
11. Review the quality and quantity of the patient's night sleep	To monitor the quality and quantity of patient's rest periods within an exercise session and between sessions to ensure adequate restorative rest and sleep
Maximize restorative rest and sleep	
Review antecedent events to bed time, mattress quality, number of pillows, the need for antisnoring devices, sleeping position, nocturnal ventilatory assistance	To monitor the quality and quantity of patient's night sleep and whether adequately restorative

Physical Therapy Diagnosis: Altered nutritional status and fluid balance

Signs and Symptoms: Too fatigued to prepare food, too fatigued to eat, too fatigued to speak in continuous sentences, inadequate intake of food and fluids, complains of reduced appetite, decreased albumen

INTERVENTIONS	RATIONALE
Obtain assessment information on the patient's nutritional status, fluid balance, weight	To provide a baseline and ongoing assessment
Define outcome criteria: reversal or mitigation of the signs and symptoms	To evaluate gastrointestinal peristalsis
Recommend patient eat foods that are easily chewed and digested	To provide a basis for defining treatment goals and criteria for discontinuing treatment
Recommend patient eat slowly	To minimize the energy cost of eating and facilitate nutrition and fluid intake
Recommend patient eat with no other competing activities	
Recommend patient eat a variety of foods at home that can be easily prepared	
Recommend occupational therapy home visit	

Continued.

INTERVENTIONS	RATIONALE
Recommend use of supplemental oxygen or increase oxygen while eating	To offset increased energy cost of eating
Assess patient's ability to shop for food	Poor eating habits in patients with airflow limitation may reflect inability to shop because of activity intolerance, as well as meal preparation and eating difficulties
Reinforce nutritionist's prescribed diet	Carbohydrates are associated with increased carbon dioxide production and may contribute to increased carbon dioxide retention in patients with chronic airflow limitation

Physical Therapy Diagnosis: **Threats to oxygen transport and gas exchange caused by her smoking history and its chronic pathological sequelae; mild obesity and general deconditioned status; respiratory muscle fatigue**

Signs and Symptoms: **Impaired alveolar ventilation, hypoxemia, hypercapnia, shortness of breath with minimal exertion, and increased work of breathing**

INTERVENTIONS	RATIONALE
Monitor threats to oxygen transport and gas exchange	To promote a baseline and ongoing assessment
Define outcome criteria: reversal or mitigation of the signs and symptoms	To provide a basis for defining treatment goals and criteria for discontinuing treatment
Breathing control and coughing maneuvers	To augment ventilation and gas exchange
Body positioning	Body positions to augment ventilation and breathing efficiency
Mobilization and exercise	To exploit effects on gas exchange and general conditioning status
Optimal activity to rest balance	To ensure oxygen demand does not exceed delivery
Pacing activities	To maximize work output

Physical Therapy Diagnosis: **Risk of the negative sequelae of recumbency**

Signs and Symptoms: **Within 6 hours reduced circulating blood volume, decreased blood pressure on sitting and standing compared with supine, light-headedness, dizziness, syncope, increased hematocrit and blood viscosity, increased work of the heart, altered fluid balance in the lung, impaired pulmonary lymphatic drainage, decreased lung volumes and capacities, decreased functional residual capacity, increased closing volume, and decreased Pao_2 and Sao_2**

INTERVENTIONS	RATIONALE
Monitor the negative sequelae of recumbency	To provide a baseline and ongoing assessment
Define outcome criteria: reversal or mitigation of the signs and symptoms	To provide a basis for defining treatment goals and criteria for discontinuing treatment
	To define treatment goals
Sitting upright position, standing and walking	The upright position is essential to shift fluid volume from central to peripheral circulation and maintain fluid volume regulating mechanisms and circulating blood volume
	The upright position maximizes effective cardiopulmonary function and minimizes closing volume
	The upright position maximizes expiratory flow rates and cough effectiveness
	The upright position optimizes the length-tension relationship of the respiratory muscles and abdominal muscles and optimizes cough effectiveness
	The upright position coupled with mobilization and breathing control and coughing maneuvers maximizes lung volumes and capacities, forced expiratory lung volumes, ventilation and perfusion matching, mucociliary transport, mucociliary clearance, and pulmonary lymphatic drainage

Physical Therapy Diagnosis: Risk of negative sequelae of restricted mobility

Signs and Symptoms: Reduced activity and exercise tolerance, muscle atrophy and reduced muscle strength, decreased tensile strength of connective tissue and cartilage, decreased bone density, decreased oxygen transport efficiency, increased heart rate, blood pressure and minute ventilation at rest and submaximal work rates, reduced respiratory muscle strength and endurance, circulatory stasis, thromboemboli (e.g., pulmonary emboli), pressure areas, skin redness, skin breakdown, and ulceration

INTERVENTIONS	RATIONALE
Determine patient's premorbid functional status and capacity	To provide a baseline and ongoing assessment
	To define treatment goals
Monitor for signs and symptoms of the sequelae of restricted mobility	To avoid unnecessary restricted mobility and its adverse effects
Define outcome criteria: reversal or mitigation of the signs and symptoms	To provide a basis for defining treatment goals and criteria for discontinuing treatment
Mobilization and exercise prescription	To exploit the *preventive* effects of mobilization and exercise (i.e., optimize cardiopulmonary conditioning, general strength, mobility, circulating blood volume) and enhance the efficiency of the steps in the oxygen transport pathway

Physical Therapy Diagnosis: Knowledge deficit

Signs and Symptoms: Lack of information about chronic airflow disease, preventative measures, relapse, or complications

INTERVENTIONS	RATIONALE
Assess specific knowledge deficits related to chronic airflow limitation and cardiopulmonary physical therapy management	To provide a baseline and ongoing assessment
Define outcome criteria: reversal or mitigation of the signs and symptoms	To provide a basis for defining treatment goals and criteria for discontinuing treatment
Promote a caring and supportive patient-therapist relationship	To focus on treating the patient with chronic airflow limitation rather than the condition
Consider every patient interaction an opportunity for patient education	
Instruct regarding avoidance of upper respiratory tract infections, nutrition, weight control, hydration and fluid balance, smoking cessation, exercise, and stress reduction	To promote patient's sense of responsibility for health, health promotion, and prevention
	To promote cooperation and active participation of patient in treatment
Reinforce effects of medications and their purpose and the medication schedule	Smoking cessation is essential to minimize further morbidity
Teach, demonstrate, and provide feedback on interventions that can be self-administered	Between-treatment interventions are as important as treatments themselves to elicit a cumulative treatment effect
Teach patient regarding balance of activity and rest	Optimal balance between activity and rest is essential to exploit short-term, long-term, and preventive effects of mobilization and exercise
Prepare information sheets for patients with the individual exercise prescription outlined	Promote continuity of care to home and follow-up
Prepare written handout for discharge with general information and specific exercise prescription and home program	
Plan for follow-up	

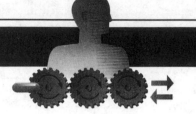

CHAPTER 5

Myocardial Infarction

PATHOPHYSIOLOGY

Myocardial infarction (MI) results from occlusion of one or more coronary arteries. The occlusion can result from thrombus or artheromatous plaque. In both cases, the lumen of the affected arteries is critically narrowed such that blood flow to the myocardium is diminished. Typically, the infarction occurs during activity and increased metabolic demand on the heart. The resulting ischemia produces varying degrees of chest, neck, and arm pain. Three levels of damage occur: ischemia, injury, and infarct. The ischemia is reversible, whereas the infarcted area does not recover. The injured area usually heals, but normal structure and function may not return. Infarcts most commonly occur in the area of the left ventricle. During the acute stages, the integrity and permeability of the cell membrane to vital electrolytes is altered and the contractility of the myocardium and cardiac output are depressed. Crackles and wheezes can be heard on auscultation. These signs and symptoms result in anxiety, pallor, diaphoresis, shortness of breath, weakness, nausea, and vomiting. About 15% to 20% of MI incidences are painless. Their occurence increases with age and in patients with diabetes mellitus. The primary complaint with this type of MI is sudden shortness of breath. Complications of MI include dysrhythmias, cardiogenic shock, congestive heart failure, ventricular aneurysm, pericarditis, and embolism. Risk factors of coronary artery disease include being male, being over 40 years of age, having high blood pressure, having smoking history, being overweight, having high cholesterol, and having stressful lifestyle.

Case Study

The patient is a 53-year-old male. He is an accountant, but is presently unemployed. He lives with his wife in a condominium townhouse. His wife is a department head in a major department store. They have three grown children who live away from home. He is about 5 feet 9 inches (176 cm) tall and weighs 191 pounds (87 kg); his body mass index is 28. The patient was admitted to the emergency room after 2 hours of severe chest pain, which began when he was working under his car. He has no history of heart disease. He was dyspneic and anxious. On auscultation, crackles were audible over his posterior bases. His chest x-ray was clear. An S3 heart sound was audible on auscultation. Ventricular tachycardia was treated with lidocaine. His blood pressure was 144/95 mm Hg. Nitroglycerine was instituted intravenously. Oxygen was administered at 2.5 L/min by nasal prongs. After 60 minutes, his arterial blood gases (ABGs) were pH 7.42, oxygen pressure (P_{O_2}) 70 mm Hg, carbon dioxide pressure (P_{CO_2}) 38 mm Hg, bicarbonate (HCO_3) 26 mEq/L, and arterial oxygen saturation (S_{aO_2}) 93%. Thrombolytic therapy was initiated (intravenous tissue plasminogen activator and oral aspirin).

Oxygen Transport Deficits: Observed and Potential

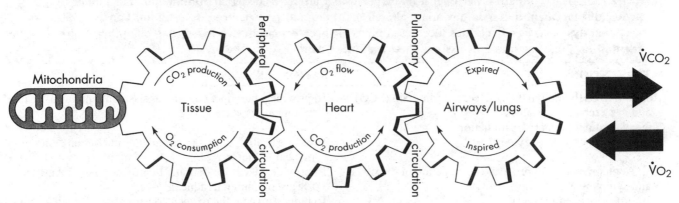

↑ Oxygen extraction

↑ Oxyhemoglobin
    dissociation
↓ Tissue perfusion
Aerobic deconditioning
Muscle weakness
↑ Submaximal ventilation
    oxygen uptake
Peripheral edema
↓ Renal insufficiency
Oliguria

Ischemia
Injury
Irreversible damage
Dysrhythmias
Hypoeffective function
↓ Stroke volume
↓ Cardiac output
Ventricular dyskinesia
Abnormal wall motion
Abnormal valve function
Pericardial effusion
Cardiac tamponade
↑ Heart rate
↑ Blood pressure
↑ Rate pressure product
↑ Myocardial oxygen
    uptake
↑ Work of the heart

Dynamic airway
    compression
Interstitial edema
Pulmonary edema
↑ Work of breathing
Basal crackles and
    wheezes
Low lung volumes
Atelectasis

↑ Vascular resistance
↑ Afterload
Hypertension

Hypoxic vasoconstriction
Shunt
↑ Vascular resistance
↑ Right ventricular work
↓ Lymphatic drainage

Blood: ↑ Catecholamines
       ↑ Red blood cells
       Polycythemia
       ↑ Hematocrit
       ↑ Viscosity
       Hypoxemia

↑ Increase
↓ Decrease

PHYSICAL THERAPY DIAGNOSES AND TREATMENT PRESCRIPTION

Physical Therapy Diagnosis: Altered cardiopulmonary function: alveolar hypoventilation and shunt, cardiac insufficiency

Signs and Symptoms: Impaired electromechanical coupling of the heart, reduced myocardial perfusion, hypoeffective cardiac pumping, reduced cardiac output, stroke volume, and ejection fraction, increased heart rate, blood pressure, and rate pressure product, increased myocardial oxygen consumption, increased work of the heart, impaired peripheral tissue perfusion, altered ventricular wall motion, cardiomegaly, cardiac displacement and axia deviation, altered breathing pattern, reduced oxygenation Pao_2 and Sao_2, exertional dyspnea, basal crackles, decreased bibasilar breath sounds, decreased lung compliance and potential for atelectasis, and decreased chest wall movement

INTERVENTIONS	RATIONALE
Monitor ABGs, hemodynamics, electrocardiogram (ECG), and gas exchange variables	To provide a baseline, ongoing assessment and measure of treatment response
Clinical cardiopulmonary examination	
Monitor serial cardiac enzymes	To assess healing of myocardium and rule out an evolving myocardial infarct
Define outcome criteria: reversal or mitigation of the signs and symptoms	To provide a basis for defining treatment goals and criteria for discontinuing treatment
Reinforce restricted mobility	To reduce myocardial oxygen consumption and work of the heart
	To promote myocardial healing
Place patient with head of bed up 10-30 degrees	To reduce work of the heart
	To optimize cardiac performance, that is maximal work output with the least cardiac stress
Place patient in high or semi-Fowler's position	To relieve positional hypoxemia with recumbency
Reposition patient in varying upright positions	To relieve effects of cardiac compression in certain positions and pulmonary edema
Modified mobilization	To ensure that oxygen demands do not exceed oxygen supply, that is, remain within oxygen delivery threshold
Body positioning	To maximize alveolar ventilation and minimize negative effects of pulmonary edema on alveolar ventilation and lung compliance
Promote self-care activities as indicated	Use of commode rather than bedpan and ability to do self-care reduce stress and oxygen demands

Physical Therapy Diagnosis: Decreased capacity to perform activities of daily living (ADL), and exercise

Signs and Symptoms: Angina, lethargy, myocardial damage, and insufficiency

INTERVENTIONS	RATIONALE
Monitor serial respiratory, hemodynamic, and gas exchange variables	To provide a baseline, ongoing assessment and measure of treatment response
Determine premorbid level of function and functional work capacity	
Define outcome criteria: reversal or mitigation of the signs and symptoms	To provide a basis for defining treatment goals and criteria for discontinuing treatment
Stage 1	
Modified mobilization exercise test	Stage 1 is instituted in consultation with the team when patient is medically stable
	To provide index of exercise responses by observing hemodynamic and gas exchange responses to routine care and procedures

INTERVENTIONS	RATIONALE
Stage 1—cont'd	
Mobilization and exercise prescription (with cardiology clearance and patient appropriately medicated)	Mobilization/exercise prescription parameters set within the capacity of the myocardium to deliver blood to the lungs and systemic circulation and within anginal threshold
Type—aerobic, rhythmic; progress from interval to continuous	
Intensity—(set according to hemodynamic stability and myocardial status); increase in heart rate < 10-20 beats per minute, increase in blood pressure < 20 mm Hg, subanginal threshold	To exploit the *acute* effects of mobilization and exercise on oxygen transport, that is, increase tidal volume and respiratory rate, increase zone of ventilation and perfusion matching, maximize alveolar ventilation, maximize functional residual capacity, reduce closing volume, optimize three-dimensional chest wall movement, stimulate normal lung movement, facilitate lymphatic drainage
Duration—short; 5-20 minutes	
Frequency—frequent; 2 to 4 times a day	
Course and progression—as indicated	
Functional activity prescription (with cardiology clearance and patient appropriately medicated)	Patient's anxiety levels decrease when permitted to perform self-care and when granted bathroom privileges instead of use of the bedpan and commode
Self-care—washing, shaving, use of bedpan and commode, combing hair, changing bed gown	
Intensity—increase in heart rate < 10-20 beats per minute, increase in blood pressure < 20 mm Hg	
Prescriptive rest	To optimize physiological restoration and healing from rest and sleep balanced with judicious, low levels of mobilization
	Minimize undue physical demands on patient; for example, double up procedures, such as conduct part of the assessment during some routine nursing procedures
Stage 2	
Modified mobilization and exercise test	To provide index of exercise responses by exposing the patient to progressive mobilization and exercise challenges, and observe and compare responses before and during exercise, and after recovery
Mobilization and exercise prescription (with cardiology clearance and patient appropriately medicated)	Exercise prescription parameters are set within the capacity of the myocardium to deliver oxygenated blood to the lungs and systemic circulation and within the anginal threshold
Type—aerobic, rhythmic, progress from interval to continuous	
Intensity—increase in heart rate < 10-20 beats per minute, increase in blood pressure < 20 mm Hg, subanginal/symptom threshold	To exploit the *long-term* effects of mobilization and exercise on oxygen transport (reduction in minute ventilation, heart rate, blood pressure, rate pressure product, oxygen consumption, perceived exertion, fatigue at submaximal work rates)
Duration—progressively increased	
Frequency—same	
Course—as indicated	
Functional activity prescription (with cardiology clearance)	As the patient's tolerance increases, the intensity and duration are increased and the frequency of sessions is reduced
Type—aerobic, rhythmic	
Intensity—increase in heart rate < 10-20 beats per minute, increase in blood pressure < 20 mm Hg, subanginal/symptom threshold	
Duration—10-30 minutes	
Frequency—2-3 times a day	
Course and progression—as indicated	
Stage 3 (predischarge)	
Graded exercise tolerance test (GXTT)	In the stress testing laboratory under the supervision of a cardiologist
Exercise prescription based on the GXTT	Carried out under the supervision of a physical therapist in the community or in a cardiac rehabilitation program
Type—aerobic, rhythmic, continuous	
Intensity—60%-75% of heart rate reserve capacity, that is, resting heart rate + (60%-75%) (peak heart rate − resting heart rate)	
Duration—15-60 minutes	
Frequency—daily to 3 times a week	

Continued.

INTERVENTIONS	RATIONALE
Stage 3—cont'd	
Course and progression—as indicated	
Counseling regarding ADL including work, leisure activities, and sexual activity	
Sexual counseling: review time of day patient is at peak energy, review positions of comfort associated with the least shortness of breath, review medication schedule to derive maximum benefit, review techniques to minimize cardiopulmonary distress	To review problems related to sexual performance (e.g., decreased tolerance and shortness of breath) and to reduce these concerns; side effects of medications

Physical Therapy Diagnosis: Discomfort and pain

Signs and Symptoms: Angina; discomfort from restricted mobility

INTERVENTIONS	RATIONALE
Monitor chest pain, ECG, and serial cardiac enzymes	To provide a baseline, ongoing assessment and treatment response
Monitor fluid and electrolyte balance	To monitor impaired cardiac output and impaired renal perfusion manifested by oliguria
Define outcome criteria: reversal or mitigation of the signs and symptoms	To provide a basis for defining treatment goals and criteria for discontinuing treatment
Ensure that patient is appropriately premedicated before treatment and appropriately monitored during treatment	Premedication is essential to optimize benefit of treatment and decrease risk
Pace mobilization and body position changes	To detect abnormal treatment responses; modify or discontinue treatment as necessary, notify team of untoward responses
Monitor ECG and other hemodynamic and respiratory variables before, during, and after treatment	
Teach breathing control and supported coughing maneuvers	Controlled breathing promotes relaxation and reduces cardiopulmonary stress
Emphasize coughing maneuvers with open glottis, (huffing)	To minimize increases in intrathoracic pressure and compromised cardiac output
Teach patient bed mobility and body repositioning	To enable patient to confidently and safely move and position self
Teach aspects of stress management	Integrate stress management and coping strategies throughout course of treatment and to provide a basis for stress management after discharge
Provide emotional support	To help patient deal with illness
Teach family about physical activity and heart disease	To promote understanding of the patient's condition and its management; identify what the patient can do and will be capable of doing physically

Physical Therapy Diagnosis: Anxiety

Signs and Symptoms: Agitation, facial tension, general tension, lack of concentration, distraction, reduced ability to retain information, and verbalization of anxiety

INTERVENTIONS	RATIONALE
Monitor signs and symptoms of anxiety	To provide a baseline and ongoing assessment
	To identify patient's anxiety and fears and consider these in treatment planning
Define outcome criteria: reversal or mitigation of the signs and symptoms	To provide a basis for defining treatment goals and criteria for discontinuing treatment
Listen to patient	To have patient identify fears and apprehensions
Talk with patient	To help patient work through fears and apprehensions
Encourage patient	To provide a positive but realistic view of patient's functional prognosis that is consistent with the team
	To help reduce reliance on anxiolytic medications
Teach relaxation procedures (breathing control, Jacobsen's progressive relaxation techniques, Benson's relaxation method, autogenic training, biofeedback, visual imagery)	To promote self-control
	To provide support and help patient manage anxiety

Physical Therapy Diagnosis: Threats to oxygen transport and gas exchange from evolving myocardial infarction, cardiac insufficiency, pulmonary congestion

Signs and Symptoms: Hypoxemia, dyspnea, increased intracardiac pressure, increased heart rate and blood pressure, increased work of the heart, pulmonary edema, decreased lung compliance, increased shunt, decreased ejection fraction, insufficiency, radiographic and clinical evidence of atelectasis

INTERVENTIONS	RATIONALE
Monitor for worsening cardiopulmonary status	To provide a baseline and ongoing assessment
Define outcome criteria: reversal or mitigation of the signs and symptoms	To provide a basis for defining treatment goals and criteria for discontinuing treatment
Need to increase Fio$_2$	Detect changes early and modify treatment accordingly
	To supplement the patient's oxygen demand and decrease work of the heart
Avoid recumbent positions with head of bed < 20-30 degrees	To reduce the patient's overall oxygen and metabolic demands
Place patient in position of comfort (least work of breathing and work of the heart)	
Continue nonresistive range-of-motion exercises with the patient monitored; coordinate with breathing	To optimize *acute* ventilatory effects of low-intensity movement, optimizing gas exchange and reducing the work of the heart
Avoid static postures and breath holding	

Physical Therapy Diagnosis: Risk of the negative sequelae of recumbency

Signs and Symptoms: Within 6 hours reduced circulating blood volume, decreased blood pressure on sitting and standing compared with supine, light-headedness, dizziness, syncope, increased hematocrit and blood viscosity, increased work of the heart, altered fluid balance in the lung, impaired pulmonary lymphatic drainage, decreased lung volumes and capacities, decreased functional residual capacity, increased closing volume, and decreased Pao$_2$ and Sao$_2$

INTERVENTIONS	RATIONALE
Monitor signs and symptoms of the negative sequelae of recumbency	To provide a baseline and ongoing assessment
Define outcome criteria: reversal or mitigation of the signs and symptoms	To provide a basis for defining treatment goals and criteria for discontinuing treatment
Sitting upright position, standing and walking	To select interventions to counter the negative sequelae of recumbency, primarily involving the upright body position
	The upright position is essential to shift fluid volume from central to peripheral circulation and maintain fluid volume and pressure-regulating mechanisms and circulating blood volume
	The upright position maximizes lung volumes and capacities and functional residual capacity; it minimizes airway closure
	The upright position maximizes expiratory flow rate and cough effectiveness
	The upright position optimizes the length-tension relationship of the respiratory muscles and abdominal muscles and optimizes cough effectiveness
	The upright position coupled with mobilization and breathing control and coughing maneuvers maximizes alveolar ventilation, ventilation and perfusion matching, mucociliary transport, and pulmonary lymphatic drainage

Continued.

Physical Therapy Diagnosis: Risk of negative sequelae of restricted mobility

Signs and Symptoms: Reduced activity and exercise tolerance, reduced circulating blood volume, muscle atrophy and reduced muscle strength, decreased oxygen transport efficiency, increased heart rate, blood pressure and minute ventilation at rest and submaximal work rates, reduced respiratory muscle strength, circulatory stasis, thromboemboli (e.g., pulmonary emboli), pressure areas, skin redness, skin breakdown, and ulceration

INTERVENTIONS	RATIONALE
Monitor the negative sequelae of restricted mobility	To provide a baseline and ongoing assessment
Determine patient's premorbid functional status and capacity	
Define outcome criteria: reversal or mitigation of the signs and symptoms	To provide a basis for defining treatment goals and criteria for discontinuing treatment
Mobilization and exercise prescription	Mobilization and exercise optimize circulating blood volume and enhance the efficiency of the steps in the oxygen transport pathway

Physical Therapy Diagnosis: Knowledge deficit

Signs and Symptoms: Lack of information about coronary artery disease, preventative measures, relapse, complications

INTERVENTIONS	RATIONALE
Assess specific knowledge deficits related to heart disease and cardiopulmonary physical therapy management	To provide a baseline and ongoing assessment
Define outcome criteria: reversal or mitigation of the signs and symptoms	To provide a basis for defining treatment goals and criteria for discontinuing treatment
Promote a caring and supportive patient-therapist relationship	To focus on treating the patient with coronary artery disease rather than the disease
Consider every patient interaction an opportunity for patient education	To promote cooperation and active participation of patient in treatment
Instruct regarding avoidance of heavy resistive exercise, stress management, nutrition, weight control, hydration, and fluid balance	Promote patient's sense of responsibility for health, health promotion, and prevention
Reinforce the purpose of medications and the medication schedule	
Teach, demonstrate, and provide feedback on interventions that can be self-administered	Between-treatment interventions are as important as treatments themselves to elicit a cumulative treatment effect
Teach patient regarding balance of activity and rest	Optimal balance between activity and rest is essential to exploit short-term, long-term, and preventive effects of mobilization and exercise
Prepare information sheets for patient with the individual exercise prescription outlined	To promote optional cumulative treatment effect by having the patient carry out a between treatment regimen
Prepare handouts, including general information, exercise prescription, and a home program for discharge	Promote continuity of care to home; follow-up by a physical therapist in the community or cardiac rehabilitation program

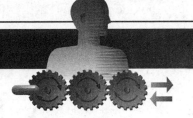

CHAPTER 6

Duchenne Muscular Dystrophy

PATHOPHYSIOLOGY

Duchenne muscular dystrophy (DMD) is a chronic progressive neuromuscular disease. Specifically, DMD is a sex-linked recessive disorder in which one of the largest human genes found in the sarcolemma of the muscle fiber, the gene responsible for producing dystrophin, mutates. The disorder is present at birth but does not manifest itself until 3 to 5 years of age. Duchenne muscular dystrophy predominantly affects males. It is characterized by delayed motor milestones, progressive weakness of muscles of the shoulder and pelvic girdles (although there is no evidence of neural degeneration), pseudohypertrophy of the calf muscles in which muscle fibers are replaced by connective tissue and fat, kyphoscoliosis, and joint contractures in the upper and lower extremities. Serum creatine kinase levels are elevated at birth (20 to 100 times normal) but decline as the disease progresses because of loss of muscle mass. These signs and symptoms result in frequent falls, a lordotic posture, and difficulty in performing activities such as running, jumping, hopping, and walking. As the disease progresses, the patient's ability to ambulate is compromised, and ultimately a wheelchair is required. Pulmonary function is impaired as a result of muscle weakness and chest deformity associated with scoliosis. Aspiration and pulmonary infections can be fatal. Mental retardation may be associated with the disease. Children with DMD have an intelligence quotient (IQ) of one standard deviation below the mean (75 to 85). The impairment is nonprogressive and appears to affect verbal ability more than performance. Cardiomyopathy is another clinical feature of DMD, but it is rarely a cause of death.

Case Study

The patient is a 26-year-old man. He works as a counselor in a residential facility for individuals with chronic disabilities. He is about 5 feet 7 inches (170 cm) tall and weighs 167 pounds (76 kg); his body mass index is 26.3. He has Duchenne muscular dystrophy and has been wheelchair dependent since the age of 14. He uses hand controls. He has lived in a group home since the age of 20. He has never smoked. He reported increased breathing difficulty at night over the past 8 months and has been having increasing difficulty with choking when eating. He has been increasingly anxious about periods of breathlessness during the night. He has been able to sleep for only 5 or 6 hours a night over the past month. Over the past 3 years, he has had two bouts of chest infections requiring antibiotics. A recent study of his arterial saturation throughout the night revealed a decrement from 95% during the day to periods of 87% during the night. Noctural ventilation (continuous positive airway pressure) is being considered. His pulmonary function test results were forced expiratory volume in a second (FEV$_1$) 73% of predicted, forced vital capacity (FVC) 77% of predicted, and FEV$_1$/FVC 95%. His arterial blood gases (ABGs) on room air were arterial oxygen pressure (Pao$_2$) 74 mm Hg, arterial carbon dioxide pressure (Paco$_2$) 40 mm Hg, pH 7.38, and bicarbonate level (HCO$_3$) 23.

Oxygen Transport Deficits: Observed and Potential

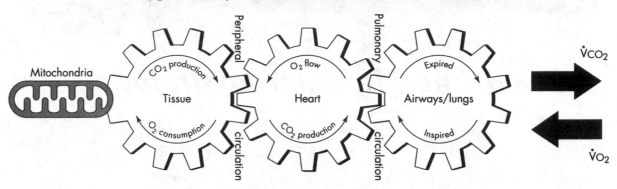

↓ Mitochondria	↓ Muscle mass	Cardiomyopathy	↓ Gag reflex
↓ Oxidative enzymes	↓ Myoglobin	↓ Myocardial mass	↓ Cough reflex
↓ Oxygen extraction	↓ Aerobic capacity	↑ Heart rate	↓ Mucociliary transport
	↓ Muscle strength	↑ Blood pressure	↑ Mucus accumulation
	↓ Tissue perfusion	↑ Fat deposits	Aspiration
		↑ Connective tissue	Hypotonic upper
		↑ Work of the heart	airway structures

Respiratory muscle
  weakness
↓ Respiratory muscle
  endurance
↓ Maximal inspiratory
  pressure
↓ Maximal expiratory
  pressure
Chest wall muscle
  hypotonia
Chest wall hyperinflation
↓ Chest wall excursion
Chest wall deformity
Impaired respiratory
  mechanics
↓ Abdominal muscle
  strength
Noctural respiratory
  insufficiency
↓ Cough effectiveness
Compression atelectasis
Low lung volumes
Closure of dependent
  airways
↑ Chest wall compliance
↓ Lung compliance

↓ Collateral circulation   Hypoxic
Circulatory stasis   Vasoconstriction
    Pulmonary hypertension
    ↓ Lymph flow

Blood: Circulatory stasis
     Thrombi formation
     Hypoxemia
     Hypercapnia

↑ Increase
↓ Decrease

PHYSICAL THERAPY DIAGNOSES AND TREATMENT PRESCRIPTION

Physical Therapy Diagnosis: Altered cardiopulmonary function caused by alveolar hypoventilation, shunt, and impaired gas exchange

Signs and Symptoms: $Pao_2 < 104.2 - 0.27$ age (± 7) mm Hg, $Pao_2 < 75$ mm Hg on room air, $Sao_2 < 90\%$ at night, increased work of breathing, increased minute ventilation and respiratory rate, increased myocardial work, increased A − a oxygen gradient, normal or low $Paco_2$, radiographic and clinical evidence of atelectasis, decreased lung compliance, decreased vital capacity, decreased tidal volume, increased respiratory rate, decreased breath sounds, decreased chest wall excursion, chest wall asymmetry, respiratory muscle weakness, and respiratory muscle fatigue

INTERVENTIONS	RATIONALE
Monitor serial ABGs, Sao_2, respiratory muscle strength and cough effectiveness, and chest x-rays	To provide a baseline, index of disease progression, ongoing assessment, and measure of treatment response
	To determine factors contributing to hypoxemia and to select appropriate interventions and prescriptions
Define outcome criteria: reversal or mitigation of the signs and symptoms	To provide a basis for defining treatment goals and criteria for discontinuing treatment
Oxygen and ventilatory support	To correct hypoxemia and reduce the work of breathing
Monitor breathing pattern; respiratory rate and tidal volume	To assess cardiopulmonary stress
Place in high or semi-Fowler's position	To facilitate breathing and diaphragmatic excursion
Place in erect sitting with legs dependent	
Sit in chair with active-assist transfer	To exploit the *acute* effects of mobilization on cardiopulmonary function in functional activities
Mobilize frequently; coordinated with activities of daily living (ADL)	
Monitor postural alignment in sitting and standing	To optimize postural alignment to enhance moment-to-moment cardiopulmonary function and to prevent chest wall deformity
Balance activity/exercise and rest	To minimize undue energy expenditure and excessive increases in oxygen demand that exceed the capacity for oxygen delivery
Monitor vital signs and electrocardiogram (ECG)	To detect myocardial strain
Assess for orthostatic hypotension	To minimize effect of orthostatic intolerance
Administer oxygen	Pao_2 should increase with increase in fraction of inspired oxygen (Fio_2)
Monitor pulmonary function and signs of deterioration and infection	To assess lung compliance and derive index of work of breathing and prognosis of patient's capacity to maintain spontaneous breathing
Teach glossopharyngeal breathing	To augment alveolar ventilation
Chest wall mobility exercises coordinated with breathing control and assisted coughing maneuvers (proprioceptive neuromuscular facilitation patterns, flexion/extension, and chest wall diagonal rotation)	To exploit the *acute* effects of mobilization and exercise on airway diameter, mucociliary transport, alveolar ventilation, distributions of ventilation, perfusion, and ventilation and perfusion matching, lung motion, lymphatic drainage
	Patient is taught self-assist coughing maneuvers to maximize cough effectiveness and reduce physical and metabolic demands of coughing
Respiratory muscle training: mobilization	Activity and exercise increases respiratory muscle strength and endurance
Intensity—low; dyspnea < 3-4 (0-10 scale)	
Duration—10-30 minutes	
Frequency—2-5 times a day	
Course and progression—as indicated	
Resistive ventilatory muscle training with flow rate control	Resisted respiratory muscle training can increase respiratory muscle strength and capacity to perform ADL
Intensity—initially low resistance	
Duration—5-10 breaths; 3 sets	
Frequency—3-5 times a day	
Course and progression—as indicated	

Continued.

INTERVENTIONS	RATIONALE
Body positioning to improve breathing efficiency and decrease the work of breathing	Upright body positioning increases lung volumes, reduces resistance of abdominal viscera on descent of the diaphragm, and increases lung compliance
Stretching and chest wall mobility exercises	To preserve the three-dimensional movement of the chest wall and minimize chest wall deformity
Prescriptive rest	Rest and ventilatory support is needed to address respiratory muscle fatigue; intermittent noninvasive mechanical ventilation is useful to rest fatigued respiratory muscles, enhance respiratory muscle strength and endurance, and postpone or delay invasive mechanical ventilation
Body positions to reduce the work of breathing	
Oxygen and ventilatory support	
Nocturnal noninvasive mechanical ventilation (continuous positive airway pressure [CPAP])	
	CPAP is a useful mode of noninvasive mechanical ventilation that can provide intermittent ventilatory assistance at night

---

Physical Therapy Diagnosis: Impaired gas exchange: airway obstruction and increased airflow resistance

Signs and Symptoms: Impaired mucociliary transport, secretion accumulation

INTERVENTIONS	RATIONALE
Monitor airflow resistance and airway obstruction	To provide a baseline and ongoing assessment
Mobilization coordinated with breathing control and assisted coughing maneuvers—rhythmic, progress from interval to continuous	To dilate airways
Intensity—dyspnea < 3 (0-10 scale)	To promote mucociliary transport and clearance
Duration—10-30 minutes	
Frequency—2-5 times a day	
Course and progression—as indicated	
Body positioning coordinated with breathing control and assisted coughing maneuvers	To stimulate exercise-induced changes in breathing pattern (rate and depth of respiration) and optimize distributions of ventilation and ventilation and perfusion matching
Body position changes coordinated with breathing control and assisted coughing maneuvers	To stimulate exercise-induced changes in breathing pattern (rate and depth of respiration) to stimulate mucociliary transport
Mobilization coordinated with breathing control and assisted coughing maneuvers—rhythmic continuous or intermittent	To mobilize secretions from peripheral to central airways
Intensity—dyspnea < 3 (0-10 scale)	
Duration—10-30 minutes	
Frequency—2-5 times a day	
Course and progression—as indicated	
Breathing control maneuvers	To augment alveolar ventilation; to stack breaths to increase peak expiratory flow rates
	To avoid breathing below normal end-tidal volume to avoid closure of dependent airways
Assisted coughing maneuvers	To enable the patient to cough effectively (productively and with the least effort)
Self-assisted—in upright seated position, patient places hands firmly over abdomen, stacks inspiratory breaths, and exhales with forward propulsive effort	To maximize inspiratory effort and forced expiratory volume during coughing
Assisted—in upright or recumbent position, physical therapist performs abdominal thrust at maximal inspiration	

Physical Therapy Diagnosis: Pulmonary aspiration

Signs and Symptoms: Hypotonia of pharyngeal and laryngeal structures and upper airway, weak respiratory muscles including abdominal muscles, diminished gag and cough reflexes, reduced ability to change position in the event of swallowing or choking problem, and increased cardiorespiratory distress during eating and around choking episodes

INTERVENTIONS	RATIONALE
Assess patient's history of aspiration and risk factors	To provide a baseline and ongoing assessment
	To establish when patient is at increased risk of aspirating
Define outcome criteria: reversal or mitigation of the signs and symptoms	To provide a basis for defining treatment goals and criteria for discontinuing treatment
Promote bronchopulmonary hygiene	To reduce the risk of aspiration
Promote oral and airway protection	To ensure that patient, friends, and family are familiar with and can apply the Heimlich maneuver
Promote increased head of bed up resting and sleep positions	
Promote side lying when recumbent	
Teach patient assisted coughing techniques (Heimlich maneuver) to dislodge airway obstruction if necessary when alone	
Promote selecting foods that do not cause swallowing problems	
Promote chewing food well	
Promote minimizing talking and laughing with food in mouth	
Teach assisted coughing techniques (e.g., abdominal thrust)	
Encourage patient to teach others how to assist with a Heimlich maneuver to relieve an airway obstruction	

Physical Therapy Diagnosis: Decreased activity and exercise tolerance resulting from neuromuscular disease and respiratory muscle weakness

Signs and Symptoms: Aerobic deconditioning and low maximal functional work capacity; increased heart rate, blood pressure, rate pressure product, and minute ventilation at rest and submaximal work rates; prolonged recovery from exercise; disproportionate exertion and fatigue during and after exercise

INTERVENTIONS	RATIONALE
Determine the patient's premorbid level of function and functional work capacity	To promote a baseline and tentative treatment goal
Define outcome criteria: reversal or mitigation of the signs and symptoms	To provide a basis for defining treatment goals and criteria for discontinuing treatment
Modified submaximal exercise test	Exercise test is modified and submaximal to avoid negative effects of a maximal test, which is invalid in patients whose maximal capacity is limited by neuromuscular or musculoskeletal dysfunction
Modified exercise training program: type—ergometer or walking, possibly hydrotherapy	To exploit the *long-term* benefits of mobilization and exercise; increase activity and exercise endurance while minimizing fatigue and exhaustion
	Water exercise increases chest wall pressure and the work of breathing and is not likely to be tolerated well
Interval training: several bouts of work and rest (e.g., 5 min work–1 min rest)	Interval training maximizes work output and minimizes cardiopulmonary and musculoskeletal stress
Intensity—dyspnea < 3 (0-10 scale) fatigue < 3-4 (0-10 scale)	To optimize cardiopulmonary reserve capacity
Duration—10-30 minutes	
Frequency—2-5 times a day	
Course and progression—as indicated	

Continued.

INTERVENTIONS	RATIONALE
Outcome measures: pulmonary function (maximal inspiratory and expiratory pressures, Sao$_2$, shortness of breath, perceived exertion, fatigue, and serial exercise retests); functional outcomes such as the ability to move or wheel purposefully in physical environment, bed mobility, transfers, ambulation, bathroom and kitchen skills	To ensure that the exercise program is achieving optimal functional outcomes, which is essential in patients with significantly reduced exercise reserve capacity that can be exploited with a mobilization/exercise stimulus
Resistive ventilatory muscle training with regulation of inspiratory flow rate	To optimize respiratory muscle strength and endurance
Prescriptive rest within and between activities and exercise sessions	To optimize energy stores and avoid energy depletion
Increased use of aids and devices (e.g., ambulation aids, electric wheelchair, chest cuirasse, scooter)	To reduce undue oxygen demands and cardiopulmonary stress
	To minimize risk of respiratory muscle fatigue, which indicates rest rather than resistive training
Monitor signs of chronic fatigue and reduced restoration from rest and sleep	Patients with neuromuscular diseases are prone to generalized chronic fatigue, which leads to further functional deterioration; exercise is prescribed to optimize a patient's remaining physiological reserve and not to maximally stress and diminish this reserve

Physical Therapy Diagnosis: Risks of impaired oxygen transport resulting from progressive neuromuscular dysfunction

Signs and Symptoms: Progressive neuromuscular deterioration, increased weakness and decreased endurance, increased shortness of breath, reduced cardiopulmonary function and deconditioning, respiratory distress, further reduction in alveolar ventilation, ability to maintain spontaneous ventilation, further reduction in functional independence, ability to perform ADL and aerobic capacity, progressive muscular weakness, functionally incapacitating respiratory distress, increased work of breathing (particularly at night and extending into the day), decreased ability to maintain a clear airway, accumulation of pulmonary secretions, and increasingly frequent episodes of aspiration

INTERVENTIONS	RATIONALE
Monitor signs and symptoms of progressive neuromuscular dysfunction	To detect signs of progressive deterioration early so treatment can be modified accordingly
Define outcome criteria: reversal or mitigation of the signs and symptoms	To provide a basis for defining treatment goals and criteria for discontinuing treatment
Modify activities and exercise training prescription so demands do not exceed patient's physiological maximal capacity	Patient can maintain an optimal level of functional work capacity and aerobic conditioning, but exercise stimulus parameters are modified
Continuous supplemental oxygen, place in high or semi-Fowler's position	To reduce cardiopulmonary work and maximize alveolar ventilation, gas exchange, mucociliary clearance, and cough effectiveness
	Patients with Duchenne muscular dystrophy primarily die from cardiopulmonary failure and infection; the goal at this stage is supportive to reduce the work of breathing, dyspnea, air hunger, and hypoxemia and maximize body position comfort
Frequent body position changes	To stimulate physiological "stir-up," ventilation; shift distribution of alveolar volume and ventilation, ventilation and perfusion matching; stimulate mucociliary transport and mobilization of secretions
Avoid supine positions, particularly with head level	Supine positions predispose the patient to aspiration and respiratory distress
	Aspiration can lead to life-threatening pneumonitis
Avoid aggressive treatments for 45 minutes after eating	To minimize the risk of gastroesophageal reflux

Physical Therapy Diagnosis: Risk of the negative sequelae of recumbency

Signs and Symptoms: Within 6 hours reduced circulating blood volume, decreased blood pressure on sitting and standing compared with supine, light-headedness, dizziness, syncope, increased hematocrit and blood viscosity, increased work of the heart, altered fluid balance in the lung, impaired pulmonary lymphatic drainage, decreased lung volumes and capacities, decreased functional residual capacity, increased closing volume, and decreased Pao_2 and Sao_2

INTERVENTIONS	RATIONALE
To monitor signs and symptoms of the negative sequelae of recumbency	To provide a baseline and ongoing assessment
	To detect orthostatic intolerance early and intervene as indicated
Define outcome criteria: reversal or mitigation of the signs and symptoms	To provide a basis for defining treatment goals and criteria for discontinuing treatment
Sitting upright position, standing and walking	The upright position is essential to shift fluid volume from central to peripheral circulation and maintain fluid volume regulating mechanisms and circulating blood volume
	The upright position maximizes lung volumes and capacities and functional residual capacity
	The upright position maximizes expiratory flow rate and cough effectiveness
	The upright position optimizes the length-tension relationship, neural stimulation of the respiratory and abdominal muscles, and cough effectiveness
	The upright position coupled with mobilization and breathing control and assisted coughing maneuvers maximizes alveolar ventilation, ventilation and perfusion matching, mucociliary transport, and pulmonary lymphatic drainage

Physical Therapy Diagnosis: Risk of negative sequelae of restricted mobility

Signs and Symptoms: Reduced activity and exercise tolerance, muscle atrophy and reduced muscle strength, decreased oxygen transport efficiency, increased heart rate, blood pressure and minute ventilation at submaximal work rates, reduced respiratory muscle strength, circulatory stasis, thromboemboli (e.g., pulmonary emboli), pressure areas, skin redness, skin breakdown, and ulceration

INTERVENTIONS	RATIONALE
Monitor the signs and symptoms of restricted mobility	To provide a baseline and ongoing assessment
	To detect the signs and symptoms of restricted mobility early and intervene as indicated
Define outcome criteria: reversal or mitigation of the signs and symptoms	To provide a basis for defining treatment goals and criteria for discontinuing treatment
Mobilization and exercise prescription	To exploit the *preventive* effects of mobilization and exercise and optimize circulating blood volume; enhance the efficiency of the steps in the oxygen transport pathway

Physical Therapy Diagnosis: Knowledge deficit

Signs and Symptoms: Lack of information about Duchenne muscular dystrophy, disease progression, and complications

INTERVENTIONS	RATIONALE
Assess knowledge deficits of disease and related cardiopulmonary physical therapy management	To direct teaching at specific deficits with respect to understanding the disease and its management

Continued.

INTERVENTIONS	RATIONALE
Define outcome criteria: reversal or mitigation of the signs and symptoms	To provide a basis for defining treatment goals and criteria for discontinuing treatment
Promote caring and supportive patient-therapist relationship	To focus on treating the patient with muscular dystrophy rather than the condition
Consider every patient interaction an opportunity for patient education	To promote cooperation and active participation of the patient in treatment
Instruct regarding avoidance of upper respiratory tract infections, nutrition, weight control, hydration and fluid balance, modified exercise, ventilatory support, breathing control, and coughing maneuvers	To promote patient's sense of responsibility for health, health promotion and prevention
Reinforce the purpose of medications and the medication schedule	
Teach, demonstrate, and provide feedback on interventions that can be self-administered	Between-treatment interventions are as important as treatments themselves to provide cumulative treatment effect
Teach patient regarding balance of activity and rest	Optimal balance between activity and rest is essential to exploit short-term, long-term, and preventive effects of mobilization and exercise

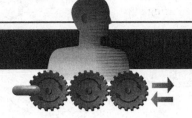

CHAPTER 7

Cerebral Palsy

PATHOPHYSIOLOGY

Cerebral palsy (CP) is a nonprogressive condition that usually results from an ischemic hypoxic injury affecting the central nervous system during the perinatal period. The location and severity of the central lesion determine the type and extent of the mental and motor deficits, the full manifestation of which may not be detected for several months or a few years after birth. Mild lesions, detectable on neurologic examination, may be associated with virtually normal cognitive and motor function. Severe cases are associated with severe mental retardation and total loss of meaningful function resulting from extreme spasticity and residual deformity. There are several patterns of movement disorders associated with CP, including rapid writhing-type movements, athetoid movements, and rapid posturing movements. Movement often alternates between flexion movements with supination and extension movements with pronation. The distribution of involvement may be localized (e.g., diplegia and hemiplegia) or may be generalized. The cardiopulmonary sequelae of CP are clinically significant. These include impaired respiratory mechanics and gas exchange caused by deformity of the chest wall and loss of normal chest wall excursion, abnormal muscle tone, discoordinated breathing pattern, esophageal reflux, poor saliva and secretion control, aspiration, impaired mucociliary clearance, secretion accumulation, ineffective cough, and increased metabolic demands. Inadequate nutrition and hydration are also complications.

Case Study

The patient is an 8-year-old girl. She has a history of moderately severe spastic cerebral palsy and mental retardation. She is confined to a wheelchair; however, she can walk (reflex stepping) with two persons assisting. She lives in a residence for multiply handicapped children. She comes from a large family that lives some distance from the center. Her family visits biweekly. The patient was admitted to hospital following an episode of ineffective coughing to clear a particulate obstruction during eating. Her right lung was completely obliterated on chest x-ray. Her arterial blood gases (ABGs) on room air were pH 7.37, oxygen pressure (Po_2) 67 mm Hg, carbon dioxide pressure (Pco_2) 45 mm Hg, bicarbonate (HCO_3) 24, and arterial oxygen saturation (Sao_2) 90%. She was placed on supplemental oxygen via nasal prongs at 2.5 L/min. The particulate matter was removed during bronchoscopy, but the right lung showed radiographic evidence of consolidation. Her temperature increased to 104°F (40.1°C). She was productive for minimal amounts of moderately thick, yellow secretions. A culture and sensitivity test was done and the appropriate antibiotic administered.

Oxygen Transport Deficits: Observed and Potential

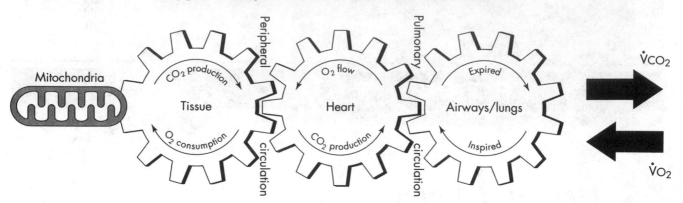

↓ Oxidative enzymes
↑ Oxygen demand

Spasticity
↑ Oxygen consumption
Abnormal muscle tone
Aerobic deconditioning
↓ Myoglobin
↓ Muscle fibers

↑ Resting heart rate
↑ Resting blood pressure

↓ Mucociliary transport
↑ Secretion accumulation
Upper airway gurgling
Drooling
↓ Gag control
↓ Cough effectiveness
↑ Saliva
Weak cough
↓ Saliva control
Aspiration
Atelectasis
Pneumonitis
Chest wall deformity
Rigid chest wall
Abnormal chest wall
   excursion
Abnormal
   thoracoabdominal
   motion
Abnormal respiratory
   muscle recruitment
Compression atelectasis
Low lung volumes
Closure of dependent
   airways
Abnormal tone of
   respiratory muscles
Discoordinated breathing
Crackles

↓ Collateral circulation
Circulatory stasis
↓ Lymph flow
Irregular lymph flow

Blood: Hypoxemia

┌─────────────┐
│ ↑ Increase │
│ ↓ Decrease │
└─────────────┘

PHYSICAL THERAPY DIAGNOSES AND TREATMENT PRESCRIPTION

Physical Therapy Diagnosis: Altered cardiorespiratory function: hypoxemia, alveolar hypoventilation, and shunt

Signs and Symptoms: Abnormal ABGs, hypoxemia, decreased Sao_2, respiratory distress, shortness of breath, radiographic evidence of obstruction in right mainstem bronchus, and radiographic evidence of whiteout of right lung

INTERVENTIONS	RATIONALE
Monitor serial ABGs, Sao_2, and signs of respiratory distress between treatments and before, during, and after treatments	To provide a baseline, ongoing assessment and measure of treatment response
Monitor changes in sputum amount, volume, and characteristics	
Define outcome criteria: reversal or mitigation of the signs and symptoms	To provide a basis for defining treatment goals and criteria for discontinuing treatment
Mobilization	To exploit the *acute* effects of mobilization; that is, maximize alveolar ventilation, ventilation perfusion matching, mucociliary transport, secretion clearance, forced expiratory flow rates, functional residual capacity, arterial saturation, reduce closing volume, and optimize respiratory muscle function
Type—dangling over bed, standing, and walking	
Intensity—within limits of Sao_2, breathlessness and heart rate	
Duration—within limits defining intensity	
Course and progression—as tolerated; as the chest x-ray resolves and the temperature decreases, ambulation in a walker is promoted as frequently as tolerated	Ambulation in the walker maximizes the cardiopulmonary benefits of being upright and moving
Range-of-motion exercises	To exploit the cardiopulmonary benefits of range-of-motion exercises
Upper extremities	
Trunk	
Lower extremities	
Body positioning to minimize further aspiration: upright, supported body positions	To optimize alveolar ventilation and the distributions of ventilation, perfusion, and ventilation and perfusion matching; and gas exchange
	To facilitate mucociliary transport, and dislodging and removing foreign material and pulmonary secretions
	To facilitate coughing and airway clearance by optimizing the length-tension relationships of the respiratory muscles in the erect, upright positions and of the abdominal muscles
	To facilitate normal thoracoabdominal motion
Postural drainage positions for the right lung	To facilitate mucociliary transport
Upper lobe: apical segment—high Fowler's position; anterior segment—supine; posterior segment—¾ prone; superior segment—prone	To mobilize secretions from the peripheral to central airways for clearance with spontaneous coughing and suctioning
Middle lobe: ¾ supine (right lung uppermost)	
Lower lobe: apical segment—prone, no tip; anterior segment—supine, head of bed down; lateral segment—left side lying, head of bed down; posterior segment—prone, head of bed down	
Promote spontaneous coughing; suction mouth and upper airway as indicated	
Frequent body position changes with least time in right side lying	To stimulate normal varied breathing pattern (changes in rate and depth) and minimize monotonous tidal ventilation
	To mobilize secretions and stimulate spontaneous coughing
	To enhance mucociliary transport and minimize bacterial colonization and multiplication
	To stimulate exercise-induced cardiopulmonary responses to optimize alveolar ventilation and airway clearance
	To promote lymphatic drainage within and around the lungs

Continued.

INTERVENTIONS	RATIONALE
Postural drainage positioning coordinated with manual techniques (e.g., percussion, shaking, and manual vibration)	To facilitate airway clearance of secretions from peripheral to central airways
	If indicated, single-handed percussion at a frequency of 1 per second minimizes the untoward effects of this intervention
	To stimulate spontaneous coughing and airway clearance
	To facilitate suctioning and maximize its effectiveness
	To monitor and detect deleterious effects of manual techniques and modify or discontinue treatment as indicated
Set up body positioning (360-degree position rotation schedule) and mobilization schedule for between treatments and during the night, and monitor to ensure positions are maintained; positions are varied; promote beneficial positions and limit deleterious positions	Cerebral palsy patients are at high risk for gastroesophageal reflux and aspiration and its life-threatening sequelae; between-treatment interventions are as important as the treatment sessions themselves
	Severely affected patients are unable to spontaneously move themselves into physiologically desirable positions or maintain such positions
	Severely affected patients may position themselves in deleterious body positions

Physical Therapy Diagnosis: Altered cardiopulmonary function: altered breathing pattern caused by decreased lung compliance

Signs and Symptoms: Increased respiratory distress, shortness of breath, and use of the accessory muscles of respiration

INTERVENTIONS	RATIONALE
Monitor breathing pattern; tidal volume and breathing rate	To provide a baseline, ongoing assessment and treatment response
Define outcome criteria: reversal or mitigation of the signs and symptoms	To provide a basis for defining treatment goals and criteria for discontinuing treatment
Range-of-motion exercises performed gradually	To stimulate a ventilatory response
	To reduce stimulation of spasticity
Stretching and passive mobilization of the upper extremities and chest wall coordinated with body positioning	To mobilize the chest wall and promote improved alveolar ventilation and symmetric breathing pattern
Body positioning: upright positions with patient secured so the position is maintained	To optimize alveolar ventilation, mucociliary transport, airway clearance, and three-dimensional chest wall movement; reduce accessory muscle use and minimize airway closure
Postural drainage positioning	To facilitate airway clearance and drainage of pulmonary secretions
Postural drainage positioning with manual techniques	If indicated, single-handed percussion at a frequency of 1 per second minimizes the untoward effects of this manual technique

Physical Therapy Diagnosis: Pulmonary aspiration and impaired airway protection

Signs and Symptoms: Increased cardiorespiratory distress, shortness of breath and use of accessory muscles of respiration, decreased Pao_2 and Sao_2, increased heart rate and blood pressure, atelectasis, intrapulmonary shunt, spasticity of the muscles of respiration, chest wall, upper airway, head and neck, abdomen, and limbs, abnormal gag and cough reflex, gurgling, gastroesophageal reflux, mental retardation and cognitive deficits, recumbency, restricted mobility, increased pulmonary secretions, pneumonia

INTERVENTIONS	RATIONALE
Monitor degree of aspiration and aspiration risk	To provide a baseline and ongoing assessment
Define outcome criteria: reversal or mitigation of the signs and symptoms	To provide a basis for defining treatment goals and criteria for discontinuing treatment

INTERVENTIONS	RATIONALE
Place patient in bed with head of bed up 10-30 degrees	To minimize the risk of oral and gastric secretions entering the upper airway
Place in high Fowler's position; secure patient	Patient may need to be secured to maintain therapeutic position and avoid moving into a deleterious position
Suction oral cavity and oropharynx frequently to remove accumulated secretions	Sustaining may be indicated if the patient is unable to adequately control mouth secretions or clear upper airway with spontaneous coughing
Suction oral cavity and oropharynx as necessary before, during, and after treatment	
Treat patient 90 minutes after feeds	To ensure that food is further down gastrointestinal tract and has the least risk of being regurgitated and aspirated
Ensure that patient is in as upright a position as possible during feeds and for 60 to 90 minutes after	
Identify triggers for gastroesophageal reflux	To avoid stimulating gastroesophageal reflux activity
Monitor patient closely to ensure that beneficial body positions are maintained and deleterious positions avoided	The patient has a limited ability to cooperate with treatment due to mental retardation

Physical Therapy Diagnosis: Threats to oxygen transport and gas exchange

Signs and Symptoms: Reduced chest wall expansion, chest wall deformity, abnormal breathing pattern, increased tone of the respiratory and chest wall muscles, discoordinated breathing pattern, aspiration, altered cough and gag reflexes, decreased cough effectiveness, poorly protected upper airway, poor saliva control, gastroesophageal reflux, chest infection, increased oxygen demands caused by spasticity, recumbency, and restricted mobility

INTERVENTIONS	RATIONALE
Monitor threats to oxygen transport and gas exchange	To provide a baseline and ongoing assessment
Define outcome criteria: prevention, reversal, or mitigation of the signs and symptoms	To provide a basis for defining treatment goals and criteria for discontinuing treatment
Body positioning schedule	To exploit the "stir-up" principle in this patient, that is, maximize alveolar ventilation, ventilation and perfusion matching, functional residual capacity, facilitate mucociliary transport, promote airway clearance, facilitate spontaneous coughing, minimize bacterial colonization and multiplication, facilitate lymphatic drainage, minimize airway closure
Maximize time in various upright rather than recumbent positions	
Frequent changes in body positions	
Reduce spasticity	Spasticity compromises oxygen transport and gas exchange via several mechanisms:
	Affects the respiratory muscles
	Affects the accessory muscles
	Affects the abdominal muscles
	Affects the oropharyngeal and laryngeal muscles
	Affects the neck, head, and face
	Affects the limbs, which impedes range-of-motion and mobilizing and positioning the patient
	Restricts chest wall movement
	Impedes airway clearance via cough or suctioning
	Significantly increases oxygen demand and the demands on the oxygen transport system
	Select positions that minimize spasticity to reduce increased oxygen demands and minimize interference with treatment and treatment effect
	Perform physical therapy interventions to inhibit spasticity
	Determine whether spasticity reduction with body positioning could be augmented with antispasticity medication; consult with team if indicated

Continued.

INTERVENTIONS	RATIONALE
Promote relaxation	Handle patient gently and with appropriate support and assistance from others as necessary
	Speak to patient in calm, reassuring manner
	Use music or other modalities to induce relaxation
	Observe what factors in the social and physical environment stimulate or reduce spasticity and incorporate this information during treatment

Physical Therapy Diagnosis: Risk of the negative sequelae of recumbency

Signs and Symptoms: Within 6 hours reduced circulating blood volume, decreased blood pressure on sitting and standing compared with supine, light-headedness, dizziness, syncope, increased hematocrit and blood viscosity, increased work of the heart, altered fluid balance in the lung, impaired pulmonary lymphatic drainage, decreased lung volumes and capacities, decreased functional residual capacity, increased closing volume, and decreased Pao_2 and Sao_2

INTERVENTIONS	RATIONALE
Monitor signs and symptoms of the sequelae of recumbency	To provide a baseline and ongoing assessment
Define outcome criteria: prevention, reversal, or mitigation of the signs and symptoms	To provide a basis for defining treatment goals and criteria for discontinuing treatment
Sitting upright position, erect standing and walking with two-person assist	To detect orthostatic intolerance early and modify treatment as indicated
	The upright position is essential to shift fluid volume from central to peripheral circulation and maintain fluid volume regulating mechanisms and circulating blood volume
	The upright position maximizes lung volumes and capacities and functional residual capacity
	The upright position maximizes expiratory flow rate and cough effectiveness
	The upright position optimizes the length-tension relationship of the respiratory muscles and abdominal muscles and optimizes cough effectiveness
	The upright position maximizes alveolar ventilation, ventilation and perfusion matching, pulmonary lymphatic drainage, mucociliary transport, mucociliary clearance

Physical Therapy Diagnosis: Risk of negative sequelae of restricted mobility

Signs and Symptoms: Reduced activity and exercise tolerance, muscle atrophy and reduced muscle strength, decreased oxygen transport efficiency, increased heart rate, blood pressure, and minute ventilation at submaximal work rates, reduced respiratory muscle strength, circulatory stasis, thromboemboli (e.g., pulmonary emboli), pressure areas, skin breakdown, and ulceration

INTERVENTIONS	RATIONALE
Monitor the negative sequelae of restricted mobility	To provide a baseline and ongoing assessment
Define outcome criteria: prevention, reversal, or mitigation of the signs and symptoms	To provide a basis for defining treatment goals and criteria for discontinuing treatment

INTERVENTIONS	RATIONALE
Mobilization and exercise prescription Type—range-of-motion exercises of the upper extremities, chest wall, and lower extremities performed in a variety of body positions, walking with assistance and with walker Coordinate with antispasticity medication as indicated	Because of the severe physical and mental deficits, mobilization consists of passive range of motion and limited standing and walking with two persons assisting to augment ventilation, flow rates, mucociliary transport, mucociliary clearance, lymphatic drainage Varying the body position simulates a "stir-up" regimen Movements are performed to minimize spasticity and detrimental body postures

Physical Therapy Diagnosis: Knowledge deficit

Signs and Symptoms: Lack of information of the caregivers about the cardiopulmonary manifestations of cerebral palsy, complications, and physical therapy management

INTERVENTIONS	RATIONALE
Assess specific knowledge deficits related to the condition and cardiopulmonary physical therapy management Define outcome criteria: reversal or mitigation of the signs and symptoms Promote a caring and supportive patient-therapist relationship Promote prevention of cardiopulmonary complications Instruct caregivers regarding avoidance of respiratory tract infections, nutrition, weight control, hydration and fluid balance, mobilization, body positioning and frequency of turning, alveolar ventilation, airway clearance, and gas exchange Reinforce medication schedule with respect to optimizing treatment response (optimizing cardiopulmonary function and gas exchange and reducing the risk of complications)	To provide a baseline and ongoing assessment To provide a basis for defining treatment goals and criteria for discontinuing treatment To focus on treating the patient with cerebral palsy rather than cerebral palsy Multiply handicapped individuals are prone to cardiopulmonary complications, which can be life-threatening Between-treatment interventions are as important as treatments themselves to provide cumulative treatment effect

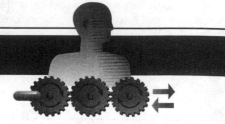

CHAPTER 8

Systemic Lupus Erythematosus

PATHOPHYSIOLOGY

Systemic lupus erythematosus (SLE) is one of the collagen vascular diseases—a group of immunologically-mediated inflammatory disorders. Although the disease predominantly affects women of childbearing age, it may also affect children, men, and the elderly. The cause of SLE is unknown; genetic and environmental factors and alterations in the immune response have been implicated. Systemic lupus erythematosus is characterized by hyperactivity of B and T lymphocytes, which results in tissue and cell destruction. Most lesions occur in the blood vessels, kidney, primary connective tissue structures, and skin; SLE may affect one or more organ systems. Depending on which systems are involved, the patient may suffer from arthritis (a nonerosive synovitis without joint deformity), glomerulonephritis, splenomegaly, hepatomegaly, pleuritis and pleural effusions, pericarditis, lymphadenopathy, peritonitis, neuritis, mild cognitive dysfunction, seizures, thrombosis, and anemia. Retinal vasculitis can develop into blindness within a few days. These pathophysiological changes result in pain, weakness, fatigue, erythema (usually in a butterfly pattern over the cheeks and bridge of the nose), photosensitivity, malaise, fever, depression, anxiety, weight loss, and anorexia.

Case Study

The patient is a 38-year-old woman. She teaches kindergarten full-time. She is married to a building contractor. They have three children. They live in a two-story home. She was diagnosed with systemic lupus erythematosus 3 years ago. Her condition had been relatively stable to the present; however, she had lost about 18 pounds (8 kg) (body mass index 21) and has been mildly anemic. Over the past 3 weeks, she developed fever and chills, which was accompanied by chest discomfort, general joint achiness, shortness of breath, and reduced exercise tolerance. She was admitted to hospital with pericarditis and arthralgia. After admission she developed a pleural effusion on the left side. Patchy acinar infiltrates were observed in the lower lobes. She is on a course of corticosteroids.

Oxygen Transport Deficits: Observed and Potential

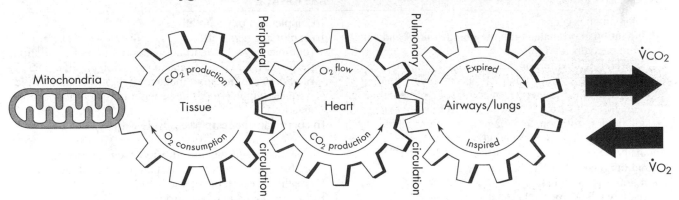

↑ Oxygen demand

↓ Muscle mass
Muscle weakness
↓ Aerobic capacity
Renal insufficiency

Right ventricular strain
Pericarditis

Closure dependent
   airways
↓ Lung compliance
Low lung volumes
Shrinking lung syndrome
↓ Chest wall excursion
↓ Breathing efficiency
↑ Energy cost of breathing
↑ Resting position of the
   diaphragm
Rapid, shallow breathing
   pattern
Compression atelectasis
Pleuritis
Pleural effusions
↓ Diffusing capacity

Vasculitis
Peripheral vasospasm
Altered regional blood
   flow

Vasculitis
↓ Lymph flow

↑	Increase
↓	Decrease

Blood: Hypoxemia

PHYSICAL THERAPY DIAGNOSES AND TREATMENT PRESCRIPTION

Physical Therapy Diagnosis: Altered cardiopulmonary function: alveolar hypoventilation and shunt

Signs and Symptoms: Respiratory infection, increased temperature, dyspnea, fever, and associated increased oxygen demand, altered arterial blood gases (ABGs), arterial hypoxemia and hypercapnia, radiographic evidence of restrictive lung pathology (i.e., shrinking lung syndrome), rigid chest wall, loss of normal chest wall excursion, arterial desaturation on exertion, increased pulmonary vascular resistance, pulmonary hypertension, increased stroke work of the heart, pleural effusions, patchy acinar infiltrates in the lower lobes on chest x-ray, elevated hemidiaphragms, pleuritic chest pain and chest wall splinting, weakness of the respiratory muscles, diffusion defect, anemia, weight loss, poor nutrition, reduced lymphatic drainage

INTERVENTIONS	RATIONALE
Monitor vital signs, hemoglobin, ABGs, arterial oxygen saturation (Sao_2) and monitor respiratory distress	To provide a baseline, ongoing assessment and measure of treatment response
Define outcome criteria: reversal or mitigation of the signs and symptoms	To provide a basis for defining treatment goals and criteria for discontinuing treatment

Continued.

INTERVENTIONS	RATIONALE
Supplemental oxygen	To supplement oxygen delivery
Mobilization coordinated with breathing control and coughing maneuvers, and tolerance	To exploit the *acute* effects of mobilization and exercise (optimize alveolar ventilation, distribution of ventilation, perfusion, and ventilation and perfusion matching, respiratory muscle function, mucociliary transport, lung fluid balance, lymphatic drainage and minimize bacterial colonization)
Type: walking, chair ergometer; aerobic rhythmic, paced; avoid isometric, static contractions and breath holding and Valsalva maneuver; sit over the edge of bed; transfer to chair; erect sitting in chair, forward flexion, extension, side flexion, rotation, and diagonal rotation; inhale on extension, exhale on flexion movements	To coordinate the respiratory cycle with movement
Intensity—Sao_2 > 90%, breathlessness < 3-5 (0-10 scale); and fatigue < 3-5 (0-10 scale)	The parameters of the mobilization/exercise prescription are based on hemodynamic stability, arterial saturation, breathlessness, fatigue, and hemoglobin levels
Duration—10-30 minutes	
Frequency—5-2 times a day	To ensure that patient is appropriately monitored so that the patient's tolerance is not exceeded and that the mobilization does not impose undue physiological stress or discomfort
Course and progression—as indicated	
Monitor the patient closely during treatment	As the patient's status improves and tolerance increases, intensity and duration are increased and the frequency of sessions is decreased
Body positioning	To reduce respiratory distress by optimizing alveolar ventilation and the distributions of ventilation, perfusion, ventilation and perfusion matching, and gas exchange
Place in high or semi-Fowler's position coordinated with breathing control and coughing maneuvers	To optimize lung compliance by reducing thoracic blood volume and abdominal pressure encroaching on diaphragmatic excursion
	To optimize chest wall excursion and compliance
	To shift pleural fluid and open previously closed alveoli
Positioning; coordinated with breathing control and coughing maneuvers (avoid breathing below end-tidal volume)	To maximize alveolar volume and resolve infiltrates in the lower lobes
Right lower lobe: anterior segment—supine, head of bed down; lateral segment—left side lying, head of bed down; posterior segment—prone, head of bed down; superior segment—prone, horizontal	
Left lower lobe: anterior segment—supine, head of bed down; lateral segment—right side lying, head of bed down; posterior segment—prone, head of bed down; superior segment—prone, horizontal	
Duration—as indicated by treatment response	
Frequency—as indicated by treatment response	
Course—monitor before, during, and after each body position, monitor before and after entire treatment session	
Select best positions for treatment, and minimize positions both in and between treatments that impair alveolar volume and ventilation and contribute to increased cardiopulmonary distress	To establish which body positions are most efficacious in maximizing alveolar volume and ventilation and overall gas exchange
360-degree positional rotation regimen (hourly) when in bed; right and left side lying; ¾ supine both sides; ¾ prone both sides; supine	To maximize three-dimensional chest wall movement by maximizing the number of body positions when recumbent and avoiding excessive time in a few positions (e.g., side lying and supine)
Stretching and range-of-motion exercises coordinated with breathing control and coughing maneuvers: upper extremities; trunk; lower extremities, including hip and knee and foot and ankle exercises	To exploit the cardiopulmonary effects of range-of-motion exercises

Physical Therapy Diagnosis: Inefficient breathing pattern: decreased lung compliance

Signs and Symptoms: Rapid shallow breathing pattern, decreased lung volumes, decreased lung compliance, chest wall rigidity, loss of normal chest wall excursion during the breathing cycle, abnormal thoracoabdominal motion, metabolically inefficient breathing pattern, and increased work of breathing

INTERVENTIONS	RATIONALE
To monitor breathing pattern at rest and during exertion	To provide a baseline, ongoing assessment and measure of treatment response
Define outcome criteria: reversal or mitigation of the signs and symptoms	To provide a basis for defining treatment goals and criteria for discontinuing treatment
Mobilization and exercise coordinated with breathing control and coughing maneuvers	To improve breathing efficiency during physical activity
Type—walking	To reduce the work of breathing and of the heart
Intensity—comfortable rhythmic erect pace, progress from interval to continuous; breathlessness < 2-3 (0-10 scale)	To minimize the negative effects of pleural effusion on ventilation
Duration—5-15 minutes to 15-30 minutes	To promote absorption and resolution of pleural fluid accumulation
Frequency—5-2 times a day	As the patient's status improves, the intensity and duration increase and the frequency of sessions decreases
Course and progression—as indicated; no undue fatigue after exercise	
Type—chair ergometer	
Intensity—comfortable rhythmic cadence; breathlessness < 2-3 (0-10 scale)	
Duration—5-15 minutes to 15-30 minutes	
Frequency—5-2 times a day	
Course and progression—as indicated; no undue fatigue after exercise	
Body positioning	Identify positions associated with improved oxygen transport and gas exchange
Positions that reduce respiratory distress and dyspnea	Identify positions associated with impaired oxygen transport and gas exchange so that duration in these positions can be minimized
Positions of relaxation (e.g., upright sitting, standing, slow walking)	
Chest wall stretching and mobility exercises coordinated with breathing control and coughing maneuvers	To optimize three-dimensional chest wall movement and chest wall compliance
In sitting and lying—trunk mobility exercises (e.g., forward flexion, extension, side flexion, rotation, diagonal rotation), upper extremity range-of-motion exercises, upper extremity and trunk rotation proprioceptive neuromuscular facilitation patterns (unresisted)	To enhance breathing efficiency
	To promote efficient and metabolically economical movement
	To reduce the work of breathing
	To reduce the work of the heart

Physical Therapy Diagnosis: Decreased activity and exercise tolerance caused by acute infection, anemia, weakness, fatigue, deconditioning, and joint pain

Signs and Symptoms: Dyspnea on exertion, desaturation on exertion, and exaggerated increase in heart rate, blood pressure, rate pressure product, minute ventilation, breathlessness, perceived exertion, and fatigue at submaximal work rates

INTERVENTIONS	RATIONALE
Determine premorbid function and functional capacity	To provide a baseline and treatment goals
Assess activity tolerance and exercise tolerance with a modified exercise test	
Monitor hemoglobin	To ensure that anemia is being optimally managed; otherwise mobilization program may place excessive demands on oxygen delivery
Define outcome criteria: reversal or mitigation of the signs and symptoms	To provide a basis for defining treatment goals and criteria for discontinuing treatment

Continued.

INTERVENTIONS	RATIONALE
Exercise prescription	To exploit the *long-term* effects of mobilization and exercise
Type—aerobic, rhythmic exercise; progress from interval to continuous schedule	
Intensity—low; Sao$_2$ > 88%; avoid undue breathlessness, fatigue, and discomfort	Exercise intensity is low commensurate with patient's physiological oxygen delivery capacity (e.g., hemoglobin)
Duration—10-30 minutes	As the patient's acute cardiopulmonary status improves, hemoglobin is controlled and tolerance increases, intensity and duration increase, and the frequency of sessions decrease
Frequency—4-1 times a day	
Course and progression—as indicated	
Type—strengthening exercise avoiding heavy resistive exercise and isometric exercise	To augment aerobic capacity capacity in functional activities
Perform repetitions slowly and coordinated with breathing; inspiration on extension and expiration on flexion	To maximize exercise tolerance
Intensity—interval training (sets interspersed with rest periods); 30%-60% of one repetition maximum	To optimize strength commensurate with functional activities
Repetitions—10	To avoid undue breathlessness and fatigue
Sets—3	
Frequency—2-1 times a day	
Course and progression—as indicated	
Type—chest wall stretching and mobility; movement in all three planes	To maintain maximal three-dimensional chest wall movement
Intensity—low, rhythmic, stretching	To minimize chest wall rigidity
Duration—as necessary	
Frequency—daily	
Course and progression—as indicated	
Teach patient chest wall stretching and mobility exercises	To promote patient's responsibility for self
Ensure restorative rest and sleep	To monitor quality and number of patient's rest periods within an exercise session and between sessions and ensure adequately restorative sleep and rest
	To monitor quality and quantity of patient's night sleep and whether adequately restorative

Physical Therapy Diagnosis: Threats to oxygen transport and gas exchange

Signs and Symptoms: Pneumonitis and pulmonary infection, increased white blood cell count, cardiopulmonary and functional manifestations of progressive collagen vascular disease, positional substernal chest pain and pericarditis, increased pleural effusions with pericardial involvement, infection resulting from long-term corticosteriod use, nutritional deficit, anemia, cardiopulmonary deconditioning, neuromuscular deconditioning, musculoskeletal deconditioning, pericardial, myocardial, endocardial, valvular, coronary artery, and electrocardiogram (ECG) abnormalities, and pleural, parenchymal, interstitial, vascular, and respiratory muscle abnormalities

INTERVENTIONS	RATIONALE
Monitor risks of impaired oxygen transport and gas exchange	To provide a baseline, detect impairment of oxygen transport, and intervene early
Serial monitoring of respiratory distress, blood work, ABGs, ECG, pulmonary function	To detect improvement and deterioration in cardiopulmonary status
Monitor complaints of substernal chest pain and signs of pericarditis	Most common clinical evidence of pericardial involvement
Define outcome criteria: prevention, reversal, or mitigation of the signs and symptoms	To provide a basis for defining treatment goals and criteria for discontinuing treatment
Promote good nutrition and balanced diet with attention to iron-rich foods and high complex carbohydrate content	To help remediate iron deficiency
	To promote glycogen stores and enhance muscle performance
Monitor response of treatment for anemia	Anemia is a primary factor contributing to reduced activity and exercise tolerance

INTERVENTIONS	RATIONALE
Exercise prescription Type—aerobic strengthening Intensity—low; breathlessness < 3-5 (0-10 scale); fatigue <3 (0-10 scale) Duration—20-40 minutes Frequency—daily Course and progression—as indicated	To exploit the *preventive* effects of exercise on oxygen transport and gas exchange To prescribe exercise within limits of breathlessness and fatigue; fatigue reflects reduced capacity secondary to anemia, thus patient should not be excessively fatigued or exhausted To enhance movement efficiency and metabolic economy to reduce untoward energy expenditure and demand on the oxygen transport system
Monitor ECG and other signs and symptoms of cardiac involvement	To detect early the cardiac manifestations of systemic lupus erythematosus and modify treatment accordingly
Monitor ABGs, pulmonary function test results, and other signs and symptoms of pulmonary involvement	To detect early the pulmonary manifestations of systemic lupus erythematosus and modify treatment accordingly

Physical Therapy Diagnosis: Nutritional and fluid deficits

Signs and Symptoms: Low body mass index, possible contribution to anemia, third spacing of fluids in pleural cavity contributes to potential fluid deficit, reduced activity/exercise tolerance, lethargy, fatigue

INTERVENTIONS	RATIONALE
Monitor input and output with respect to solids and fluids	To establish the degree to which nutritional and fluid deficits contribute to cardiopulmonary distress and activity/exercise intolerance To establish the degree to which dyspnea, shortness of breath, and fatigue contribute to nutritional and fluid deficits
Define outcome criteria: prevention, reversal, or migitation of the signs and symptoms	To provide a basis for defining treatment goals and criteria for discontinuing treatment
Encourage optional nutrition and fluid intake	Optimal nutrition and hydration essential for homeostasis, optimal health, and treatment response

Physical Therapy Diagnosis: Risk of the negative sequelae of recumbency

Signs and Symptoms: Within 6 hours reduced circulating blood volume, decreased blood pressure on sitting and standing compared with supine, light-headedness, dizziness, syncope, increased hematocrit and blood viscosity, increased work of the heart, altered fluid balance in the lung, impaired pulmonary lymphatic drainage, decreased lung volumes and capacities, decreased functional residual capacity, increased closing volume, and decreased Pao_2 and Sao_2

INTERVENTIONS	RATIONALE
Monitor signs and symptoms of negative sequelae of recumbency	To provide a baseline and ongoing assessment To detect such sequelae early and intervene accordingly
Define outcome criteria: prevention, reversal, or mitigation of the signs and symptoms	To provide a basis for defining treatment goals and criteria for discontinuing treatment
Sitting upright position, standing and walking	The upright position is essential to shift fluid volume from central to peripheral circulation and maintain fluid volume regulating mechanisms and circulating blood volume The upright position maximizes lung volumes and capacities and functional residual capacity The upright position maximizes expiratory flow rate and cough effectiveness The upright position optimizes the length-tension relationship, neural stimulation of the respiratory muscles, and abdominal muscles, and cough effectiveness

Continued.

INTERVENTIONS	RATIONALE
	The upright position coupled with mobilization and breathing control and coughing maneuvers maximizes alveolar ventilation, ventilation and perfusion matching, and pulmonary lymphatic drainage

Physical Therapy Diagnosis: Risk of negative sequelae of restricted mobility

Signs and Symptoms: Reduced activity and exercise tolerance, muscle atrophy and reduced muscle strength, decreased oxygen transport efficiency, increased heart rate, blood pressure, and minute ventilation at submaximal work rates, reduced respiratory muscle strength, circulatory stasis, thromboemboli (e.g., pulmonary emboli), pressure areas, skin breakdown, and ulceration

INTERVENTIONS	RATIONALE
To monitor the signs and symptoms of the negative sequelae of restricted mobility	To provide a baseline and ongoing assessment
	To detect such sequelae early and intervene accordingly
Define outcome criteria: reversal or mitigation of the signs and symptoms	To provide a basis for defining treatment goals and criteria for discontinuing treatment
Mobilization and exercise prescription	Mobilization and exercise optimize circulating blood volume, enhance the efficiency of all steps in the oxygen transport pathway
	To exploit the *preventive* effects of mobilization and exercise

Physical Therapy Diagnosis: Knowledge deficit

Signs and Symptoms: Lack of information about systemic lupus erythematosus, exacerbations, infections, and complications

INTERVENTIONS	RATIONALE
Assess specific knowledge deficits related to systemic lupus erythematosus and cardiopulmonary physical therapy management	To provide a baseline of specific knowledge deficits and ongoing assessment
Define outcome criteria: reversal or mitigation of the signs and symptoms	To provide a basis for defining treatment goals and criteria for discontinuing treatment
Promote a caring and supportive patient-therapist relationship	To treat the patient with lupus rather than the condition
Consider every patient interaction an opportunity for patient education	To promote cooperation and active participation of the patient in treatment
Instruct regarding avoidance of respiratory tract infections, nutrition, weight control, hydration and fluid balance, exercise, fatigue management, stress management	Promote patient's sense of responsibility for health, health promotion, and prevention
Reinforce medications, their purpose, and medication schedule	
Teach, demonstrate, and provide feedback on interventions that can be self-administered	Between-treatment interventions are as important as treatments themselves to provide cumulative treatment effect
Teach patient regarding balance of activity and rest	Optimal balance between activity and rest is essential to exploit short-term, long-term, and preventive effects of mobilization and exercise
Provide individualized written handout on general information, treatment, and treatment prescription	To promote cumulative benefit of treatments
Provide a handout at discharge on general information, exercise prescription, and home program	To promote continuity of care and follow-up with a community physical therapist

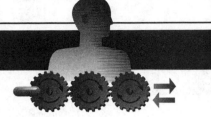

CHAPTER 9

Crohn's Disease

PATHOPHYSIOLOGY

Crohn's disease is a form of inflammatory bowel disease primarily affecting young men between the ages of 30 and 50. The cause of Crohn's disease is not known. Various environmental factors, infectious agents, diet, stress, and emotional factors have been implicated. Crohn's disease may occur anywhere in the gastrointestinal tract but is most commonly found in the proximal colon and ileocecal junction. The rectum is usually spared. Crohn's disease is characterized by chronic inflammation that affects the mesentery and lymph nodes. It extends through all layers of the intestinal wall in a discontinuous, "cobblestone" pattern in which affected portions of the intestine are separated by normal intestine. In the early stage, the intestine is edematous but still pliable. In later stages the intestine becomes thick and leathery; the lumen is narrowed and eventually becomes obstructed. Ulcerations of the mucosa may penetrate into the submucosa and muscularis to form fistulas and fissures. The inflamed and scarred intestinal wall interferes with the absorption of nutrients. These changes cause fever, abdominal pain, diarrhea (without blood), steatorrhea, generalized fatigue, anorexia, nausea, vomiting, and weight loss. Complications associated with Crohn's disease are intestinal obstruction, fistula formation, gastric and duodenal involvement, small intestine and colonic malignancy, and less commonly intestinal perforation and secondary amyloidosis. Bile salt malabsorption and gallstones are associated with advanced and extensive stages of the disease.

Case Study

The patient is a 26-year-old man. He is a welder. He has been trying to put in overtime to help reduce the mortgage on his house. He has had a 10-year history of gastrointestinal complaints and severe abdominal pain; he was diagnosed with Crohn's disease. Surgery was advised last year but he was reluctant to go through with it. Over the past year, his symptoms have become more persistent to the point where he has missed considerable time from work. His medications have been less effective during this time. He smokes half a pack of cigarettes a day and has done so for the past 10 years. He is a moderately heavy drinker. He is about 20 pounds (9 kg) underweight. He has been admitted to hospital for workup of his bowel disease. In addition, he has a lower respiratory tract infection with productive cough. His chest x-ray showed small lung volumes, elevated hemidiaphragms bilaterally, and bilateral infiltrates.

Oxygen Transport Deficits: Observed and Potential

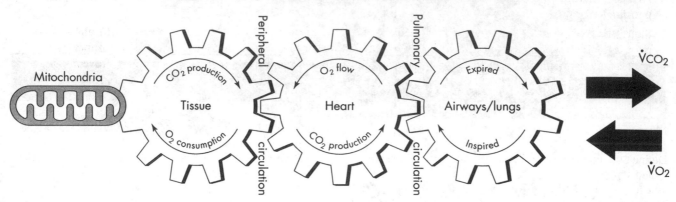

↑ Oxygen demand

↓ Aerobic capacity
↓ Muscle strength

Pericardial effusions

↑ Airway closure
Low lung volumes
Atelectasis
Altered thoracoabdominal
    motion

Pleural effusions
↓ Lymph flow
↓ Lymphatic drainage

| ↑ Increase |
| ↓ Decrease |

PHYSICAL THERAPY DIAGNOSES AND TREATMENT PRESCRIPTION

Physical Therapy Diagnosis: Pain

Signs and Symptoms: Verbalization of pain, grimacing, abdominal guarding, cramps, restlessness, favoring fetal position with abdominal guarding during acute pain episodes, rigid posture and hesitation to change body position, avoidance of activity and exercise, reduced tolerance for activity and exercise, impaired sleep, and nonrestorative rest and sleep

INTERVENTIONS	RATIONALE
Monitor pain type, location, characteristics, duration, intensity, and relationship to diet; monitor activity and elimination	To provide a baseline, ongoing assessment and measure of treatment response
	To establish causative and contributing factors to pain and ameliorating factors
Define outcome criteria: reversal or mitigation of the signs and symptoms	To provide a basis for defining treatment and criteria for discontinuing treatment
Promote patient's sense of control over pain	To promote pain management interventions that the patient can self-administer
Ensure that medications taken as indicated (e.g., analgesics and antiinflammatories)	To ensure that patient understands importance of medication in relieving symptoms and need to take them as prescribed
Teach relaxation procedures (e.g., breathing control, Jacobsen's relaxation technique, Benson's relaxation method, autogenic training, visual imagery, biofeedback)	To enable patient to reduce stress and avoid or mitigate exacerbations of the disease and pain
	To reduce patient's suffering
Encourage frequent use of relaxation procedures between exacerbations	To reduce the patient's reliance on medication for pain control
Encourage frequent use of relaxation procedures during acute pain episodes	To promote habitual use of relaxation procedures between and during acute exacerbations; during acute exacerbations, relaxation may assist patient to alter body positions and reduce muscular guarding and tension
	Pain control is a priority to reduce patient's suffering and to promote patient's ability to cooperate with treatment

Physical Therapy Diagnosis: Inefficient breathing pattern caused by lower respiratory tract infection and pain and its anticipation

Signs and Symptoms: Guarding and splinting secondary to acute and long-term experience with abdominal pain, impaired thoracoabdominal wall movement, reduced chest wall excursion, chest wall asymmetry, stooped, forward flexion posture, rigid posture during ambulation, avoidance of activity and movement, and slow ambulation

INTERVENTIONS	RATIONALE
Monitor breathing pattern	To provide a baseline, ongoing assessment and measure of treatment response
Define outcome criteria: reversal or mitigation of the signs and symptoms	To provide a basis for defining treatment goals and criteria for discontinuing treatment
Teach avoidance of aggravating factors	Promote patient's control over symptoms
Teach relaxation and its integration into activities of daily life (ADL)	
Teach breathing control; integrate into ADL and relaxation sessions	
Teach breathing control in conjunction with corrected posture and gait	
Teach postural correction and normal, efficient walking gait	
Prescribe an exercise program based on an exercise or types of exercise selected by the patient	Maximize patient's involvement with exercise prescription to maximize long-term adherence to the program
Promote appropriate use of medications to maximize function and disease control	Promote general physical and mental health and wellness

Physical Therapy Diagnosis: Nutritional and fluid deficits

Signs and Symptoms: Inability to ingest and absorb nutrients and water, pain, lack of appetite, fear of eating, weight loss, diarrhea, nausea and vomiting, anorexia, dehydration

INTERVENTIONS	RATIONALE
Monitor serial blood work and clinical indicators of nutritional status and fluid balance	To provide a baseline, ongoing assessment and measure of treatment response
Monitor nutritional and fluid status, body weight, activity level, and sense of well-being	Modify treatment prescription of particular exercise and other metabolically demanding activities with exacerbations and remissions of symptoms
Define outcome criteria: reversal or mitigation of the signs and symptoms	To provide a basis for defining treatment goals and criteria for discontinuing treatment
Determine severity of nutritional and fluid deficits	Reinforce optimal nutrition, optimal food choices for the patient's condition at different stages for maximal health, functional performance, and symptom reduction
Reinforce avoidance of exacerbating foods and alcohol	
Assess eating behaviors; encourage preparing interesting meals of nonaggravating foods, eating small meals frequently, consuming fluids plentifully; eat in a pleasant environment; avoid stress around mealtimes; avoid physical activity and exercise for 60 minutes after meals	Optional nutrition and hydration are essential for the patient to maximally benefit from the short-term and long-term benefits of treatment
Reinforce the need for adherence to preprandial and postprandial medication schedule	Adherence to preprandial and postprandial medication schedule is essential to maximize digestion and absorption of nutrients and to promote the absorption of supplemental vitamins and minerals

Continued.

Physical Therapy Diagnosis: Risks of impaired oxygen transport and gas exchange caused by exacerbations of inflammatory bowel episodes; pain; medications, recumbency, inactivity

Signs and Symptoms: Exacerbation of inflammatory bowel disease with pain, cramps, guarding and splinting, inadequate intake of nutrients and fluids, diarrhea, nausea, lack of appetite, anorexia, intestinal obstruction, nutrition and fluid deficits, fluid and electrolyte imbalance, anemia, restricted mobility, recumbency

INTERVENTIONS	RATIONALE
Monitor oxygen transport status and cardiopulmonary function	To provide a baseline to indicate improvement or deterioration and ongoing assessment
Define outcome criteria: prevention, reversal, or mitigation of the signs and symptoms	To provide a basis for defining treatment goals and criteria for discontinuing treatment
Promote a healthy lifestyle (exercise; balanced diet; nonaggravating foods; adequate hydration; adequate sleep and rest; avoidance of smoking, alcohol intake, and substance abuse; balanced social life; good social support network; stress management)	To minimize risk of exacerbation of bowel inflammation To minimize severity of exacerbation To enhance recovery from an exacerbation
Modify treatment prescription with fluctuations in condition	

Physical Therapy Diagnosis: Altered cardiopulmonary function: alveolar hypoventilation and abnormal breathing pattern

Signs and Symptoms: Breathing at low lung volumes, monotonous tidal ventilation, irregular breathing pattern with pain and its anticipation, maintaining static body positions, diffuse bilateral infiltrates

INTERVENTIONS	RATIONALE
Monitor alveolar ventilation and breathing pattern	To provide a baseline and ongoing assessment
Define outcome criteria: reversal or mitigation of the signs and symptoms	To provide a basis for defining treatment goals and criteria for discontinuing treatment
Coordinate breathing control with mobilization and ADL	To promote normal ventilatory pattern To promote regular respiratory cycle with sighs interspersed
Promote breathing control during relaxed upright postures and walking	To optimize chest wall expansion and excursion
Relax chest wall and abdominal musculature	To relax the chest wall muscles to effect a normal breathing pattern

Stretching and chest wall mobility exercises
  Upper extremity
  Trunk
  Lower extremity
	To practice coordinating relaxation and breathing control between bouts of acute abdominal pain so this skill is easier to perform during episodes of pain
	To maximize chest wall mobility and optimize excursion

360-degree positional rotation schedule when recumbent (coordinate with breathing control and coughing maneuvers)	To maximize physiological "stir-up" and exploit the *acute* effects of mobilization and positioning on alveolar volume, alveolar ventilation, and gas exchange
Duration—less than 1-2 hours in any position	
Frequency—at least every 1-2 hours	
Course and progression—as indicated	

Physical Therapy Diagnosis: Decreased activity and exercise tolerance

Signs and Symptoms: General malaise, lethargy, fatigue, reduced ability to perform ADL, reduced aerobic capacity and muscle strength, and reduced efficiency of the oxygen transport system

INTERVENTIONS	RATIONALE
Establish premorbid activity level and functional work capacity	To provide a baseline, ongoing assessment and treatment goal

INTERVENTIONS	RATIONALE
Define outcome criteria: reversal or mitigation of the signs and symptoms	To provide a basis for defining treatment goals and criteria for discontinuing treatment
Exercise prescription	To exploit the *long-term* effects of exercise (i.e., maximize functional capacity and efficiency of the oxygen transport system) and optimize functional capacity and physical and psychological well-being
Preexercise conditions: feeling well; minimal acute pain; peak energy time of day; medicated as required	
Type—aerobic, rhythmic exercise (e.g., walking, or cycling)	To optimize functional capacity and cardiopulmonary reserve to enable patient's body to deal with disease, or ensure optimal conditioning should surgery be indicated
Intensity—pain < 3 (0-10 scale); fatigue < 2-3 (0-10 scale); heart rate 60%-75% of age-predicted maximum, or 60%-75% of heart rate reserve (resting heart rate + [0.60-0.75] peak heart rate); peak heart rate determined from a symptom-limited graded exercise tolerance test	As the patient's tolerance improves, the intensity and duration increase and the frequency of sessions decreases
Duration—15-40 minutes	
Frequency—3 times a day to daily	
Course and progression—as indicated	
Type—general muscle strengthening; upper and lower extremities and trunk	To optimize general muscle strength to enhance functional capacity, general conditioning, and well-being
Intensity—mild to moderate intensity; not heavy resistance	
Duration—15-60 minutes total	
Frequency—2 times daily to once daily	
Course and progression—as indicated	
Assess quality and quantity of patient's night sleep	Factors that exacerbate physical symptoms are identified to help empower patient to exercise control over exacerbating factors
Discuss with patient what factors trigger pain and impair sleep; timing of meals, events of day, presleep activity, worrying	Other factors that can impair sleep are also examined to help promote better-quality sleep (e.g., presleep habits, firmness of mattress, reading, music, television, hot drinks, avoidance of caffeine and alcohol)
Examine quality of mattress; use of pillows, presleep routine	Encourage patient to determine what factors induce sleep

Physical Therapy Diagnosis: Impaired coping skills and stress management

Signs and Symptoms: Engaging in high-risk behaviors that can exacerbate inflammatory bowel symptoms, agitation, anxiety, distraction, lack of concentration, lethargy, depression, social withdrawal

INTERVENTIONS	RATIONALE
Assess coping skills and stress management	To provide a baseline and ongoing assessment
Define outcome criteria: reversal or mitigation of the signs and symptoms	To provide a basis for defining treatment goals and criteria for discontinuing treatment
Reinforce a healthy lifestyle (exercise, nutrition, fluid intake, adequate sleep and rest, stress management)	To minimize exacerbations of episodes of bowel inflammation
Teach relaxation procedures	To minimize the severity of an exacerbation and speed recovery
Reinforce integration of relaxation procedures into lifestyle	To reinforce the patient's medical and nursing management and integrate into physical therapy management
Reinforce stress management and coping strategies	
Reinforce taking medications as indicated	
Reinforce having a social support network (e.g., friends, Crohn's disease support group)	Patients with chronic diseases can benefit from participation in a support group; source of information to help empower the patient and source of social support

Continued.

Physical Therapy Diagnosis: Risk of the negative sequelae of recumbency

Signs and Symptoms: Within 6 hours reduced circulating blood volume, decreased blood pressure on sitting and standing compared with supine, light-headedness, dizziness, syncope, increased hematocrit and blood viscosity, increased work of the heart, altered fluid balance in the lung, impaired pulmonary lymphatic drainage, decreased lung volumes and capacities, decreased functional residual capacity, increased closing volume, and decreased Pao_2 and Sao_2

INTERVENTIONS	RATIONALE
Monitor signs and symptoms of the negative sequelae of recumbency	To provide a baseline, ongoing assessment and measure of treatment response
Define outcome criteria: prevention, reversal, or mitigation of the signs and symptoms	To provide a basis for defining treatment goals and criteria for discontinuing treatment
Sitting upright position, standing and walking	The upright position is essential to shift fluid volume from central to peripheral circulation and maintain fluid volume regulating mechanisms and circulating blood volume
	The upright position maximizes lung volumes and capacities and functional residual capacity
	The upright position maximizes expiratory flow rate and cough effectiveness
	The upright position optimizes the length-tension relationship, neural stimulation of the respiratory and abdominal muscles, and cough effectiveness
	The upright position coupled with mobilization and breathing control and coughing maneuvers maximizes alveolar ventilation, ventilation and perfusion matching, and pulmonary lymphatic drainage
Avoid excessive duration in recumbent and restricted positions (i.e., minimal position changes) during acute exacerbations	Excessive duration in restricted body positions with abdominal guarding contributes to breathing at low lung volumes, airway closure, atelectasis, impaired mucociliary transport

Physical Therapy Diagnosis: Risk of negative sequelae of restricted mobility

Signs and Symptoms: Reduced activity and exercise tolerance, muscle atrophy and reduced muscle strength, decreased oxygen transport efficiency, increased heart rate, blood pressure, and minute ventilation at submaximal work rates, reduced respiratory muscle strength, increased fatigue and reduced endurance at submaximal work rates, circulatory stasis, thromboemboli (e.g., pulmonary emboli), pressure areas, skin breakdown, and ulceration

INTERVENTIONS	RATIONALE
Monitor signs and symptoms of the negative sequelae of restricted mobility	To provide a baseline and ongoing assessment
Define outcome criteria: prevention, reversal, or mitigation of the signs and symptoms	To provide a basis for defining treatment goals and criteria for discontinuing treatment
Mobilization and exercise prescription	To prescribe exercise for its *preventive* effects
	Mobilization and exercise optimize circulating blood volume, enhance the efficiency of all steps in the oxygen transport pathway
Modify exercise prescription with exacerbations and remission of symptoms (e.g., reduce intensity and duration), increase frequency	Exercise may need to be significantly reduced during acute exacerbation of symptoms in favor of stretching and low-intensity mobilization coordinated with breathing-control functional activity
	As mobilization/exercise sessions decrease in intensity and duration, the frequency of sessions is increased

Physical Therapy Diagnosis: Knowledge deficit

Signs and Symptoms: Lack of information about Crohn's disease, exacerbations, complications, and management

INTERVENTIONS	RATIONALE
Assess specific knowledge deficits related to disease and cardiopulmonary physical therapy management	To provide a baseline and ongoing assessment
Define outcome criteria: reversal or mitigation of the signs and symptoms	To provide a basis for defining treatment goals and criteria for discontinuing treatment
Promote a caring and supportive patient-therapist relationship	To treat the patient with Crohn's disease rather than the condition
Consider every patient interaction an opportunity for patient education	
Reinforce knowledge and information about disease and its relationship to lifestyle, exercise, diet, and stress	To promote patient's sense of responsibility for health, health promotion, and prevention of exacerbations as much as possible
Reinforce optimal diet and nutrition, weight control, hydration and fluid balance, exercise, stress reduction, smoking cessation, and drinking reduction	
Reinforce knowledge of medications and medication schedule	
Teach, demonstrate, and provide feedback on interventions that can be self-administered	Between-treatment interventions are as important as treatments themselves to provide cumulative treatment effect
Teach patient to balance activity and rest	Optimal balance between activity and rest essential to exploit short-term, long-term, and preventive effects of mobilization and exercise
Provide written information about treatment and exercise program	To promote continuity of care and follow-up with a physical therapist in a clinic or in the community
Provide written handouts at discharge with general information, exercise prescription, and home program	

PART III

Surgical Case Studies

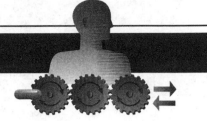

CHAPTER 10

Orthopedic Surgery: Pelvic Fracture Fixation

PATHOPHYSIOLOGY

One or more fractures of the pelvis is a common result of severe trauma or minor trauma in patients with osteoporosis. If such fractures are unstable or unlikely to heal without stabilization, internal fixation is indication. Pelvic fractures are complicated by acetabular involvement and internal injuries. Preservation of the integrity of the pelvis and acetabulum is essential for normal weight bearing and ambulation and to minimize degenerative joint changes and deformity over the long term. Additional complications of pelvic trauma and surgery include damage to the internal organs (particularly the bladder), blood loss, thrombus formation, and thromboemboli.

Case Study

The patient is a 58-year-old man. He is a consultant specializing in international aid projects and spends several months of the year working in underdeveloped countries. He is 6 feet 2 inches (188 cm) tall and weighs 176 pounds (80 kg); his body mass index is 22.5. He is divorced and lives in an apartment in his daughter's home. The patient is an active individual; he runs and is a proficient cyclist. His past medical history is unremarkable other than a recently diagnosed supraventricular dysrhythmia, specifically premature atrial contractions, for which he is taking medication. While cycling at moderately high speed, he hit a curb. He sustained facial lacerations but no head injury; he was wearing a helmet. He was cleared of spinal cord involvement. A Foley catheter and intravenous line were inserted. He required surgical fixation of two pelvic fractures, including a fracture of the left acetabulum. He underwent several hours of surgery, lost a moderate amount of blood, and required 4 hours to sustain spontaneous breathing after surgery. He required 5 U of blood replacement. Initially, morphine was administered intravenously for pain control. On day 2, morphine administration was patient controlled. In addition, he was on anticoagulant therapy. Over the first 2 days, he was lethargic and fatigued. On day 5, he complained of tenderness over the left lower thigh. Serial ultrasound scans revealed thrombus formation at two sites. Thrombolytic therapy was instituted. His hemoglobin was 10 gm/dl. His arterial blood gases (ABGs) on supplemental oxygen via nasal cannula, flow rate 2 L/min, were pH 7.43, oxygen pressure (Po_2) 83 mm Hg, carbon dioxide pressure (Pco_2) 39 mm Hg, bicarbonate (HCO_3) 24 mEq/L, and arterial oxygen saturation (Sao_2) 93%.

Oxygen Transport Deficits: Observed and Potential

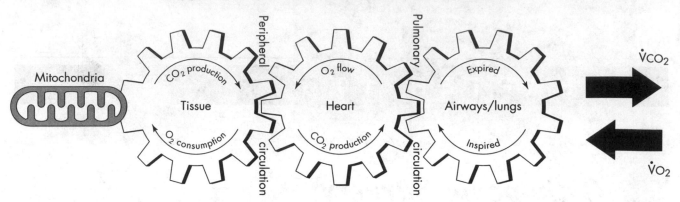

↓ Aerobic efficiency
Muscle deconditioning
↑ Oxygen demand

Atrial dysrhythmia

↑ Airway closure of
    dependent airways
↓ Mucociliary transport
↓ Ciliary motion due to
    supplemental oxygen
↓ Respiratory drive due
    to narcotics
↓ Lung volumes and
    capacities
Monotonous tidal
    ventilation
Breathing at low lung
    volumes
↓ Functional residual
    capacity
↓ Surfactant production
↓ Surfactant distribution
↓ Forced expiratory
    flow rates
Weak cough
Atelectasis
Shunt

Circulatory stasis
Venous thrombosis
thrombophlebitis

↓ Lymphatic motion
↓ Lymphatic drainage

Blood: ↓ Blood volume
    Anemia
    Hypoxemia
    Arterial desaturation

↑	Increase
↓	Decrease

PHYSICAL THERAPY DIAGNOSES AND TREATMENT PRESCRIPTION

Physical Therapy Diagnosis: Altered cardiopulmonary function: alveolar hypoventilation and shunt

Signs and Symptoms: $Pao_2 < 104.2 - 0.27$ age (± 7) mm Hg, $Sao_2 < 98\%$, hypermetabolic; febrile, decreased arousal, depressed cough, monotonous tidal ventilation, increased work of breathing, increased minute ventilation, decreased lung volumes and capacities, reduced functional residual capacity, increased closing volume of dependent airways, increased work of the heart, increased cardiac output, decreased urinary output, decreased air entry, decreased mucociliary transport, prolonged surgery, prolonged anesthesia and sedation, blood loss, 5 U of blood and blood products transfused, prolonged supine positioning during surgery, prolonged weaning off ventilatory support, restricted mobility and position turns, restricted left hip flexion to 90°, anemia, fluid shifts, and third spacing

INTERVENTIONS	RATIONALE
Monitor ABGs, hemoglobin, ECG, chest x-rays, pulmonary function, vital signs, Sao_2 Perform serial clinical cardiopulmonary assessments	To provide a baseline, ongoing assessment and measure of treatment response
Define outcome criteria: reversal or mitigation of the signs and symptoms	To provide a basis for defining treatment goals and criteria for discontinuing treatment
Reinforce use of supplemental oxygen and appropriate fit of face mask or nasal prongs	To ensure that the oxygen mask or nasal prongs are positioned such that oxygen delivery to the patient is maximized and not wasted
Mobilization prescription coordinated with breathing control and coughing maneuvers Medications — analgesia at peak potency, supplemental oxygen Mobilization coordinated with the upright position, non–weight bearing on the left leg Bed mobility and bed exercises using monkey bar, weights, and pulleys Dangling, self-supported, erect, feet on floor Transfers; active assist to active transfers Chair exercises; sitting erect, upper extremity, trunk, and right leg exercises; modified movement and positioning of the left leg Walker; non–weight bearing Crutches; non–weight bearing Functional activities, bathroom, washing, shaving, hair care, changing bed wear	To exploit the *acute* effects of mobilization on cardiopulmonary function and oxygen transport (i.e., increase arousal, optimize alveolar volume, functional residual capacity, the distributions of ventilation, perfusion, and ventilation and perfusion matching; gas exchange; three-dimensional chest wall movement, efficient and coordinated thoracoabdominal movement, mucociliary transport, decrease secretion accumulation, optimize lung movement and lymphatic drainage, increase surfactant production and distribution, reduce the work of breathing and the work of the heart, and augment peripheral circulation) To counter the negative effects of surgery: lung volumes are significantly reduced by anesthesia, surgery, pain, recumbency, and restricted mobility; functional residual capacity is reduced by up to 50% when supine and is reduced further by anesthesia To minimize the risk of deep vein thrombosis, which is a high risk following pelvic surgery; the need for thrombolytic therapy given in this type of surgery is associated with a high risk of postsurgical bleeding
Breathing control and coughing maneuvers; optimal starting position—seated or high Fowler's position Maximal inspiration–hold–passive expiration to normal end-tidal volume Frequency—10 times every hour coordinated with movement and position changes Course and progression—decrease breathing control and coughing maneuvers commensurate with increased mobilization, frequent position changes, and ambulation Intensity — interval schedule (i.e., paced to minimize pain, undue cardiopulmonary stress, fatigue) $Sao_2 > 90\%$ Duration—15-30 minutes Frequency—every 4-6 hr Course and progression—as indicated	Breathing control and coughing maneuvers performed frequently in all positions initially and less frequently with increased time upright and moving Breathing control and coughing maneuvers combined with the upright position and movement are prescribed to optimize alveolar volume, functional residual capacity, ventilation, ventilation and perfusion matching, mucociliary transport, surfactant production and distribution, lymphatic drainage, neural stimulation of the diaphragm, respiratory mechanics, and cough effectiveness To promote alveolar ventilation and gas exchange by optimizing lung compliance and decreasing airway resistance

Continued.

INTERVENTIONS	RATIONALE

Aids and devices:
  Monkey bar for bed mobility and to be independent in frequent position changes
  Free weights, pulley system
	To maximize functional independence and maintain strength of the unaffected limbs and trunk

Promote optimal body position and alignment during mobilization and exercise	Optimal alignment promotes optimal cardiopulmonary function and minimizes biomechanical compensations for injuries and surgical incisions, which can lead to long-term complications
Intersperse rest periods within treatments; encourage slow controlled movement and body repositioning coordinated with breathing control	To promote quality rest periods and sleep between treatments to maximize treatment effect
Modify mobilization prescription when patient develops thrombi in the left leg and place on course of thrombolytic agents	To minimize the risk of dislodging thrombi and pulmonary emboli

Correction of postural alignment (erect posture, upright, minimal sway or list, relaxed shoulders, upper extremities, upper body, and chest wall):
  At rest
  In the chair
  Standing
  Walking with walker and crutch walking (non–weight bearing)
	To optimize breathing pattern, chest wall excursion, and distribution of ventilation; to minimize compression atelectasis and suboptimal alveolar filling, gas mixing, and gas exchange
	To relieve musculoskeletal stiffness and rigidity and long-term cardiopulmonary sequelae of impaired postural alignment
	To enhance breathing and movement efficiency and movement economy

Body positioning coordinated with breathing control, coughing maneuvers, and pain control strategies:
  Place in as high a Fowler's position as possible based on patient's tolerance and response
  Reverse-Trendelenburg position (head up with feet down)
  Body positioning in the horizontal plane and variants with head of bed up and down
  Side lying on either side; modify left side lying
  ¾ prone to each side; modify to left side
  Supine
  Frequency — when in bed, frequent body position changes at least every 1-2 hr; promote frequent body position changes by patient coordinated with breathing control and coughing maneuvers
  Course and progression—as indicated
Minimize duration recumbent, particularly supine
	To optimize alveolar volume and distribution of ventilation, ventilation and perfusion matching, lung volumes and capacities, functional residual capacity; minimize airway closure of the dependent airways, redistribute thoracic blood volume; increase lung compliance; minimize cephalad displacement of the diaphragm by the viscera; increase arousal; stimulate deep breaths; increase lung movement, mucociliary transport, and lymphatic drainage; promote effective coughing; minimize intraabdominal pressure and encroachment on the thoracic cavity; maintain fluid volume regulation, which can only be maintained with the upright position
	Dependency of the feet is permitted provided swelling is not a problem; minimize the risk of pulmonary aspiration, and stimulate bowel and bladder functions
	
	Supine is a particularly deleterious position; supine is included in the turning schedule, but duration should not exceed 1-2 hr; supine compromises expansion of the dependent lung fields, significantly reduces functional residual capacity, increases closing volume, and reduces lung compliance because of increased thoracic blood volume and encroachment of the abdominal viscera

Encourage patient not to favor any single position, and stress importance of position changes to simulate the changes that would occur when mobile	To optimize turning frequency to augment cardiopulmonary function, the distribution of ventilation, and ventilation and perfusion matching, mucociliary transport, lung movement, and lymphatic drainage
Encourage patient to perform pain control strategies and request medication if necessary to provide comfort, reduce suffering, and facilitate movement; frequent position changes	To place the patient in as many positions as possible; extreme positions (e.g., prone) are modified within the patient's limits of comfort and in consideration of fractures To change the patient's body position frequently with optimal assist from the patient at least every 1-2 hr Avoid excessive duration in *any* single position because the dependent lung fields will be compromised after 1-2 hr

INTERVENTIONS	RATIONALE

Range-of-motion exercises (active and active assist) coordinated with breathing control and coughing maneuvers:
  Upper extremities
  Trunk
  Lower extremities, especially hips and knees (left hip < 90°) and feet and ankles
	To exploit the cardiopulmonary benefits of range-of-motion exercises (i.e., ventilatory and peripheral vascular benefits)

Physical Therapy Diagnosis: Pain: fractures of left pelvis and acetabulum, internal trauma, surgical trauma, and incisional pain

Signs and Symptoms: Complaints of discomfort and pain, grimacing, guarding, holding body rigid, moaning, reluctance to move and change body position, distracted, lack of concentration, fatigue and lethargy, disturbed rest and sleep, loss of appetite, reduced ability to cooperate with treatment

INTERVENTIONS	RATIONALE
Monitor pain; its quality, quantity and location; and factors that increase and decrease pain	To provide a baseline, ongoing assessment and measure of treatment response
Define outcome criteria: reversal or mitigation of the signs and symptoms	To provide a basis for defining treatment goals and criteria for discontinuing treatment
Ensure that patient is appropriately medicated for treatments (preferably alternative agents to narcotics when possible) and medications are at peak efficacy	To minimize pain, suffering, and distress To promote pain self-management
Reinforce the appropriate use of patient-controlled analgesia	Patient weaned from scheduled narcotics, to patient-controlled narcotic analgesia, to nonnarcotic pain management
Teach relaxation procedures (e.g., breathing control, Jacobsen's relaxation procedure, Benson's relaxation method, autogenic training, biofeedback, visual imagery)	To maximize patient arousal during treatments To minimize pain and discomfort by encouraging gentle movement and frequent body position changes while performing relaxation procedures
Coordinate treatments with breathing control and coughing maneuvers	To maximize tolerance of mobility exercises and body position changes with rest periods (i.e., these interventions are performed in stages and with optimal assistance such
Pace treatments	that the patient has the physiological benefits of actively
Intersperse rest periods within and between treatments	participating within the limits of pain and discomfort)
Respond to patient's complaints of pain; consider patient's comfort at all times	Although weaning off pain medication is encouraged, the patient is encouraged to request analgesia before pain is excessive and unduly interferes with breathing, mobility, positioning, and ability to rest effectively
Promote good body alignment in sitting and standing as well as when lying in bed	To minimize discomfort associated with stiffness
Frequent body position changes	

Physical Therapy Diagnosis: Decreased tolerance for physical activity and exercise

Signs and Symptoms: Physical activity restricted by complaints of pain, discomfort, apprehension about moving left hip, fatigue, weakness and loss of endurance, increased metabolic and oxygen demands because of injuries, surgery, and healing and repair

INTERVENTIONS	RATIONALE
Assess ability to perform activities of daily living (ADL), dangle over bed, transfer, walk (non–weight bearing) with walker	To provide a baseline, ongoing assessment and measure of treatment response
Determine premorbid level of function and functional capacity	Patient had high premorbid aerobic capacity, optimal weight and nutritional habits; these factors are protective and enhance recovery
Define outcome criteria: reversal or mitigation of the signs and symptoms	To provide a basis for defining treatment goals and criteria for discontinuing treatment

Continued.

INTERVENTIONS	RATIONALE

Mobilization and exercise prescription (coordinated with breathing control maneuvers):
  Walking with walker—non–weight bearing and progressing to crutches
  Intensity: low to moderate; < 60%-75% of age predicted maximal heart rate or fatigue < 4-5 (0-10 scale); pace within tolerance of strength, endurance, and pain
  Duration: 15-45 minutes
  Intersperse with sitting and standing rest periods
  Monitor signs and symptoms of orthostatic intolerance with standing rests
  Monitor tolerance
  Frequency: up to several times daily; activities include ADL, bathroom, hallway walks
  Course and progression: increase duration, speed; reduce rest periods; increase frequency
	To exploit the *long-term* effects of mobilization and exercise on cardiopulmonary function and oxygen transport (e.g., reduce minute ventilation, perceived exertion, fatigue, rate pressure product, cardiac output at rest and submaximal work rates; increase peripheral collateral circulation and increase extraction and uptake of oxygen at the tissue level)

Monitor for signs and symptoms of postural hypotension; record heart rate and blood pressure before and after lying supine and assuming an upright seated or standing position Monitor responses to mobilization, e.g., heart rate, blood pressure, exertion	Patient is susceptible to postural hypotension; a chair must be available initially when walking in case patient becomes light-headed or fatigued Intensity of mobilization and exercise is low to moderate to avoid exceeding patient's capacity for oxygen delivery, given his anemia Patient's ability to tolerate treatment varies initially, thus treatment is modified accordingly; treatment frequency may be increased to offset short treatment durations

General strengthening (coordinated with breathing control):
  Weights and pulleys
  Upper extremities
  Left leg strengthening modified commensurate with pain < 3-5 (0-10 scale); stability of fractures and episode of thrombus formation and recovery
  Right leg
  Intensity—3 sets of 5-10 repetitions submaximal
  Duration—20 minutes
  Frequency—1-2 times daily
  Course and progression—as indicated
	To improve overall conditioning and oxygen transport efficiency
	Resistance set at low intensity; movements are rhythmic and coordinated; do not elicit undue cardiopulmonary/hemodynamic stress, and avoid straining, breath holding, Valsalva maneuver, and static contractions

Optimize patient's movement efficiency and metabolic economy Minimize hand strain during crutch walking; metal crutches preferred by patient over wood crutch with hand cushions	To reduce excessive physical demands of physical activity and ADL associated with inefficient movement
Prescriptive rest periods within treatments Prescriptive rest periods between treatments Promote quality rest and sleep periods Schedule treatments as much as possible after rest and sleep periods	The patient is in a hypermetabolic state because of trauma, recovery from extensive surgery, anesthesia, sedation and narcotics, blood loss, anemia, healing and repair, inadequate nutrition and fluid intake; quality rest and sleep periods between treatments are essential to promote healing and repair, restore energy, and reduce fatigue and thereby enhance functional activity and work output Rest and sleep are priorities in conjunction with active therapy; patient is prone to fatigue and exhaustion because of reduced oxygen-carrying capacity of the blood, thus undue levels of fatigue are avoided

Physical Therapy Diagnosis: Thrombophlebitis and thrombus formation in left leg

Signs and Symptoms: Soreness and pain, redness, swelling, and restricted movement of left leg

INTERVENTIONS	RATIONALE
Monitor for signs of phlebitis (e.g., redness, swelling, pain)	To provide a baseline, ongoing assessment and measure of treatment response
Define outcome criteria: reversal or mitigation of the signs and symptoms	To provide a basis for defining treatment goals and criteria for discontinuing treatment
Monitor thrombolytic therapy and its course	To be knowledgable about thrombolytic therapy and its indications, contraindications, and side effects
Follow serial ultrasound scans	To modify treatment accordingly once thrombolytic agents are prescribed
	To monitor resolution or worsening of thrombi
	To monitor for signs of emboli, particularly to the lungs
Teach signs of breathing distress associated with pulmonary emboli and position call button close to patient	To ensure that patient can notify nursing staff immediately if signs of pulmonary embolus occur
Ensure that compression stockings fit properly (i.e., over full length of the legs), are unwrinkled, and are reapplied several times daily	To maximize the effect of physical measures to control thrombi formation and minimize contributing to thrombi formation
Ensure that intermittent compression device is attached to lower limbs and the inflation boots are attached adequately so that appropriate pressure transmitted to limbs	
Minimize left hip, knee, foot, and ankle movements	While patient is on course of thrombolytic agents, reduce left leg movement to prevent dislodging of clots
Continue hip and knee and foot and ankle exercises on the right leg (hourly)	To minimize further thrombus formation
Minimize reciprocal left leg movement during right leg exercise	Avoid excessive movement of left leg

Physical Therapy Diagnosis: Reduced emotional and psychological well-being

Signs and Symptoms: Depression, emotional instability, fearful and frightened, insecurity, frustration, anger

INTERVENTIONS	RATIONALE
Monitor emotional and psychological well-being	To provide a baseline and ongoing assessment
Comfort, reassurance, empathy	To promote psychological well-being
Caring	To promote patient's sense of control
Listen to patient	To promote self-responsibility
Encouragement	
Involve patient in decision making	
Support patient and family members	To help patient and family deal with the accident and its short-term and long-term consequences
Discuss early transition to home and work and performance of ADL and mobility issues	To facilitate rehabilitation planning in preparation for discharge
Initiate discharge planning early (e.g., with other team members); prepare handouts of exercise regimens; communicate with home health care agency or public health, home care, or community physical therapist	To promote continuity of care and follow-up care

Continued.

Physical Therapy Diagnosis: Threats to oxygen transport and gas exchange

Signs and Symptoms: History of premature atrial contraction, age-related airway closure in sitting, age-related closure of dependent airways in recumbent positions, age-related inhomogeneity of ventilation, age-related decrease of mucociliary clearance rate, age-related depression of cough reflex, anemia, blood transfusions; (whole blood and blood products), circulatory stasis, venous thrombosis, pulmonary embolism, restricted mobility, recumbency

INTERVENTIONS	RATIONALE
Monitor for signs and symptoms related to factors threatening oxygen transport	To provide a baseline and ongoing assessment
Monitor ABGs, electrocardiogram (ECG), fluid and electrolyte balance, respiratory, hemodynamic and gas exchange variables, ultrasound scans for thrombi	
Define outcome criteria: prevention, reversal, or mitigation of the signs and symptoms	To provide a basis for defining treatment goals and criteria for discontinuing treatment
Preoperative teaching includes the disease pathology and surgery (type, body position, anesthesia and sedation, incision, duration, and dressings), and pain to be expected	Basic background regarding the disease and surgery provides a basis for understanding treatment, which enhances cooperation with the treatment program when supervised and when not directly supervised
Preoperative teaching includes a description of when the patient will be seen by the physical therapist after surgery, the postoperative assessment, and treatment interventions (including breathing control and supported coughing coordinated with positioning, frequent position changes, and mobilization and relaxation procedures)	Preoperative teaching reduces postoperative complications, morbidity, and length of hospital stay
Mobilization, walking erect	To exploit the *preventive* effects of mobilization/exercise coupled with breathing control and coughing maneuvers (e.g., optimize alveolar volume and ventilation and minimize atelectasis, particularly of the dependent lung fields), optimize mucociliary transport, minimize mucociliary accumulation, maximize functional residual capacity, minimize airway closure, minimize circulatory stasis, and maximize circulating blood volume
Intensity — within limits of pain, endurance, and fatigue	
Duration — 5-20 minutes	
Frequency — increase to several times daily	
Course and progression — as tolerated	
Breathing control and coughing maneuvers (relaxed deep inhalations and exhalation to end-tidal volume and coughing)	
Perform hourly	
Coordinate before, during, and after each position change	
Coordinate before, during, and after mobilization	
Chair exercises:	
Upper extremities	
Chest wall	
Lower extremities with left leg restricted to 90° flexion (hip and knee and foot and ankle exercises hourly)	
Varied and extreme body positions when lying down	Patients favor lying in restricted positions (e.g., the less painful side) for prolonged periods, thus are at risk of developing cardiopulmonary complications in the dependent lung fields
Frequent body position changes (hourly)	
Avoid excessive time in right side lying	
Monitor for signs of deep vein thrombosis	Patient developed thrombi in his left leg, which places him at additional risk of developing further thrombi and pulmonary emboli
Monitor for signs of pulmonary emboli	
Teach patient the symptoms associated with pulmonary emboli and instruct to alert team member immediately	
Monitor ECG status	History of premature atrial contractions increases the patient's risk of more serious dysrhythmias given the insults associated with trauma, prolonged and major surgery, anesthesia, impaired oxygen transport, hypoxemia, and associated stress, and anxiety

Physical Therapy Diagnosis: Risk of the negative sequelae of recumbency

Signs and Symptoms: Within 6 hours reduced circulating blood volume, decreased blood pressure on sitting and standing compared with supine, light-headedness, dizziness, syncope, increased hematocrit and blood viscoscity, increased work of the heart, altered pulmonary fluid balance, impaired pulmonary lymphatic drainage, decreased lung volumes and capacities, decreased forced expiratory flow rates, decreased functional residual capacity, decreased pulmonary compliance, increased closing volume, increased airflow resistance, and decreased Pao_2 and Sao_2

INTERVENTIONS	RATIONALE
Monitor signs and symptoms of the negative sequelae of recumbency	To provide a baseline and ongoing assessment
Define outcome criteria: prevention, avoidance, reversal, or mitigation of the signs and symptoms	To provide a basis for defining treatment goals and criteria for discontinuing treatment
Sitting upright position, preferably with feet dependent, standing and walking	To exploit the benefits of the upright position on hemodynamics and plasma volume regulation
Coordinate physical activity and mobilization with breathing control and coughing maneuvers	The upright position is essential to shift fluid volume from central to peripheral circulation and maintain fluid volume regulating mechanisms and circulating blood volume
	The upright position maximizes lung volumes and capacities (especially functional residual capacity) and minimizes airway closure; these factors are adversely affected by anesthesia and surgery
	The upright position maximizes expiratory flow rates and cough effectiveness
	The upright position optimizes the length-tension relationship of the respiratory muscles and abdominal muscles, neural stimulation of the respiratory muscles, and cough effectiveness
	The upright position coupled with mobilization and breathing control and coughing maneuvers maximizes alveolar ventilation, ventilation and perfusion matching, mucociliary transport, and pulmonary lymphatic drainage

Physical Therapy Diagnosis: Risk of negative sequelae of restricted mobility: secondary to trauma, surgery, fatigue, and thrombus formation

Signs and Symptoms: Reduced activity and exercise tolerance, muscle atrophy and reduced muscle strength, decreased oxygen transport efficiency, increased heart rate, blood pressure, and minute ventilation at rest and submaximal work rates, reduced respiratory muscle strength and endurance, circulatory stasis, thromboemboli (e.g., pulmonary emboli), pressure areas, skin redness, skin breakdown and ulceration, and cognitive dysfunction

INTERVENTIONS	RATIONALE
Monitor the negative sequelae of restricted mobility	To provide a baseline of oxygen transport efficiency and cardiopulmonary status and ongoing assessment
Determine premorbid cardiopulmonary status	
Monitor areas of redness and soreness over sacrum and right hip; the patient's positions of comfort are toward the unaffected side	
Define outcome criteria: prevention, avoidance, reversal, or mitigation of the signs and symptoms	To provide a basis for defining treatment goals and criteria for discontinuing treatment
Mobilization and exercise prescription	To exploit the *preventive* effects of mobilization and exercise (e.g., optimize circulating blood volume and enhance the efficiency of all steps in the oxygen transport pathway)

Continued.

Physical Therapy Diagnosis: Knowledge deficit

Signs and Symptoms: Lack of information about injuries, surgery, implications of surgery on physical therapy, complications, and prognosis, and issues related to discharge and resumption of ADL and work

INTERVENTIONS	RATIONALE
Determine specific knowledge deficits related to injury, surgery, and cardiopulmonary physical therapy management	To address specific knowledge deficits
Define outcome criteria: reversal or mitigation of the signs and symptoms	To provide a basis for defining treatment goods and criteria for discontinuing interventions
Promote a caring and supportive patient-therapist relationship	To focus on treating the patient with a pelvic fracture fixation rather than the pelvic fracture fixation
Consider every patient interaction an opportunity for education	To promote patient's sense of responsibility for full recovery, wellness, and health promotion
Instruct regarding avoidance of respiratory tract infections, nutrition, hydration and fluid balance, exercise, stress management, and quality sleep	To promote cooperation and active participation in treatment
Reinforce medications, their purposes, and medication schedule	
Reinforce knowledge provided by other team members	
Patient is given a personalized handout with a listing and description of exercises and their prescription parameters; precautions are emphasized	The patient can follow the handout instructions on his own between supervised treatments; he does not have to rely on memory, which will be impaired because of the distractions of his postsurgical state and the hospital environment
	The content of the handout is reviewed with the patient
Provide handout of mobilization and exercise schedule, body positioning guidelines, and breathing control and supported coughing maneuvers	On subsequent treatments, the physical therapist makes sure the patient knows how to follow the handout and perform the exercises as prescribed
Teach, demonstrate, and provide feedback on interventions that can be self-administered	Between-treatment interventions are as important as treatments themselves to provide cumulative treatment effect
Teach patient regarding balance of activity and rest	Optimal balance between activity and rest is essential to exploit short-term, long-term, and preventive effects of mobilization and exercise
Provide written handouts and information sheets, including exercise program and prescription parameters, which are modified frequently during the inpatient stay, and information about specific activity and exercise restriction involving the left hip	Information and the exercise prescriptions the patient is expected to perform on his own between supervised treatments are documented in written and pictorial form to ensure that the patient performs the appropriate exercises in accordance with their specific prescription; the handout also includes the signs and symptoms that indicate discontinuing an exercise and alerting the physical therapist, nurse, or physician
Identify functional outcome goals with patient that should be achieved before discharge	To review home and work settings (e.g., stairs, walking distances, walking surfaces, lifting, driving, and architectural barriers) so that the patient is maximally prepared for discharge
Practice specific crutch walking skills, (e.g., transfers, stairs)	
Prepare a revised handout for discharge, including general information, exercise prescriptions, and home treatment plan	To promote continuity of care and follow-up by a physical therapist in a clinic or in the community

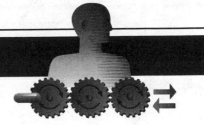

CHAPTER 11

Lower Abdominal Surgery: Partial Hysterectomy

PATHOPHYSIOLOGY

A partial hysterectomy is usually indicated to remove a localized growth or an area of chronic irritation in the uterus while sparing the cervix. These conditions are frequently heralded by menstrual irregularities, including menorrhagia (excessive bleeding), and pain. Anemia and fatigue are often associated with these conditions. Because the anemia is a result of blood loss, it does not respond to iron supplementation. A laparatomy is performed with the incision over the lower abdomen and through the layers of abdominal muscles.

Case Study

The patient is a 38-year-old woman. She is a lawyer and lives in her family home with her mother. She is 48.5 pounds (22 kg) overweight and has a protruding abdomen. She describes herself as a light smoker; she has smoked for 20 years. Her medical history includes anemia despite iron supplementation. Six weeks ago she experienced considerable fatigue caused by unremitting abdominal pain associated with sleep loss and anemia. She was diagnosed with myoma of the uterus and scheduled for a partial hysterectomy. The surgery lasted 45 minutes and was uneventful.

Oxygen Transport Deficits: Observed and Potential

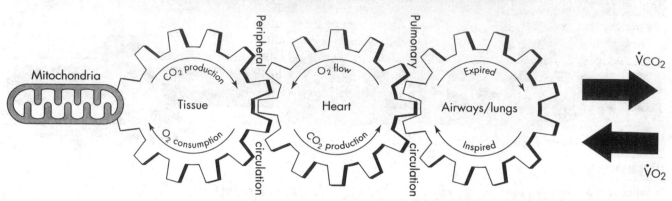

Generalized deconditioning and inefficient oxygen transport
↑ Oxygen demand

↑ Work of the heart

↑ Airway closure
↓ Mucociliary transport
↓ Ciliary function due to smoking history and surgery
↓ Lung volumes and capacities
↓ Functional residual capacity
↓ Forced expiratory, flow rates
Monotonous tidal ventilation
Breathing at low lung volumes
Avoidance of deep breathing
Avoidance of coughing
Atelectasis
↑ Abdominal pressure from obesity
Encroachment of the diaphragm and reduced descent
↑ Work of breathing

Hypertension

↓ Lymphatic motion
↓ Lymphatic drainage

↑ Increase
↓ Decrease

PHYSICAL THERAPY DIAGNOSES AND TREATMENT PRESCRIPTION

Physical Therapy Diagnosis: Altered cardiopulmonary function: alveolar hypoventilation and shunt due to surgery, ie, laparotomy, duration, supine surgical position, anesthesia and sedation, smoking history, obesity, incision of the abdominal musculature, incisional pain, and anemia

Signs and Symptoms: Arterial oxygen saturation (Sao_2) < 98%, body mass index > 25; 48.5 pounds overweight, increased minute ventilation, monotonous tidal ventilation, reduced functional residual capacity, increased closing volume, radiographic evidence of basal atelectasis, reduced arousal, depressed cough and cough effectiveness, breathing at low lung volumes, decreased air entry, lack of spontaneous movement and position changes, arterial desaturation, lethargy

INTERVENTIONS	RATIONALE
Monitor arterial blood gases (ABGs), hemoglobin, electrocardiogram (ECG), pulmonary function, fluid balance, chest x-ray, pulmonary function	To provide a baseline, ongoing assessment and measure of treatment response
Perform serial cardiopulmonary assessments	To assess presence and severity of hypoxemia, its causative factors, and select optimal interventions
Define outcome criteria: reversal or mitigation of the signs and symptoms	To provide a basis for defining treatment goals and criteria for discontinuing treatment
Mobilization and activity coordinated with breathing control and supported coughing maneuvers	This patient warrants being upright and mobile several times daily because her complicating factors could rapidly precipitate cardiopulmonary insufficiency
Type—dangle, stand, walking, transfer to chair, chair exercises, bed mobility, and bed exercises	No particular contraindications to an aggressive mobilization treatment program with appropriate monitoring
Intensity—within limits of fatigue, < 3 (0-10 scale), increase in heart rate < 30 beats per minute; increase in blood pressure < 30 mm Hg; commensurate increase in rate and depth of breathing, Sao_2 > 90%	To exploit the *acute* effects of mobilization: increased arousal, ventilation, ventilation and perfusion matching, forced expiratory flow rates, lung movement and lymphatic drainage, and mucociliary transport; decreased airway resistance and airway closure
Duration—pace session so that responses are within preset parameters	To emphasize maximal inspirations to total lung capacity, the inspiratory hold to optimize gas exchange, and passive expiration to avoid airway closure of the dependent airways
Course and progression—as indicated	
Teach breathing control and coughing maneuvers	
Erect high Fowler's position	This patient should be able to tolerate coughing with closed glottis if the incision site is well supported; coughing maneuvers with a closed glottis are associated with greater intrathoracic pressure and expulsive force compared with open glottis maneuvers
Maximal inspiration, 3-5 seconds hold, and passive expiration to normal end-tidal volume	
Supported coughing with pillow or hand support over incision	
Coughing with closed glottis	
Type of mobilization: Walking Chair ergometer (minimal resistance) Erect postures in walking and chair sitting	
Intensity: comfortable walking pace and cycling cadence	
Interval schedule progressed to continuous exercise schedule	
Increase minute ventilation (breathing depth and rate)	
Increase heart rate < 30 beats per minute	
Increase blood pressure < 30 mm Hg	
Exertion < 3-5 (0-10 scale)	
Fatigue < 3-4 (0-10 scale)	
Pain control; coordinate treatment with medications, teach integration of breathing control into physical activity, activities of daily living (ADL), and ambulation; teach relaxation procedures and integration of these during physical activity	To promote a sense of self-control To reduce discomfort, pain, and suffering

Continued.

INTERVENTIONS	RATIONALE
Self or assisted support over incision site (e.g., pillow) during bed mobility and in conjunction with coughing maneuvers	Supported coughing relieves strain on the incision site
Teach modified coughing procedures (e.g., stacking breaths in preparation for cough) and huffing	Modified coughing reduces recruitment of the abdominal muscles incised during surgery, reduces intraabdominal pressure, relieves pain, avoids excessive increases in intrathoracic pressures and airway closure

Teach the use of the incentive spirometer
Incentive spirometer prescription:
    Type—volume controlled spirometer
    Body position—sitting erect, preferably dangling over bed or chair sitting
    Parameters—inhale maximally, 3-5 second inspiratory hold, passively expire, rest 20-30 seconds, repeat 10 times, at least every 1-2 hr; ensure that the device is being used correctly
    Course and progression—wean and discontinue with increased ambulation, improved ventilatory volume, and when airway closure and desaturation no longer occur
	The incentive spirometer serves as an adjunct to mobilization, body positioning, and breathing control maneuvers in patients whose ventilatory volumes are suboptimal (e.g., patients after thoracic or abdominal surgery, obese patients, and patients who are hesitant to perform maximal inspirations)
	Monitor Sao_2 and vital signs before, during, and after treatment to determine treatment effect and modify the incentive spirometer prescription

Body positioning coordinated with breathing control and supported coughing maneuvers:
    Place in erect high Fowler's position
    Place in reverse-Trendelenburg position (head up and feet down)
Place in horizontal plane with variants in the head up and head down positions:
    ¾ supine to each side
    ¾ prone to each side
    Side lying to either side
    Supine
Change positions frequently (at least every 1-2 hr); encourage active and active assist position changes
Minimize positions in which the weight of the abdomen encroaches on and further impedes diaphragmatic excursion
	To stimulate the physiological effects of normal gravitational stress in the upright position: increased arousal, alveolar volume, distribution of ventilation, perfusion, and ventilation-perfusion matching, three-dimensional chest wall motion, increased minute ventilation, increased lung volumes and capacities, increased functional residual capacity, reduced closing volumes, increased expiratory flow rates, reduced thoracic blood volume, reduced encroachment of abdominal viscera on the underside of the diaphragm; optimize the length-tension relationships of the respiratory muscles and abdominal muscles, optimize neural stimulation of the respiratory muscles, optimize mucociliary transport, maximize airway clearance and cough effectiveness, maximize lymphatic drainage, reduce compression of the heart on the adjacent lung parenchyma
	Obese patients are prone to ventilatory insufficiency, particularly after surgery and with recumbency, due to the increased chest wall mass and increased work of breathing to effect normal diaphragmatic descent
	The ¾-prone positions are beneficial positions when the patient is not erect; these positions optimize alveolar volume in the posterior lung fields and facilitate diaphragmatic descent because the abdominal viscera are displaced forward and away from the diaphragm

Range-of-motion exercises coordinated with breathing control and supported coughing maneuvers (maximal inspiration on extension movements, expiration to normal end-tidal volume on flexion movements) in upright and recumbent positions Upper extremities Chest wall; thoracic forward flexion, back extension, side flexion, rotation, diagonal rotation Lower extremities, including hip, knee, and foot and ankle exercises	To exploit the cardiopulmonary benefits of range-of-motion exercises; range-of-motion exercises simulate in part the cardiopulmonary benefits of mobilization

INTERVENTIONS	RATIONALE
Proprioceptive neuromuscular facilitation patterns—active, with minimal resistance as tolerated; coordinated with breathing control	To promote three-dimensional chest wall excursion, including normal bucket handle and pump handle movements, and optimize lung volumes
Weights and pulleys in axial and rotational patterns of movement; coordinated with breathing control	Resistance set at low intensity; movements are rhythmic and coordinated, do not elicit significant cardiopulmonary/hemodynamic stress, and avoid straining, breath holding, Valsalva maneuver, and static contractions

Physical Therapy Diagnosis: Altered breathing pattern caused by pain, surgical incision, fluid shifts and third spacing, and increased body mass

Signs and Symptoms: Decreased chest wall excursion, monotonous ventilation, rapid shallow breathing, lack of spontaneous deep breaths, diminished breath sounds to the bases and dependent lung fields, crackles in the bases and dependent lung fields, and bouts of irregular breathing with pain

INTERVENTIONS	RATIONALE
Monitor breathing pattern; tidal volume, respiratory rate, chest wall movement, and symmetry	To provide a baseline, ongoing assessment and measure of treatment response
Define outcome criteria: reversal or mitigation of the signs and symptoms	To provide a basis for defining treatment goals and criteria for discontinuing treatment
Breathing control and coughing maneuvers in erect upright postures	To promote a normal relaxed breathing pattern in positions associated with maximal lung volumes and capacities
Emphasize a normal breathing pattern	
Emphasize erect postures between and during treatments	
Promote coordination of relaxation procedures with breathing control and coughing maneuvers	
Coordinate treatments with medications and peak effectiveness of analgesics	To optimize breathing pattern with respect to optimal rate and depth, three-dimensional chest wall movement, and optimal cough effectiveness
Promote pain control strategies	To optimize comfort and minimize pain and suffering
Promote adequate sleep and rest	To optimize efficiency of breathing and physical work output
Pace treatments	
Protect and support incision site	
Teach patient to protect and support incision site	
Coordinate breathing control with slow, rhythmic, and unstrained movement	
Optimize postural alignment in sitting, standing, walking, and recumbent positions	
Schedule treatments at peak energy times and not when patient unduly fatigued	
Schedule treatments 45-60 minutes after meals	

Physical Therapy Diagnosis: Pain

Signs and Symptoms: Complaints of pain and discomfort, grimacing, guarding, splinting, moaning, reluctance to cooperate with treatment, reluctance to move spontaneously and reposition herself

INTERVENTIONS	RATIONALE
Monitor pain quality, quantity, and location	To provide a baseline, ongoing assessment and measure of treatment response
Monitor increase and decrease in pain, including the effects of medication	
Define outcome criteria: reversal or mitigation of the signs and symptoms	To provide a basis for defining treatment goals and criteria for discontinuing treatment
Consult with patient about pain control	To involve patient in pain management strategies to promote her sense of control

Continued.

INTERVENTIONS	RATIONALE
Provide information about treatment and rationale and the integration of pain control strategies	To inform patient about importance of active treatment participation, carrying out treatments between treatments
Provide reassurance and stress the goal of pain control	To reassure patient that her comfort during treatment is a priority
Ensure that patient is medicated appropriately before treatments (analgesia at peak effectiveness)	Although the goal is to wean the patient off analgesia as soon as possible, particularly narcotic analgesia, the effect of medication is augmented with noninvasive, non-pharmacological interventions, to reduce the amount of medication needed, to promote weaning, and to minimize the side effects of the drugs
Pace treatments with adequate rest between	
Prescribe exercise on an interval schedule, (i.e., work to rest phases, high- to low-intensity phases)	
Provide pillow and teach hand support for coughing maneuvers	
Reduce undue fatigue	Fatigue increases pain perception and decreases the patient's ability to fully cooperate and participate in treatment

Physical Therapy Diagnosis: Decreased tolerance for physical activity and exercise because of fatigue, low functional work capacity, decreased muscle strength, pain, obesity, smoking history, and anemia

Signs and Symptoms: Increased heart rate, blood pressure, minute ventilation, and perceived exertion at rest and submaximal work rates, reduced capacity to perform ADL and physical activity, muscle weakness, and reduced endurance

INTERVENTIONS	RATIONALE
Monitor patient's ability to perform ADL and responses to physical activity	To provide a baseline, ongoing assessment and measure of treatment response
Monitor anemia and hemoglobin levels	
Establish patient's premorbid functional level and functional capacity	
Serial monitoring of ABGs, blood work, Sao_2, pulmonary function, ECG changes, chest x-rays, and responses to activity	
Serial monitoring of subjective parameters of discomfort, fatigue, and pain	
Define outcome criteria: reversal or mitigation of the signs and symptoms	To provide a basis for defining treatment goals and criteria for discontinuing treatment
Mobilization and exercise prescription: Types—walking Intensity—within limits of comfort, low intensity to 65%-80% maximal age-predicted heart rate Duration—5-20 minutes Frequency—3-10 times a day Course and progression—as indicated, progress to cycle ergometry commensurate with incision healing	To exploit the *long-term* effects of mobilization and exercise on cardiopulmonary function, oxygen transport, and gas exchange, to enhance the efficiency of oxygen delivery, uptake, and extraction along the oxygen transport pathway To modify mobilization and exercise prescription according to anemia status To provide exercise to promote weight loss
Provide handout on discharge summary and treatment plan; exercise prescription with precautions and when to notify the physical therapist, community nurse, or physician	To maximize long-term benefit of cardiopulmonary physical therapy and continuity of care at discharge
Comprehensive discharge planning includes a smoking reduction and cessation program, nutritional program and weight loss program, stress management, and a program of regular physical (aerobic) exercise	Commitment to long-term lifestyle changes is imperative for this patient's physical and mental health, well-being, and health promotion

Physical Therapy Diagnosis: Threats to oxygen transport and gas exchange: obesity, nutritional deficits, smoking history, stress, muscular weakness, postsurgical status (including type and duration of sedation), fluid shifts and third spacing, recumbency, and restricted mobility

Signs and Symptoms: Decreased lung volumes (particularly functional residual capacity and vital capacity), hypoxemia, decreased ventilation and perfusion matching, monotonous tidal ventilation, decreased diffusing capacity, decreased lung compliance, increased airway resistance, decreased mucociliary transport, decreased secretion clearance, decreased cough effectiveness, decreased expiratory flow rates, circulatory status, thrombus formation, thromboemboli (e.g., pulmonary emboli), and skin breakdown

INTERVENTIONS	RATIONALE
Assess patient's risk factors	To provide a baseline and ongoing assessment
Monitor signs and symptoms of impaired oxygen transport related to threats	
Define outcome criteria: prevention, reversal, or mitigation of the signs and symptoms	To provide a basis for defining treatment goals and criteria for discontinuing treatment
Preoperative cardiopulmonary physical therapy assessment, including history and clinical examination based on inspection, palpation, percussion, and auscultation	To exploit the *preventive* effects of mobilization and exercise before and after surgery
Integrate the results of relevant preoperative tests and investigations into the treatment plan	
Preoperative exercise program, smoking cessation, and optimal nutrition program several weeks before surgery	A preoperative exercise program and smoking cessation/reduction can significantly reduce perioperative complications, morbidity, and length of hospital stay
Preoperative teaching includes the pathology and surgery (type, body position, anesthesia and sedation, incision, duration, and dressings), pain to be expected, medication, and when the physical therapist will be seen postoperatively	Preoperative teaching and patient preparation minimizes cardiopulmonary complications, morbidity, and length of hospital stay
	Basic background regarding the underlying disease and surgery provides a basis for understanding treatment, which enhances cooperation with the treatment program when supervised and when not directly supervised
Preoperative teaching directly related to physical therapy includes breathing control and supported coughing maneuvers, bed mobility and positioning, range-of-motion exercises, mobilization, transferring, ambulation, pain control, and relaxation procedures	A preoperative exercise program can significantly reduce perioperative complications, morbidity, and length of hospital stay

Physical Therapy Diagnosis: Risk of the negative sequelae of recumbency

Signs and Symptoms: Within 6 hours reduced circulating blood volume, decreased blood pressure on sitting and standing compared with supine, light-headedness, dizziness, syncope, increased hematocrit and blood viscosity, increased work of the heart, altered fluid balance in the lung, impaired pulmonary lymphatic drainage, decreased lung volumes and capacities, decreased functional residual capacity, increased closing volume, and decreased Pao_2 and Sao_2

INTERVENTIONS	RATIONALE
Monitor signs and symptoms of the negative sequelae of recumbency	To provide a baseline and ongoing assessment
Define outcome criteria: prevention, avoidance, reversal, or mitigation of the signs and symptoms	To provide a basis for defining treatment goals and criteria for discontinuing treatment
Sitting upright position, standing and walking	The upright position is essential to shift fluid volume from central to peripheral circulation and maintain fluid volume regulating mechanisms and circulating blood volume
	The upright position maximizes lung volumes and capacities and functional residual capacity

Continued.

INTERVENTIONS	RATIONALE
	The upright position maximizes expiratory flow rates and cough effectiveness
	The upright position optimizes the length tension relationship of the respiratory muscles and abdominal muscles, and neural stimulation of the respiratory muscles, and optimizes cough effectiveness
	The upright position coupled with mobilization and breathing control and supported coughing maneuvers maximizes alveolar ventilation, ventilation and perfusion matching, and pulmonary lymphatic drainage

Physical Therapy Diagnosis: Risk of negative sequelae of restricted mobility

Signs and Symptoms: Reduced activity and exercise tolerance, muscle atrophy and reduced muscle strength, decreased oxygen transport efficiency, increased heart rate, blood pressure, and minute ventilation at submaximal work rates, reduced respiratory muscle strength and endurance, circulatory stasis, thromboemboli (e.g., pulmonary emboli), pressure areas, skin redness, skin breakdown and ulceration, cognitive dysfunction, impaired circadian rhythms, and impaired sleep patterns

INTERVENTIONS	RATIONALE
Monitor signs and symptoms of the negative sequelae of restricted mobility	To provide a baseline and ongoing assessment
Define outcome criteria: prevention, avoidance, reversal, or mitigation of the signs and symptoms	To provide a basis for defining treatment goals and criteria for discontinuing treatment
Mobilization and exercise prescription	Mobilization and exercise optimize circulating blood volume and enhance the efficiency of all steps in the oxygen transport pathway

Physical Therapy Diagnosis: Knowledge deficit

Signs and Symptoms: Lack of information about medical status, surgery, perioperative course, and complications

INTERVENTIONS	RATIONALE
Assess specific knowledge deficits related to the patient's condition, surgery, and cardiopulmonary physical therapy management	To address patient's specific knowledge deficits
Define outcome criteria: reversal or mitigation of the signs and symptoms	To provide a basis for defining treatment goals
Promote a caring and supportive patient-therapist relationship	To focus on treating the patient with a partial hysterectomy rather than a partial hysterectomy
Consider every patient interaction an opportunity for education	
Reinforce knowledge related to role of other health care team members	
Patient is given a personalized handout with a listing and description of exercises and their prescription parameters; precautions are emphasized	The content of the handout is reviewed with the patient
Provide handout of mobilization and exercise schedule, body positioning guidelines, and breathing control and supported coughing maneuvers	The patient can follow the handout instructions on her own between supervised treatments; she does not have to rely on memory, which will be impaired because of the distractions of her postsurgical state and the hospital environment
	On subsequent treatments, the physical therapist makes sure the patient knows how to follow the handout and perform the exercises as prescribed

INTERVENTIONS	RATIONALE
Instruct regarding avoidance of respiratory tract infections, nutrition, weight control, hydration and fluid balance, smoking cessation, exercise, and stress management	Promote patient's sense of responsibility for full recovery, health, and health promotion
Reinforce purposes of medication, their prescription parameters, and schedule	To promote cooperation and active participation in treatment
Teach, demonstrate, and provide feedback on interventions that can be self-administered	Between-treatment interventions are as important as treatments themselves to provide cumulative treatment effect
Teach patient regarding balance of activity and rest	Optimal balance between activity and rest is essential to exploit short-term, long-term, and preventive effects of mobilization and exercise
Identify functional outcomes with patient that should be achieved before discharge	To align treatment goals with patient's specific needs
Provide written handouts that are specific to the patient with general and specific information and between-treatment prescriptions	To promote an optimal cumulative treatment response by providing the patient with individualized treatment and exercise prescription parameters in written form
Plan for discharge early; prepare handouts, including home exercise program, precautions	To promote smooth transition from hospital to home; promote continuity of care with physician, community health, and family; and follow-up
Assess home and work physical environments to ensure that patient can function optimally	

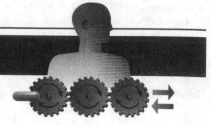

CHAPTER 12

Upper Abdominal Surgery: Cholecystectomy

PATHOPHYSIOLOGY

Inflammation of the gall bladder, cholecystitis, has a predilection for women, who are overweight and over 40 years of age. The gall bladder is responsible for the production of bile, an important substance in the digestion of fats. Excessive fat in the diet exacerbates gall bladder irritation and obstruction of the cystic duct by a stone. Pain can be extremely severe. Although usually localized to the right upper quadrant, the pain may be referred to the back under the scapula and to the right shoulder. Surgery involves a small incision over the right upper quadrant of the abdomen through which the gall bladder is excised. During surgery the right phrenic nerve is irritated, resulting in reflex phrenic nerve inhibition. The resulting diaphragmatic dysfunction can persist for a week following surgery. If no complications arise, patients can be discharged within 3 days after surgery.

Case Study

The patient is a 53-year-old woman. She is an engineer for a large commercial building firm. She lives with her partner in a single-family home in a city suburb. She is 5 feet (154 cm) tall and weighs 95 pounds (43 kg); her body mass index is 18. She is a nonsmoker. Her medical history is unremarkable except for occasional migraine headaches, hypothyroidism, and several bouts of cholecystitis. She was admitted to the emergency room in severe distress: extreme pain, nausea, and vomiting. She had signs of intravascular and extravascular volume depletion. An emergency cholecystectomy was performed. No intraoperative complications were encountered, and she was returned to the ward within 3 hours with a Foley catheter and nasogastric tube in place. Her vital signs were stable, but she was nauseated and not very alert.

Oxygen Transport Deficits: Observed and Potential

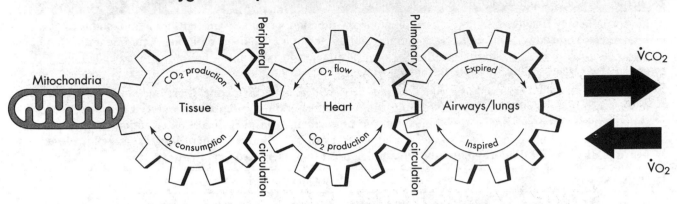

Generalized deconditioning
  and inefficient oxygen
  transport
↑ Oxygen demand

↓ Cardiac reserve;
  deconditioned

↑ Airway closure
↓ Mucociliary transport
↑ Secretion accumulation
Intravascular volume
  depletion
↓ Lung volumes and
  capacities
↓ Functional residual
  capacity
↓ Forced expiratory flow
  rates
Monotonous tidal
  ventilation
Breathing at low
  lung volumes
Avoidance of deep
  breathing
Avoidance of coughing
Diaphragmatic paresis
  due to phrenic nerve
  inhibition
Elevated right
  hemidiaphragm
Atelectasis
Basal atelectasis (R>L)

Shunt
↓ Lymphatic motion
↓ Lymphatic drainage

↑ Increase
↓ Decrease

PHYSICAL THERAPY DIAGNOSES TREATMENT AND PRESCRIPTION

Physical Therapy Diagnosis: Altered cardiopulmonary function: alveolar hypoventilation and shunt caused by surgery, right lower lobe compression/manipulation, trauma to right phrenic nerve and hemidiaphragm, anesthesia and sedation, supine surgical position, reduced arousal, pain, depressed cough and cough effectiveness, fluid shifts, hypovolemia

Signs and Symptoms: Arterial oxygen saturation $Sao_2 < 98\%$, hypermetabolic, increased work of breathing, increased minute ventilation, decreased lung volume, decreased lung compliance, reduced functional residual capacity, increased closing volume, reduced mucociliary transport, secretion retention, radiographic evidence of basal atelectasis (R > L), decreased air entry to bases and dependent lung fields, reflex phrenic nerve inhibition and diaphragmatic dysfunction, hypotension, increased heart rate

INTERVENTIONS	RATIONALE
Monitor arterial blood gases (ABGs), hemoglobin, electrocardiogram (ECG), chest x-rays, pulmonary function, vital signs, Sao_2	To provide a baseline, ongoing assessment and measure of treatment response
Perform serial cardiopulmonary assessments	
Monitor patient's thyroid status	To determine the degree to which the patient's hypothyroidism contributes to the patient's endurance and fatigue and limits treatment response
Define outcome criteria: reversal or mitigation of the signs and symptoms	To provide a basis for defining treatment goals and criteria for discontinuing treatment
Breathing control and supported coughing maneuvers: breathing control with relaxed lateral costal expansion (maximal inspiration—3-5 second hold; exhalation to resting end-tidal volume)	Lung volumes are significantly reduced by anesthesia and surgery
	Postsurgically, vital capacity decreased to 50%; a 10% decrease in vital capacity is associated with 5% increase in oxygen cost, increasing demand on the oxygen transport system
Supported coughing with the use of a pillow or other support (by patient or assisted)	Functional residual capacity is reduced up to 50% when supine and reduced further by anesthesia
Strong effective coughs	Reflex phrenic nerve inhibition and diaphragmatic dysfunction is a complication of upper abdominal surgery and may persist for several days
	Anesthesia decreases central and peripheral drives to breathe, alters breathing pattern, contributes to monotonous tidal ventilation, loss of the sign mechanism, reduced mucociliary transport, reduced surfactant production and distribution, increased airway closure, secretion accumulation, and atelectasis
	Abdominal surgery and pain inhibit effective coughing
Upright body positioning coordinated with breathing control and supported coughing maneuvers	To exploit the effects of gravity with body position changes on cardiopulmonary function and gas exchange
	To optimize respiratory muscle function and neural stimulation of the respiratory muscles
	Phrenic nerve inhibition contributes to loss of diaphragmatic tone, elevation of the affected hemidiaphragm, and basal atelectasis
	Upright positioning coupled with breathing control maximizes functional residual capacity and minimizes the negative effects of phrenic nerve inhibition on airway closure and atelectasis

INTERVENTIONS	RATIONALE
Mobilization prescription coordinated with medications; analgesia at peak potency	To exploit the *acute* effects of mobilization on cardiopulmonary function and oxygen transport (i.e., increase arousal, optimize alveolar volume, functional residual capacity, the distributions of ventilation, perfusion, and ventilation and perfusion matching; gas exchange; three-dimensional chest wall movement, efficient and coordinated thoracoabdominal movement, mucociliary transport, decrease secretion accumulation, increase lung movement, increase surfactant production and distribution, promote lymphatic drainage, and reduce the work of breathing and the work of the heart)
Mobilization coordinated with the upright position, breathing control, and supported coughing maneuvers	
Bed mobility and bed exercises	
Dangling, self-supported, erect, feet on floor/stool	
Transfers; active assist to active transfers	
Chair exercises; sitting erect, upper extremity, trunk, and leg exercises	
Functional activities, bathroom, washing, hair care, changing gown	
Intensity—paced to minimize pain and cardiopulmonary stress (i.e., heart rate increase < 30 beats/min, blood pressure increase < 30 mm Hg, pain < 3-5 [0-10 scale] and fatigue < 3-5 [0-10 scale])	To promote alveolar ventilation and gas exchange by optimizing lung compliance and decreasing airway resistance
Sao_2 > 95%	To ensure that the patient is not unduly fatigued given the patient's hypothyroid condition; she tolerates short, frequent treatments better than longer, less frequent treatments
Duration—10-30 minutes; extended to minimize pain throughout the session	
Frequency—at least every 2-3 hr	
Course and progression—as indicated	
Promote optimal body position and alignment during mobilization and exercise as well as at rest, sitting, or recumbent	
Intersperse rest periods within treatments; encourage movement and body repositioning to be done in a slow, controlled fashion coordinated with breathing control	
Patient is cautioned to avoid resistive exercise, breath holding, and straining	Resistive exercise, breath holding, and straining place undue strain on the incision site and elicit pain
Promote quality rest periods and sleep between treatments	Quality rest and sleep are essential for optimal healing and treatment response
	To optimize breathing pattern, chest wall excursion, and distribution of ventilation; minimize compression atelectasis and suboptimal alveolar filling, gas mixing, and gas exchange

Correction of postural alignment:
  At rest
  In the chair
  Standing
  Walking
	To relieve musculoskeletal rigidity and long-term cardiopulmonary sequelae of impaired postural alignment

	To enhance breathing and movement efficiency
Frequent body position changes (hourly) coordinated with breathing control and supported coughing maneuvers when the patient is in bed	Favoring the right side by persistently lying on the left can lead to atelectasis in the dependent lung fields as a result of physical compression, reduced chest wall excursion, and monotonous tidal ventilation

Type:
  High and semi Fowler's positions
  Body positioning in the horizontal plane and variants of side to side positions
	To increase arousal, optimize alveolar volume and distribution of ventilation, lung volumes and capacities, functional residual capacity, and three-dimensional chest wall movement, and minimize airway closure of the dependent airways and cephalad displacement of the diaphragm by the viscera

Minimize favoring right side
  Side lying on either side
  ¾ prone to each side; modified to right side if poorly tolerated
  Supine
	To stimulate deep breaths, increase lung movement, surfactant production and distribution, mucociliary transport and lymphatic drainage, to promote effective coughing, to minimize intraabdominal pressure and encroachment on the thoracic cavity, to minimize thoracic blood volume and optimize lung compliance, to maintain fluid volume regulation (which can only be maintained with the upright position), to minimize the risk of pulmonary aspiration, to stimulate bowel and bladder functions, and reduce intraabdominal pressure

Continued.

INTERVENTIONS	RATIONALE
	The neural drive to the diaphragm is increased in the upright position to offset shortened diaphragmatic position and the reduced force generated in this position
	To encourage patient not to favor any single position; stress importance of position changes to simulate the changes that would occur when mobile
	To encourage patient to perform pain control strategies and request medication if necessary to provide comfort, reduce suffering, and facilitate movement, and frequent position changes
	Supine is a deleterious position particularly in the postsurgical patient; supine is included in the turning schedule, but duration should not exceed 1-2 hr; supine compromises expansion of the chest wall and dependent lung fields and reduces lung compliance because of increased thoracic blood volume and encroachment of the abdominal viscera
Frequency—when in bed, frequent body position changes at least every 1-2 hr; promote frequent body position changes by patient coordinated with breathing control and coughing maneuvers	To optimize turning frequency to augment cardiopulmonary function, ventilation, mucociliary transport, lung movement, and lymphatic drainage
Course—as indicated by monitoring patient closely	To place the patient in as many positions as possible; extreme positions (e.g., prone) are modified within the patient's limits of comfort
	To change the patient's body position frequently with maximal assist from the patient (every 1-2 hr); maximal assist provides an exercise stimulus so that patient has the advantage of the new position, the position change, and the *acute* effects of the mobilization stimulus on ventilation
	To avoid excessive duration in *any* single position, even those with initially favorable outcomes, because the dependent lung fields will be compromised within 1-2 hr
Range-of-motion exercises (active and active assist) coordinated with breathing control and supported coughing: Upper extremities Trunk Lower extremities, especially hips and knees and feet and ankles	To exploit the cardiopulmonary benefits of range-of-motion exercises, and peripheral circulatory effects
360° positional rotation schedule when recumbent Coordinate body position changes with breathing control and supported coughing Promote active or active-assist turns Frequent body positions changes at least every 1-2 hr	To promote physiological "stir-up"; alters the distribution of ventilation, lung volumes, mucociliary clearance; stimulates spontaneous deep breaths and coughing; stimulates lymphatic drainage
Promote log rolling (i.e., shoulders and hips turn simultaneously to avoid trunk and abdominal stress)	To avoid trunk and abdominal stress on surgical incision
Pain control: coordinate treatments with medication as required; ensure that patient is adequately premedicated before treatment; ensure that analgesics are at peak effectiveness during treatment; breathing control and supported coughing maneuvers; relaxation procedures	Pain reduction and the normal physiological stresses imposed by gravity and movement help restore normal breathing pattern

Physical Therapy Diagnosis: Ineffective breathing pattern: diaphragmatic dysfunction, reflex phrenic nerve inhibition, pain, decreased lung compliance, increased airway, resistance; recumbency, reluctance to change body position, restricted mobility

Signs and Symptoms: Avoidance of deep breathing, reduced chest wall excursion, loss of normal chest wall motion, chest wall asymmetry, radiographic evidence of elevated right hemidiaphragm, radiographic evidence of right lower lobe atelectasis, increased minute ventilation, monotonous tidal ventilation, absent sigh mechanism, suppressed cough

INTERVENTIONS	RATIONALE
Monitor breathing pattern, chest wall excursion, chest x-rays, and thoracoabdominal motion	To provide a baseline ongoing assessment and measure a treatment response
Define outcome criteria: reversal or mitigation of the signs and symptoms	To provide a basis for defining treatment goals and criteria for discontinuing treatment
Erect upright positioning	To maximize fluid shifts to the dependent areas and optimize fluid volume regulating mechanisms, reducing bed rest deconditioning and orthostatic intolerance
Upright positioning with legs dependent	
Mobilization, body positioning, and range-of-motion exercises coordinated with breathing control and supported coughing maneuvers	In the upright position, the rib cage assumes its maximal anteroposterior diameter, the inspiratory intercostals and scalene muscles are lengthened, and the diaphragmatic muscle fibers are shortened as a result of descent and displacement of the abdominal viscera
	The neural drive to the diaphragm is increased in the upright position to offset shortened diaphragmatic position and the reduced force generated in this position
Pain control: coordinate treatments with medication as required; ensure that patient is adequately premedicated before treatment; ensure that analgesics are at peak effectiveness during treatment; breathing control and supported coughing maneuvers; relaxation procedures	Pain reduction and the normal physiological stresses imposed by gravity and movement help restore normal breathing pattern

Physical Therapy Diagnosis: Pain: incision and internal surgical trauma

Signs and Symptoms: Verbal complaints of discomfort and pain, grimacing, guarding, splinting, holding body rigid, and moaning, reluctance to move and change body position, distracted, restless, reduced ability to cooperate with treatment, fatigue and lethargy, loss of sleep, disturbed rest and sleep, loss of appetite and interest in eating

INTERVENTIONS	RATIONALE
Monitor quality, quantity, and location of pain; factors that improve or worsen pain, including pain medications	To provide a baseline, ongoing assessment and measure of treatment response
Define outcome criteria: reversal or mitigation of the signs and symptoms	To provide a basis for defining treatment goals and criteria for discontinuing treatment
Ensure that patient is appropriately medicated for treatments (preferably alternative agents to narcotics when possible) and medications are at peak efficacy	To minimize pain, suffering, and distress
	To promote pain self-management
Teach relaxation procedures (e.g., breathing control, Jacobsen's relaxation procedure, Benson's relaxation method, autogenic training, biofeedback, visual imagery)	To minimize pain and discomfort by encouraging gentle movement and frequent body position changes within limits of comfort
Breathing control and supported coughing maneuvers	Breathing control maneuvers help release muscle tension, release guarding and static posturing, and induce relaxation
Teach supported coughing; patient provides pillow or hand support over incision site	To minimize pain and undue stress on the incision site and facilitate healing
Coordinate treatments with breathing control and supported coughing maneuvers	
Pace treatments	

Continued.

INTERVENTIONS	RATIONALE
Intersperse rest periods within and between treatments	To maximize tolerance of mobility exercises and body position changes with rest periods (i.e., these interventions are performed in stages and with optimal assistance such that the patient has the physiological benefits of actively, physically participating within limits of pain and discomfort)
Respond to patient's complaints of pain and make the patient as comfortable as possible	
	Although weaning off pain medication is encouraged, the patient is encouraged to request analgesia before pain is excessive and unduly interferes with breathing, mobility, positioning, and ability to rest effectively
Promote good body alignment when sitting and standing, as well as when lying in bed	To minimize residual postural deficits secondary to abdominal surgery
Frequent body position changes	To minimize stiffness and associated discomfort

Physical Therapy Diagnosis: Decreased tolerance for physical activity and exercise resulting from illness, surgery, hypovolemia, premorbid aerobic deconditioning, inadequate nutrition, and hypothyroidism

Signs and Symptoms: Decreased physical activity, complaints of pain, discomfort, fatigue, weakness, and loss of endurance

INTERVENTIONS	RATIONALE
Assess tolerance for physical activity and exercise	To provide a baseline, ongoing assessment and measure of treatment response
Determine premorbid functional capacity	
	To provide a basis for defining treatment goals and for discontinuing treatment
Monitor thyroid function	Hypothyroidism contributes to fatigue and reduced exercise tolerance
Monitor nutrition and fluid intake	To determine to what degree poor nutritional status contributes to reduced activity and exercise tolerance
	Patient's capacity to respond to exercise depends on optimal nutrition and fluid intake
Define outcome criteria: reversal or mitigation of the signs and symptoms	To provide a basis for defining treatment goals and criteria for discontinuing treatment
Mobilization and exercise prescription:	To exploit the *long-term* effects of mobilization and exercise on cardiopulmonary function and oxygen transport (e.g., adaptation of lung parenchyma, pulmonary circulation, lymphatics, reduced minute ventilation and reduced perceived exertion and fatigue, rate pressure product, and cardiac output at rest and submaximal work rates, increased peripheral collateral circulation, and increased extraction and uptake of oxygen at the tissue level)
Type—walking; monitor posture and gait, activities of daily life (ADL), and bathroom	
Intensity—low to moderate, pace within limits of pain and fatigue; heart rate increase < 30 beats per minute, blood pressure increase < 30 mm Hg	
Duration—intersperse with sitting and standing rest periods	
Frequency—several times daily	
Course and progression—increase duration, speed; reduce rest periods	
Monitor signs and symptoms of orthostatic intolerance	
Prescriptive rest periods within treatments	The patient is in a hypermetabolic state caused by surgery and surgical trauma, recovery from surgery, anesthesia, sedation and narcotics, healing and repair, inadequate nutrition and fluid intake; thus quality rest and sleep periods between treatments are essential to promote healing and repair, restore energy, and reduce fatigue, thereby enhancing functional activity and work output
Prescriptive rest periods between treatments	

Physical Therapy Diagnosis: Perioperative anxiety

Signs and Symptoms: Worried, agitated, inattentive, distracted, preoccupied with readiness to return to work and perform ADL

INTERVENTIONS	RATIONALE
Monitor signs and symptoms of anxiety	To provide a baseline and ongoing assessment
Identify factors that increase and decrease anxiety	
Define outcome criteria: reversal or mitigation of the signs and symptoms	To provide a basis for defining treatment goals
Comfort, reassurance, empathy	To improve psychological well-being
Caring	To promote internal locus of control
Listen and be attentive to patient	To promote self-responsibility
Be encouraging	
Provide knowledge about condition, surgery, and what can be expected	
Provide an atmosphere that facilitates patient's questions and expressing concerns	
Provide sufficient time for preoperative preparation and teaching	
Involve patient in decision making	
As soon as patient is ready, discuss transition to home and work	To facilitate continuity of rehabilitation after discharge
Initiate discharge planning early (e.g., with other team members)	To promote continuity of care after discharge and follow-up care
Prepare handouts of exercise regimens	To provide patient with written information on exercise prescription

Physical Therapy Diagnosis: Threats to oxygen transport and gas exchange because of postsurgical status, type and duration of surgery, supine position during surgery, anesthesia and sedation, decreased arousal, fluid shifts and third spacing, poorly controlled hypothyroidism, increased body mass, recumbency, restricted mobility

Signs and Symptoms: Hypoxemia, decreased lung volumes (particularly functional residual capacity), decreased expiratory flow rates, decreased ventilation and perfusion matching, decreased lung compliance, increased airway resistance, monotonous tidal ventilation, impaired mucociliary transport, depressed cough reflex, hypotension, increased heart rate, decreased cough effectiveness, circulatory stasis, thrombus formation, thromboemboli (e.g., pulmonary emboli), skin breakdown, age-related airway closure in sitting, age-related closure of dependent airways in recumbent positions, age-related inhomogeneity of ventilation, restricted mobility, recumbency, circulatory stasis, venous thrombosis, pulmonary embolism, age-related decrease of mucociliary clearance rate, age-related depression of cough reflex, premorbid aerobic deconditioning, reduced thyroid level

INTERVENTIONS	RATIONALE
Assess patient's risk factors	To provide a baseline and ongoing assessment
Monitor oxygen transport status	
Define outcome criteria: prevention, reversal, or mitigation of the signs and symptoms	To provide a basis for defining treatment goals and criteria for discontinuing treatment
Preoperative cardiopulmonary physical therapy assessment, including history and clinical examination based on inspection, palpation, percussion, and auscultation	The preoperative assessment includes a review of risk factors threatening cardiopulmonary function and oxygen transport, lab tests, and investigations
Integrate the results of relevant preoperative tests and investigations	

Continued.

INTERVENTIONS	RATIONALE
Preoperative teaching includes the disease pathology and surgery (type, body position, anesthesia and sedation, incision, duration, and dressings), pain to be expected, medication, and when the physical therapist will be seen postoperatively	Preoperative teaching and patient preparation minimize cardiopulmonary complications, morbidity, and length of hospital stay
	A preoperative exercise program can significantly reduce perioperative complications, morbidity, and length of hospital stay
	To explain the *preventive* effects of mobilization and exercise before and after surgery
Preoperative teaching directly related to physical therapy includes breathing control and supported coughing maneuvers, bed mobility and positioning, range-of-motion exercises, transferring, ambulation, pain control, and the rationale for these interventions, including prevention	Basic background regarding the disease and surgery provides a basis for understanding treatment, which enhances cooperation with treatment program when supervised and when not directly supervised
Preoperative teaching includes a description of when the patient will be seen by the physical therapist after surgery, the postoperative assessment, and treatment interventions, including breathing control and supported coughing coordinated with positioning, frequent position changes and mobilization, and relaxation procedures	The patient is more cooperative and able to actively participate in treatment when exposed to the postoperative regimen before surgery
Teach preoperatively bed mobility exercises, transfers, changing body positions, mobilizing, walking, and supporting the incision site	
Teach the patient to coordinate the preceding activities with breathing control and supported coughing maneuvers	
Frequent body position changes when lying down (hourly)	To promote physiological "stir-up"
Coordinate breathing control and coughing maneuvers during position changes	
Avoid excessive time in left side lying	Patients favor lying in restricted positions (e.g., the less painful side) for prolonged periods, thus are at risk of developing cardiopulmonary complications in the dependent lung fields
Monitor for signs of deep vein thrombosis	Surgical patients are at risk of thrombus formation
Monitor for signs of pulmonary emboli	
Monitor thyroid status and medication effectiveness	Hypothyroidism contributes to lethargy and fatigue and interferes with ADL and exercise performance, hence functional work capacity

Physical Therapy Diagnosis: Risk of the negative sequelae of recumbency

Signs and Symptoms: Within 6 hours reduced circulating blood volume, decreased blood pressure on sitting and standing compared with supine, light-headedness, dizziness, syncope hypotension, increased hematocrit and blood viscosity, increased work of the heart, altered fluid balance in the lung, impaired pulmonary lymphatic drainage, decreased lung volumes and capacities, decreased functional residual capacity, increased closing volume, and decreased Pao_2 and Sao_2

INTERVENTIONS	RATIONALE
Monitor signs and symptoms of the negative sequelae of recumbency	To provide a baseline and ongoing assessment
Define outcome criteria: prevention, reversal, or mitigation of the signs and symptoms	To provide a basis for defining treatment goals and criteria for discontinuing treatment
Place patient in upright sitting position, preferably with feet dependent; standing and walking	The upright position minimizes the adverse effects of recumbency on reflex phrenic nerve inhibition

INTERVENTIONS	RATIONALE
Coordinate physical activity and mobilization in the upright position and with breathing control maneuvers	The upright position is essential to shift fluid volume from central to peripheral circulation and maintain fluid volume regulating mechanisms and circulating blood volume
	The upright position maximizes lung volumes and capacities (especially functional residual capacity) and minimizes airway closure; these factors are adversely affected by anesthesia and surgery
	The upright position maximizes expiratory flow rates and cough effectiveness
	The upright position optimizes the length-tension relationship of the respiratory muscles and abdominal muscles, neural stimulation of the respiratory muscles, and cough effectiveness
	The upright position coupled with mobilization and breathing control and supported coughing maneuvers maximizes alveolar ventilation, ventilation and perfusion matching, and pulmonary lymphatic drainage

Physical Therapy Diagnosis: Risk of negative sequelae of restricted mobility

Signs and Symptoms: Reduced activity and exercise tolerance, muscle atrophy and reduced muscle strength and endurance, decreased oxygen transport efficiency, increased heart rate, blood pressure, and minute ventilation at rest and submaximal work rates, reduced respiratory muscle strength and endurance, circulatory stasis, thromboemboli (e.g., pulmonary emboli), pressure areas, skin redness, skin breakdown and ulceration, cognitive dysfunction, impaired circadian rhythms, and impaired sleep patterns

INTERVENTIONS	RATIONALE
Monitor the signs and symptoms of the negative sequelae of restricted mobility	To provide a baseline and ongoing assessment
Define outcome criteria: prevention, reversal, or mitigation of the signs and symptoms	To provide a basis for defining treatment goals and criteria for discontinuing treatment
Mobilization and exercise prescription	To exploit the *preventive* effects of mobilization and exercise (e.g., optimize circulating blood volume and enhance the efficiency of all steps in the oxygen transport pathway)

Physical Therapy Diagnosis: Knowledge deficit

Signs and Symptoms: Lack of information about cholecystitis, surgery, complications, and recovery

INTERVENTIONS	RATIONALE
Assess patient's specific knowledge deficits related to her condition and cardiopulmonary physical therapy management	To address patient's specific knowledge deficits
Define outcome criteria: reversal or mitigation of the signs and symptoms	To provide a basis for defining treatment goals and criteria for discontinuing interventions
Promote a caring and supportive patient-therapist relationship	To focus on treating the patient with a cholecystectomy rather than a cholecystectomy
Consider every patient interaction an opportunity for education	To promote patient's sense of responsibility for full recovery, wellness, and health promotion
Instruct regarding avoidance of respiratory tract infection, nutrition, hydration and fluid balance, exercise, stress management, and quality sleep	To promote cooperation and active participation in treatment

Continued.

INTERVENTIONS	RATIONALE
Reinforce knowledge related to the roles of other health care team members	
Reinforce purposes of medication, their prescription parameters, and schedule	
Teach, demonstrate, and provide feedback on interventions that can be self-administered	Between-treatment interventions are as important as treatments themselves to provide cumulative treatment effect
Teach patient regarding balance of activity and rest	Optimal balance between activity and rest is essential to exploit short-term, long-term, and preventive effects of mobilization and exercise
Patient is given a personalized handout with a listing and description of exercises and their prescription parameters; precautions are emphasized	The patient can follow the handout instructions on her own between treatments; she does not have to rely on memory, which will be impaired because of the distractions of her postsurgical state and the hospital environment
The content of the handout is reviewed with the patient	
Provide handout of mobilization and exercise schedule, body positioning guidelines, and breathing control and supported coughing maneuvers	On subsequent treatments, the physical therapist makes sure the patient knows how to follow the handout and perform the exercises as prescribed
Prepare patient for functioning at home and work after discharge	To review home and work settings (e.g., stairs, walking distances, lifting, driving, ADL and work) so that patient is maximally prepared for discharge
Identify functional outcome goals with patient that should be achieved before discharge	
Provide written handouts that are specific to the patient with general and specific information and between-treatment prescriptions	To promote transition to home
Plan for discharge early; prepare handouts, including home exercise program and precautions	

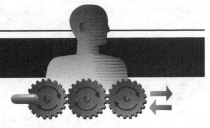

CHAPTER 13

Cardiovascular Thoracic Surgery: Lung Resection

PATHOPHYSIOLOGY

Lung resections include the excision of a single bronchopulmonary segment (segmentectomy), a complete lobe (lobectomy), or an entire lung (pneumonectomy). Lung resection is indicated to excise lung tissue that has been irreversibly damaged from recurrent chest infections and has lost its structural integrity and ability to participate in gas exchange, and to excise lung tumors and affected lymphatic tissue. Surgical incision depends on the site of the area to be resected; large areas require thoracotomy incisions over the anterolateral or posterolateral chest wall. These incisions are particularly painful because they are extensive and penetrate extensive areas of chest wall muscles. Once the lung tissue has been removed, the vacated space is occupied by fluid and expansion of adjacent lung tissue into the area. Also, depending on the amount of lung tissue removed, the mediastinal structures will shift toward the operated side. Chest tubes are inserted into the pleural space to facilitate the drainage of fluid and blood from the surgical site.

Case Study

The patient is a 34-year-old man. He is a fisherman by trade and runs a business with his brother. He is 5 feet 8.5 inches (174 cm) tall and weighs 123 pounds (56 kg); his body mass index is 18. He has a history of chronic lung infections since childhood and has been hospitalized twice in the past 15 months. He was diagnosed with bronchiectasis. The patient smoked a pack a day for 18 years but gradually quit 2 years ago because he was becoming increasingly short of breath. The patient underwent a lobectomy on the left side (lingula and left base). He had a posterolateral thoracotomy incision. Two chest tubes were inserted. After 4 days, his condition began to deteriorate. His arterial blood gases (ABGs) at a fractional inspired oxygen concentration (Fio_2) of 0.35 were pH 7.41, oxygen pressure (Po_2) 77 mm Hg, carbon dioxide pressure (Pco_2) 42 mm Hg, bicarbonate (HCO_3) 27, and arterial oxygen saturation (Sao_2) 89%. His chest x-ray showed whiteout on the right side. He also had an infection of his incision site.

Oxygen Transport Deficits: Observed and Potential

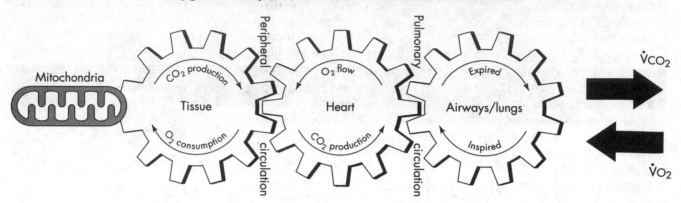

↑ Oxygen demand

Hemodynamic instability

↑ Airway closure
↓ Mucociliary transport
↓ Ciliary motion due to
   supplemental oxygen
↑ Secretion accumulation
Bronchovesicular breath
   sounds
↑ Airway resistance
↓ Chest wall excursion
Restricted chest wall motion
   (L>R)
Chest wall asymmetry
↓ Lung volumes and
   capacities
↓ Functional residual
   capacity
↑ Closing volume
Monotonous tidal
   ventilation
Breathing at low lung
   volumes
↓ Forced expiratory flow
   rates
Compression atelectasis
↓ Compliance
Pleural effusion
Diffusion defect
Weak cough
End expiratory crackles
Postural deviation; lists
   to the left
↑ Work of breathing

Blood: Hypoxemia
       Fluid shifts
       Central fluid accumulation
       Third spacing

Hypoxic vasoconstriction
Shunt
↓ Lymph flow
↓ Lymphatic drainage

| ↑ Increase |
| ↓ Decrease |

PHYSICAL THERAPY DIAGNOSES TREATMENT AND PRESCRIPTION

Physical Therapy Diagnosis: Altered cardiopulmonary function: hypoxemia, alveolar hypoventilation, and shunt due to lung pathology, lung resection, type of surgery, duration, right side lying, surgical position, anesthesia, sedation, medication, fluid and blood loss, fluid and blood replacement, ventilatory support, compression of the heart and lungs during the surgical procedure, recumbency, and restricted mobility

Signs and Symptoms: $Pao_2 < 104.2 - 0.27$ age ($\pm$ 7) mm Hg, $Sao_2 < 90\%$, hypermetabolic, fever, decreased arousal, increased work of breathing, increased minute ventilation, decreased lung volumes and capacities, reduced functional residual capacity, increased closing volume, depressed cough reflex, depressed cough effectiveness, depressed ciliary action, reduced mucociliary transport, secretion retention, decreased lung compliance, increased airway resistance, third spacing of fluid in thoracic cavity, alveolar-capillary fluid leak and impaired diffusing capacity, increased work of the heart, decreased urinary output, fluid accumulation requiring chest tube drainage, and orthostatic intolerance

INTERVENTIONS	RATIONALE
Monitor serial ABGs, hemoglobin, electrocardiogram (ECG), hemodynamics, fluid and electrolyte balance, chest x-rays, pulmonary function, vital signs, Sao_2 Perform serial cardiopulmonary assessments	To provide a baseline, ongoing assessment and measure of treatment response
Define outcome criteria: reversal or mitigation of the signs and symptoms	To provide a basis for defining treatment goals and criteria for discontinuing treatment
Reinforce use of supplemental oxygen and appropriate fit of face mask or nasal prongs	Ensure that the oxygen mask or nasal prongs are positioned so that oxygen delivery to the patient is maximized and not wasted
High Fowler's position and dangling over edge of bed with feet supported coordinated with breathing control and supported coughing maneuvers: breathing control with lateral costal expansion (maximal inspiration 3-5 second hold, exhalation to resting end-tidal volume)	To exploit the effect of gravity with body position changes on cardiopulmonary function and gas exchange Lung volumes are significantly reduced by anesthesia and surgery Vital capacity decreases to 50%; increases over a few days Further reduction in vital capacity caused by excised lung tissue
Supported coughing with the use of a pillow or other firm support (by patient or with assist)	Functional residual capacity is reduced by up to 50% when supine and is reduced further by anesthesia Airway closure is promoted with recumbency and further by anesthesia Each 10% decrease in vital capacity is associated with a 5% increase in energy expenditure, increasing demand on the oxygen transport system Anesthesia depresses central and peripheral drives to breathe, alters breathing pattern, contributes to monotonous tidal ventilation, loss of the sigh mechanism, reduced surfactant production and distribution, and atelectasis
Mobilization prescription coordinated with breathing control and supported coughing maneuvers: medications—analgesia at peak potency, supplemental oxygen Mobilization coordinated with the upright position, breathing control, and supported coughing maneuvers Bed mobility and bed exercises Dangling, self-supported, erect, feet on floor Transfers; active assist to active transfers Chair exercises; sitting erect, upper extremity, trunk, and leg exercises Functional activities, bathroom, washing, shaving, hair care, changing bed wear Intensity—paced to minimize pain and cardiopulmonary stress; $Sao_2 > 90\%$	To exploit the *acute* effects of mobilization on cardiopulmonary function and oxygen transport (i.e., increase arousal, optimize alveolar volume, functional residual capacity, the distributions of ventilation, perfusion, and ventilation and perfusion matching; gas exchange; reduce airway resistance; optimize three-dimensional chest wall movement, efficient and coordinated thoracoabdominal movement, mucociliary transport, decrease secretion accumulation, lung movement, increase surfactant production and distribution and lymphatic drainage, and reduce the work of breathing and the work of the heart) To promote lung movement and chest tube drainage

Continued.

INTERVENTIONS	RATIONALE
Duration—5-30 minutes	
Frequency—several times daily	
Course and progression—as indicated	
Intersperse rest periods within treatments; encourage movement and body repositioning to be done in a slow, controlled fashion coordinated with breathing control	Cycles of mobilization and rest increase patient's treatment tolerance, duration, and benefit
Promote quality rest periods and sleep between treatments	Optimal rest between treatments optimizes treatment response
	A balance of rest/sleep/recumbency to activity is essential; excessive rest/sleep/recumbency reduces ventilation and lung volumes and contributes to airway closure
Patient cautioned to avoid resistive movement/exercise, breath holding, and straining	Resistive exercises, breath holding, and straining place undue strain on the incision site and elicit pain
Patient is given a personalized handout with a listing and description of exercises and their prescription parameters; precautions are emphasized	The patient can follow the handout instructions on his own between supervised treatments; he does not have to rely on memory, which will be impaired because of the distractions of his postsurgical state and the hospital environment
	The content of the handout is reviewed with the patient
	On subsequent treatments, the physical therapist makes sure the patient can follow the handout and perform the exercises as prescribed
In bed, frequent body position changes (hourly) coordinated with breathing control and supported coughing maneuvers	Favoring the left side by persistently lying on the right can lead to atelectasis in the dependent lung fields because of physical compression, reduced chest wall excursion, and monotonous tidal ventilation
Body positioning coordinated with breathing control and supported coughing maneuvers before, during, and after treatment:	To optimize alveolar volume and distribution of ventilation, lung volumes and capacities, lung compliance, functional residual capacity, increase arousal, and minimize airway closure of the dependent airways, thoracic blood volume, and displacement of the diaphragm cephalad by the viscera
Place in as high a semi-Fowler's position as possible based on patient's tolerance and response	
Reverse-Trendelenburg position (head up with feet down)	
Body positioning in the horizontal plane and variants with head of bed up and down	To stimulate deep breaths, increase lung movement, surfactant production and distribution, mucociliary transport, and lymphatic drainage
Minimize favoring the left side	To promote strong, effective coughing
	To minimize intraabdominal pressure and encroachment on the thoracic cavity
	To minimize thoracic blood volume and reduced lung compliance
	To maintain fluid volume regulation, which can only be maintained with upright positioning
	To minimize the risk of pulmonary aspiration
	To stimulate bowel activity and minimize intraabdominal pressure
Side lying on either side; modify left side lying	To encourage patient not to favor any single position; stress importance of position changes to simulate physiological perturbations associated with mobilization
¾ prone to each side; modify to left side if poorly tolerated	
Supine	To encourage patient to perform pain control strategies and request medication if necessary to provide comfort, reduce suffering, and facilitate movement; frequent position changes
	Supine is a deleterious position particularly in the postsurgical patient; supine is included in the turning schedule, but duration should not exceed 1-2 hr; supine compromises expansion of the dependent lung fields and reduces lung compliance because of increased thoracic blood volume and encroachment of the abdominal viscera

INTERVENTIONS	RATIONALE
Frequency—when in bed, frequent body position changes every 1-2 hr; promote frequent body position changes by patient coordinated with breathing control and coughing maneuvers	Optimize turning frequency to augment cardiopulmonary function, ventilation, mucociliary transport, lung movement, and lymphatic drainage
Course—as indicated by monitoring patient closely	
Place the patient in as many positions as possible; extreme positions (e.g., prone) are modified within the patient's limits of comfort	
Promote active position changes	
Increase duration in positions with favorable outcomes	
Minimize the duration in positions with unfavorable outcomes	
Avoid excessive duration in *any* single position	Even body positions with initially favorable outcomes will become unfavorable because the dependent lung fields will be compromised after 1-2 hr
Range-of-motion exercises (active and active assist) coordinated with breathing control and supported coughing:	To exploit the cardiopulmonary effects of range-of-motion exercises primarily; secondarily to maintain joint range and muscle length and reduce stiffness
Upper extremities	
Trunk	
Lower extremities especially hips and knees and feet and ankles	
Postural drainage positions for right lung:	Postural drainage positions are specific to the bronchopulmonary segments; the specific position and degree of tilt is necessary to effect maximal drainage; a modified position is indicated if the patient cannot tolerate the position or is too hemodynamically unstable
Upper lobe: apical segment—high Fowler's position; anterior segment—supine; posterior segment—¾; prone to the right	
Middle lobe: ¾ supine; on right side; head of bed down 30 degrees if tolerated	
Lower lobe: apical segment—prone, bed level; anterior segment—supine, head of bed down 30-45 degrees; lateral segment—left side lying, head of bed down 30-45 degrees; posterior segment—prone, head of bed down 30-45 degrees	
Postural drainage positions with manual techniques (i.e., percussion, shaking, and vibration)	If indicated, single-handed percussion at a frequency of 1 per second minimizes the adverse effects of this intervention
Monitor continuously the patient's tolerance in the tipped positions	Patients in the early postoperative stage or who are hemodynamically unstable may not tolerate tipped positions; modify degree of tip as necessary

Physical Therapy Diagnosis: Pain: incisional and internal surgical trauma

Signs and Symptoms: Complaints of pain, grimacing, guarding, splinting, holding body rigid, moaning, reluctance to move and change body position, distracted, reduced ability to cooperate with treatment, fatigue and lethargy, disturbed rest and sleep, and loss of appetite

INTERVENTIONS	RATIONALE
Monitor pain quality, quantity, and location	To provide a baseline and ongoing assessment
Monitor factors that improve and worsen the pain	
Define outcome criteria: reversal or mitigation of the signs and symptoms	To provide a basis for defining treatment goals and criteria for discontinuing treatment
Ensure that patient is appropriately medicated for treatments (preferably alternative agents to narcotics when possible) and medications are at peak efficacy	To minimize pain, suffering, and distress
	To promote pain self-management

Continued.

INTERVENTIONS	RATIONALE
Teach relaxation procedures (e.g., breathing control, Jacobsen's relaxation procedure, Benson's relaxation method, autogenic training, biofeedback, visual imagery)	To minimize pain and discomfort by encouraging gentle movement and frequent body position changes Breathing control maneuvers help release muscle tension, relieve guarding and static posturing, and induce relaxation
Transcutaneous electrical nerve stimulation (TENS) for incisional pain	Posterolateral thoracotomy incisions are particularly painful because of extensive incision through muscle; TENS may provide some relief of incisional pain
Pace treatments Intersperse rest periods within and between treatments	To maximize tolerance of mobility exercises and body position changes with rest periods (i.e., these interventions are performed in stages and with optimal assistance such that the patient has the physiological benefits of actively, physically participating within his limits of pain and discomfort)
Promote good body alignment when sitting and standing, as well as when lying in bed Frequent body position changes	In addition to the direct effects positioning and frequent body position changes have on oxygen transport, these interventions minimize stiffness, associated discomfort, and long-term chest wall deformity
Respond to patient's complaints of pain and make the patient as comfortable as possible	Although weaning off pain medication is encouraged, the patient is encouraged to request analgesic before pain is excessive and unduly interferes with breathing, mobility, positioning, and ability to rest effectively

Physical Therapy Diagnosis: Ineffective breathing pattern: extensive left posterolateral thoracotomy incision, pain, decreased lung compliance, increased airway resistance, recumbency, reluctance to change body position, and restricted mobility

Signs and Symptoms: Loss of normal chest wall motion, reduced chest wall excursion, chest wall asymmetry, increased minute ventilation, radiographic evidence of atelectasis, absent sigh mechanism, monotonous tidal ventilation, breathing at low lung volumes, decreased breath sounds, and listing to the affected side when lying, sitting, standing, and ambulating

INTERVENTIONS	RATIONALE
Monitor breathing pattern Monitor chest wall excursion, chest x-rays, and thoracoabdominal motion	To provide a baseline, ongoing assessment and measure of treatment response
Define outcome criteria: reversal or mitigation of the signs and symptoms	To provide a basis for defining treatment goals and criteria for discontinuing treatment
Mobilization, body positioning, and range-of-motion exercises coordinated with breathing control maneuvers and pain control Upright positioning	In the upright position, the rib cage assumes its maximal anteroposterior diameter, optimal transverse diameter; the inspiratory intercostals and scalene muscles are lengthened and the diaphragmatic muscle fibers are shortened by descent and displacement of the abdominal viscera The neural drive to the diaphragm is increased in the upright position to offset the shortened diaphragmatic position and the reduced force generated in this position

Coordinate treatments with medication as required:
  Ensure the patient is adequately premedicated before treatment
  Ensure that analgesics are at peak effectiveness during treatment
  Breathing control and supported coughing maneuvers
  Relaxation procedures
	Normal breathing pattern will be restored with pain reduction and with the normal physiological stresses imposed by gravity and movement

INTERVENTIONS	RATIONALE

Body alignment, postural correction, and chest wall stretching and mobility exercises
Correction of postural alignment:
  At rest
  In the chair
  Standing
  Walking
	To optimize three-dimensional chest wall movement, including bucket handle and pump handle motions
	To optimize breathing pattern, chest wall excursion, and distribution of ventilation; minimize compression atelectasis and suboptimal alveolar filling, gas mixing, and gas exchange
	To relieve musculoskeletal rigidity and long-term cardiopulmonary sequelae of impaired postural alignment
	To enhance breathing and movement efficiency and movement economy metabolically

Upright positioning with legs dependent	To maximize fluid shifts to the periphery and optimize fluid regulation; this will reduce intrathoracic blood volume and maximize chest wall motion, lung movement, lung compliance, lymphatic drainage, orthostatic intolerance, and bed rest deconditioning

Physical Therapy Diagnosis: Decreased tolerance for physical activity and exercise resulting from prolonged history of lung disease and its sequelae; surgery and its sequelae

Signs and Symptoms: Physical activity restricted by complaints of pain, discomfort, apprehension about incision line, fatigue, weakness, loss of endurance

INTERVENTIONS	RATIONALE
Assess tolerance for physical activity and exercise	To provide a baseline, ongoing assessment and measure of treatment response
Define outcome criteria: reversal or mitigation of the signs and symptoms	To provide a basis for defining treatment goals and criteria for discontinuing treatment
Mobilization and exercise prescription Type—walking; monitor posture and gait, activities of daily living (ADL), and bathroom Intensity—low to moderate, pace within tolerance, pain < 3-4 (0-10 scale), dyspnea < 3-4 (0-10 scale), heart rate increase < 20-30 beats per minute; blood pressure increase < 30 mm Hg Duration—intersperse with sitting and standing rest periods Monitor signs and symptoms of orthostatic intolerance Frequency—every 1-2 hr Course and progression—increase duration, speed; reduce rest periods; increase frequency of sessions	To exploit the *long-term* effects of mobilization and exercise on cardiopulmonary function and oxygen transport (e.g., adaptation of lung parenchyma, pulmonary circulation, lymphatics, increased strength and endurance of the respiratory muscles, reduced minute ventilation and reduced perceived exertion and fatigue, rate pressure product, cardiac output at submaximal work rates, increased peripheral collateral circulation, and increased extraction and uptake of oxygen at the tissue level)
Monitor for signs and symptoms of postural hypotension; record heart rate and blood pressure before and after lying supine and assuming an upright seated or standing position	Patient is susceptible to postural hypotension; a chair must be available initially when walking in case patient becomes light-headed or fatigued
Prescriptive rest periods within treatments Prescriptive rest periods between treatments	The patient is in a hypermetabolic state, that is, has an increased oxygen demand, due to surgery and surgical trauma, recovery from extensive surgery, anesthesia, sedation and narcotics, blood loss, anemia, healing and repair, and inadequate nutrition and fluid intake; thus quality rest and sleep periods between treatments are essential to promote healing and repair, restore energy, reduce fatigue, and thereby enhance functional activity and work output To ensure prescription parameters are set so oxygen demand does not exceed the capacity of oxygen delivery

Continued.

INTERVENTIONS	RATIONALE
Correct postural alignment during ambulation, as well as sitting and lying down	To optimize postural alignment (i.e., erect posture with no list to the left) to optimize movement efficiency and reduce energy cost and oxygen demand of ambulation

Physical Therapy Diagnosis: Perioperative anxiety

Signs and Symptoms: Depression, emotional lability, being frightened, insecurity, worry, agitation, inattentiveness, and concern regarding return to work

INTERVENTIONS	RATIONALE
Monitor level of anxiety	To provide a baseline and ongoing assessment
Define outcome criteria: reversal or mitigation of the signs and symptoms	To provide a basis for defining treatment goals
Provide comfort, reassurance, and empathy	To improve psychological well-being
Caring	To promote patient's sense of control
Listen and be attentive to patient	To promote self-responsibility
Be encouraging	
Involve patient in decision making	
Support patient and family members	
Discuss transition to home and work early	To facilitate rehabilitation planning when patient is discharged
Initiate discharge planning early (e.g., with other team members); prepare handouts of exercise regimens; communicate with home health care agency or public health or home care physical therapist	To promote continuity of care after discharge and follow-up care

Physical Therapy Diagnosis: Threats to oxygen transport and gas exchange from cardiopulmonary disease, smoking history, age-related changes in cardiopulmonary function, type of surgery, incision, position during surgery, surgery duration, chest tubes, blood and fluid loss, blood and fluid resuscitation, anesthesia, sedation, infection, medications, recumbency, restricted mobility

Signs and Symptoms: Hypoxemia, arterial desaturation, increased work of breathing, increased work of the heart, increased vital signs, decreased pulmonary function, restricted mobility, recumbency, circulatory stasis, and venous thrombosis

INTERVENTIONS	RATIONALE
Assess perioperative risks of compromised oxygen transport and gas exchange	To provide a baseline and ongoing assessment
Preoperative and ongoing postoperative cardiopulmonary physical therapy assessment	The preoperative assessment includes a review of risk factors threatening cardiopulmonary function and oxygen transport, lab tests and investigations, premorbid pulmonary function tests and cardiac function tests, and the clinical examination
Define outcome criteria: prevention, reversal, or mitigation of the signs and symptoms	To provide a basis for defining treatment goals and criteria for discontinuing treatment
Preoperative teaching includes the disease pathology and surgery (type, body position, anesthesia and sedation, incision, duration, and dressings), pain to be expected, and the rationale for the interventions and prevention	Basic background regarding the disease and surgery provides a basis for understanding treatment, which enhances cooperation with the treatment program when supervised and when not directly supervised
Preoperative teaching includes a description of when the patient will be seen by the physical therapist after surgery, the postoperative assessment, and treatment interventions (including breathing control and supported coughing coordinated with positioning, frequent position changes, and mobilization and relaxation procedures)	Preoperative teaching and patient preparation minimize cardiopulmonary complications, morbidity, and length of hospital stay
	A preoperative exercise program can significantly reduce perioperative complications, morbidity, and length of hospital stay

INTERVENTIONS	RATIONALE
Teach the patient bed mobility exercises, transfers, changing body positions, mobilizing, and walking while supporting the incision site	The patient is more cooperative and able to actively participate in treatment when exposed to the postoperative regimen before surgery
Teach the patient to coordinate these activities with breathing control and coughing maneuvers	
Mobilization, walking erect	To exploit the *preventive* effects of mobilization and exercise (i.e., to optimize alveolar volume and ventilation and minimize atelectasis, particularly of the dependent lung fields, to optimize mucociliary transport, to minimize secretion accumulation, to maximize functional residual capacity, to minimize airway closure, to minimize circulatory stasis, and to maximize circulating blood volume)
Intensity—within limits of pain, breathlessness, and fatigue	
Duration—5-20 minutes	
Frequency—several times daily	
Course and progression—as tolerated	
Breathing control and coughing maneuvers (relaxed deep inhalation, inspiratory hold, and exhalation to end tidal volume) and supported coughing	
Perform hourly	
Coordinate before, during, and after each position change	
Coordinate before, during, and after mobilization	
Chair exercises	
Upper extremities	
Chest wall	
Lower extremities (hip and knee and foot and ankle exercises hourly)	
Frequent body position changes when lying down (hourly)	Patients favor lying in restricted positions (e.g., the less painful side) for prolonged periods, thus are at risk of developing cardiopulmonary complications in the dependent lung fields
Avoid excessive time on left side	
Monitor for signs of thrombophlebitis and deep vein thrombosis	To minimize risk of thromboemboli (e.g., to lungs, kidneys and brain)
Monitor for signs of pulmonary emboli	
Monitor areas of redness and soreness over sacrum, hips, and heels; the patient's positions of comfort are away from the left side	To detect pressure areas early and avoid skin breakdown
Promote smoking cessation	Smoking is highly injurious to this patient during his recovery, as well as to his long-term health and well-being

Physical Therapy Diagnosis: Risk of the negative sequelae of recumbency

Signs and Symptoms: Within 6 hours reduced circulating blood volume, decreased blood pressure on sitting and standing compared with supine, light-headedness, dizziness, syncope, increased hematocrit and blood viscosity, increased work of the heart, altered fluid balance in the lung, impaired pulmonary lymphatic drainage, decreased lung volumes and capacities, decreased functional residual capacity, increased closing volume, increased airway resistance, decreased Pao_2 and Sao_2

INTERVENTIONS	RATIONALE
Monitor the negative sequelae of recumbency	To provide a baseline and ongoing assessment
Define outcome criteria: prevention, reversal, or mitigation of the signs and symptoms	To provide a basis for defining treatment goals and criteria for discontinuing treatment
Sitting upright position, preferably with feet dependent, standing and walking	The upright position is essential to shift fluid volume from central to peripheral circulation and maintain fluid volume regulating mechanisms and circulating blood volume
Coordinate physical activity and mobilization with breathing control and supported coughing maneuvers	The upright position maximizes lung volumes and capacities, especially functional residual capacity, and minimizes airway closure; these factors are adversely affected by anesthesia and surgery

Continued.

INTERVENTIONS	RATIONALE
	The upright position maximizes expiratory flow rates and cough effectiveness
	The upright position optimizes the length-tension relationship of the respiratory muscles and abdominal muscles, neural stimulation of the inspiratory muscles, and cough effectiveness
	The upright position coupled with mobilization and breathing control and supported coughing maneuvers maximizes alveolar ventilation, ventilation and perfusion matching, and pulmonary lymphatic drainage

Physical Therapy Diagnosis: Risk of negative sequelae of restricted mobility

Signs and Symptoms: Reduced activity and exercise tolerance, muscle atrophy and reduced muscle strength, decreased oxygen transport efficiency, increased heart rate, blood pressure, and minute ventilation at rest and submaximal work rates, reduced respiratory muscle strength, circulatory stasis, thromboemboli (e.g., pulmonary emboli) pressure areas, skin redness, skin breakdown and ulceration, and cognitive dysfunction

INTERVENTIONS	RATIONALE
Monitor the negative sequelae of restricted mobility	To provide a baseline and ongoing assessment
Define outcome criteria: prevention, reversal, or mitigation of the signs and symptoms	To provide a basis for defining treatment goals and criteria for discontinuing treatment
Mobilization and exercise prescription	To exploit the *preventive* effects of mobilization and exercise (e.g., optimize circulating blood volume and enhance the efficiency of all steps in the oxygen transport pathway)

Physical Therapy Diagnosis: Knowledge deficit

Signs and Symptoms: Lack of information about bronchiectasis, surgery, complications, and recovery

INTERVENTIONS	RATIONALE
Assess patient's specific knowledge deficits related to bronchiectasis, surgical lung resection, and cardiopulmonary physical therapy management	To address patient's specific knowledge deficits
Define outcome criteria: reversal or mitigation of the signs and symptoms	To provide a basis for defining treatment goals and criteria for discontinuing intervention
Promote a caring and supportive patient-therapist relationship	To focus on treating the patient with a lung resection rather than a lung resection
Consider every patient interaction an opportunity for education	To promote cooperative and active participation in treatment
Instruct regarding avoidance of respiratory tract infections, nutrition, hydration and fluid balance, exercise, stress management, and quality sleep	To promote patient's sense of responsibility for full recovery, wellness, and health promotion
Reinforce knowledge related to the roles of other health care team members	
Reinforce purposes of medication, their prescription parameters, and schedule	
Patient is given a personalized handout with a listing and description of exercises and their prescription parameters; precautions are emphasized	The patient can follow the handout instructions on his own between supervised treatments; he does not have to rely on memory, which will be impaired by the distractions of his postsurgical state and the hospital environment
	The content of the handout is reviewed with the patient

INTERVENTIONS	RATIONALE
Provide handout of mobilization and exercise schedule, body positioning guidelines, and breathing control and supported coughing maneuvers	On subsequent treatments, the physical therapist makes sure the patient can follow the handout and perform the exercises as prescribed
Teach, demonstrate, and provide feedback on interventions that can be self-administered	Between-treatment interventions are as important as treatments themselves to provide cumulative treatment effect
Teach patient balance of activity and rest	Optimal balance between activity and rest is essential to exploit short-term, long-term, and preventive effects of mobilization and exercise
Prepare patient for functioning at home and work after discharge	Review home and work settings (e.g., stairs, walking distances, lifting, driving, ADL, and work) so that patient is maximally prepared for discharge
Identify functional outcome goals with patient that should be achieved prior to discharge	
Provide written hand-outs that are specific to the patient regarding general and specific information and 'between-treatment' prescriptions	To promote smooth transition to home; promote continuity of care with physician, community health, and family; and follow-up
Plan for discharge early; prepare handouts including home exercise program, precautions	
Assess home and work physical environments to ensure patient can function optimally	

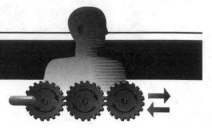

CHAPTER 14

Open Heart Surgery: Coronary Artery Bypass

PATHOPHYSIOLOGY

Coronary artery bypass surgery is performed to bypass stenosed or occluded coronary arteries. Coronary artery disease, the leading cause of death in the Western world, is hallmarked by stenosis or occlusion of the coronary arteries by atheromatous plaques that narrow the vessel lumen and impair coronary perfusion. Myocardial ischemia and infarction result when myocardial oxygen demand exceeds supply. Angina, chest pain triggered by coronary ischemia, is frequently associated with coronary insufficiency and infarction. Angina is commonly induced during exercise in which there is increased demand on the heart. Risk factors for coronary artery disease include elevated cholesterol and triglyceride levels, being male, being older, hypertension, obesity, sedentary lifestyle, stress, and having a family history of heart disease. The condition may be medically managed with coronary vasodilators, exercise, and diet. If the stenosis is severe, surgery is indicated. Surgery has not been shown to increase life expectancy, but it is associated with improved quality of life and reduced morbidity.

Case Study

The patient is a 55-year-old man. He is a pilot for a major commercial international airline. He lives with his wife and two of his four children. He is 5 feet 9 inches (176 cm) tall and weighs 132 pounds (60 kg); his body mass index is 19.4. He has never smoked. He had been experiencing chest tightness over the past 2 months since he started lifting weights. He went for a routine annual examination and underwent a cardiac stress test, at which time myocardial ischemia was apparent on electrocardiogram (ECG) at moderate exercise intensities. Although he had not experienced classic angina and had been relatively asymptomatic up to this time, he had extensive occlusion of his coronary arteries. He was scheduled for surgery, specifically, triple coronary artery bypass grafts. A median sternotomy was performed and the anterior chest wall retracted. Graft material was excised from his left saphenous vein. Intraoperative complications extended the length of time in surgery and on the cardiopulmonary bypass machine to 6 hours. He left the operating room with three chest tubes in place: intrapleural, mediastinal, and pericardial. On a fractional inspired oxygen concentration (Fio_2) of 100%, his arterial blood gases (ABGs) were oxygen pressure (Po_2) 200 mm Hg, carbon dioxide pressure (Pco_2) 38 mm Hg, bicarbonate (HCO_3) 28 mEq/L, pH 7.30, and arterial oxygen saturation (Sao_2) 99%. His hemoglobin was low normal. Chest x-ray showed basal atelectasis, especially on the left side. By the morning of the second day, he was hemodynamically stable. He has just been extubated.

Oxygen Transport Deficits: Observed and Potential

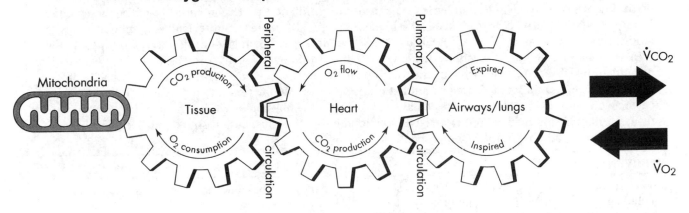

↓ Kidney perfusion
↓ Urinary output
↑ Oxygen demand

Trauma from surgical
   procedure
Blood and fluid around
   surgical site
Pericardial effusion
Dysrhythmias
↑ Work of the heart

↓ Mucociliary transport
↓ Ciliary motion due to
   supplemental oxygen
↑ Mucus accumulation
↑ Airway resistance
↓ Chest wall excursion
Restricted chest wall motion
   (L>R)
Chest wall asymmetry
Monotonous tidal
   ventilation
Breathing at low lung
   volumes
Weak cough
Left lower lobe atelectasis
↓ Lung compliance
Postural deviation
   (i.e., lists to left)
↑ Work of breathing

↑ Risk of atherosclerosis
   of large arteries (i.e.,
   abdominal aorta,
   femoral arteries, and
   popliteal arteries)
Hypotension

Hypoxic vasoconstriction
Shunt
↑ Demand on lymph
   drainage system
↓ Lymphatic drainage

Blood: ↓ Blood volume
   ↓ Hemoglobin
   Electrolyte disturbance
   Damage to red blood cells
      due to prolonged period
      on coronary artery bypass
      machine

↑ Increase
↓ Decrease

PHYSICAL THERAPY DIAGNOSES TREATMENT AND PRESCRIPTION

Physical Therapy Diagnosis: Altered cardiopulmonary function: hypoxemia, alveolar hypoventilation, and shunt resulting from type of surgery, duration, position during surgery, anesthesia, sedation, compression of heart and adjacent lung parenchyma during surgery, medications, blood loss, fluid replacement, intubation and mechanical ventilation, prolonged duration on cardiopulmonary bypass machine and trauma to blood cells, blood transfusions, extubation, recumbency, and restricted mobility

Signs and Symptoms: Arterial oxygen pressure (Pao_2) $< 104.2 - 0.27$ age (±7) mm Hg, $Pao_2 < 75$ mm Hg on room air, $Sao_2 < 98\%$, hypermetabolic, fever, increased work of breathing, increased minute ventilation, breathing at low lung volumes, increased regions of low ventilation perfusion ratios in lungs, increased shunt fraction, radiographic evidence of basal atelectasis (L>R), increased afterload (i.e., increased systemic vascular resistance), increased work of the heart, decreased urinary output, decreased arousal, decreased lung volumes and capacities, decreased functional residual capacity, increased closing volume of dependent airways, effects of prolonged cardiopulmonary bypass (i.e., decreased diffusing capacity, increased A-a oxygen difference, venous admixture, right-to-left shunt, ventilation perfusion mismatch, noncardiogenic pulmonary edema), pericardial effusion, hypovolemia, impaired cough caused by irritation from intubation and medication, restricted mobility and position turns, fluid shifts and third spacing into thoracic cavity, and orthostatic intolerance

INTERVENTIONS	RATIONALE
Monitor serial ABGs, hemoglobin, hemodynamic status including central venous pressure, pulmonary artery pressures and wedge pressure, fluid and electrolyte balance, red blood cell count, white blood cell count, ECG, chest x-rays, pulmonary function, vital signs, Sao_2 Perform serial cardiopulmonary assessments	To provide a baseline, ongoing assessment and measure of treatment response Ongoing monitoring of cardiopulmonary and hemodynamic status is essential during physical therapy treatments, including heart rate, blood pressure, rate pressure product, ECG, Sao_2; and breathlessness, chest pain, and fatigue
Define outcome criteria: reversal or mitigation of the signs and symptoms Coordinate interventions with pain control strategies	To provide a basis for defining treatment goals and criteria for discontinuing treatment To encourage patient to perform pain control strategies and request medication if necessary to provide comfort, reduce suffering and facilitate movement, and frequent position changes
Reinforce supplemental oxygen and appropriate fit of face mask or nasal prongs	To ensure that the oxygen mask or nasal prongs are positioned such that oxygen delivery to the patient is maximized and not wasted
Phase I (initial) Medications—analgesia at peak potency, supplemental oxygen Mobilization coordinated with breathing control (maximal inspiration—3-5 second inspiratory hold, passive expiration to resting end-tidal volume) and supported coughing maneuvers Maximal inspiration on extension movements and passive expiration to resting end-tidal volume on flexion movements Range-of-motion exercises Dangling, self-supported, erect, feet on floor Transfers; active assist to active transfers Chair exercises; sitting erect, upper extremity trunk and right leg exercises; modified movement and positioning of the left leg Functional activities, bathroom, washing, shaving, hair care, changing bed wear Intensity—heart rate increase <20 beats per minute; paced to minimize pain and cardiopulmonary stress $Sao_2>90\%$	To exploit the *acute* effects of mobilization on cardiopulmonary function and oxygen transport (i.e., increase arousal, optimize alveolar volume, functional residual capacity, the distributions of ventilation, perfusion, and ventilation and perfusion matching; increased surfactant production and distribution; gas exchange; three-dimensional chest wall movement, efficient and coordinated thoracoabdominal movement, mucociliary transport, decrease secretion accumulation, lung movement, and lymphatic drainage, and reduce the work of breathing and the work of the heart) To promote alveolar ventilation and gas exchange by optimizing lung compliance and decreasing airway resistance To promote surfactant production and distribution To minimize the risk of deep vein thrombosis To increase exercise stress and the volume of work the patient can perform; lower-intensity, shorter-duration exercise sessions are performed more frequently than higher-intensity, longer-duration exercise sessions

INTERVENTIONS	RATIONALE

Duration—5-20 minutes
Frequency—3-5 times daily
Course and progression—as indicated

Phase II
   Mobilization prescription coordinated with breathing control and supported coughing maneuvers
   Mobilization coordinated with the upright position and breathing control and supported coughing maneuvers
   Bed mobility and bed exercises
   Intensity—heart rate increase <20 beats per minute; to 60%-75% age-predicted heart rate
   Duration—15-60 minutes
   Frequency—3 to 1 time a day
   Course and progression—as indicated

Promote optimal body position and alignment during mobilization and exercise

Correction of postural alignment:
   At rest
   In the chair
   Standing

             Optimal alignment is essential to maximize chest wall excursion and minimize cardiopulmonary compromise

To optimize breathing pattern, chest wall excursion, and distribution of ventilation; minimize compression atelectasis and suboptimal alveolar filling, gas mixing, and gas exchange

To relieve musculoskeletal rigidity and long-term cardiopulmonary sequelae of impaired postural alignment

To enhance breathing and movement efficiency and movement economy metabolically

Optimal treatment response depends on optimal balance with rest and sleep

Intersperse rest periods within treatments; encourage movement and body repositioning to be done in a slow, controlled fashion coordinated with breathing control

Promote quality rest periods and sleep between treatments

Body positioning (coordinated with breathing control and supported coughing maneuvers before, during, and after treatment)

Place in high Fowler's position

Reverse-Trendelenburg position (head up with feet down)

Body positioning in the horizontal plane and varying angles of head of bed up

Maintain head of bed at 15-30 degrees or higher when supine

Side lying on either side; modify left side lying

¾ prone to each side; modified to left side

Supine

Encourage patient not to favor any single position, and stress importance of position changes to simulate the changes that would occur when mobile

To optimize alveolar volume and distribution of ventilation, lung volumes and capacities, functional residual capacity, increase arousal and minimize airway closure of the dependent airways, thoracic blood volume and reduced lung compliance, and displacement of the diaphragm cephalad by the viscera

To stimulate deep breaths, increase lung movement, mucociliary transport, and lymphatic drainage

To promote effective coughing

To minimize intraabdominal pressure and encroachment on the thoracic cavity

To maintain fluid volume regulation, which can only be maintained with the upright position; dependency of the feet is permitted provided swelling is not significant

To promote chest tube drainage; mediastinal, pleural, and pericardial tubes

To minimize the risk of pulmonary aspiration

To promote urinary drainage

To stimulate bowel activity

Supine is a particularly deleterious position; supine is included in the turning schedule, but duration should not exceed 1-2 hours; supine compromises expansion of the dependent lung fields and reduces lung compliance because of increased thoracic blood volume and encroachment of the abdominal viscera

Continued.

INTERVENTIONS	RATIONALE
Frequency—when in bed, frequent body position changes at least every 1-2 hr; promote frequent body position changes by patient coordinated with breathing control and supported coughing maneuvers	When patient is not erect, optimize turning frequency to augment cardiopulmonary function, ventilation, muco-ciliary transport, lung movement, and lymphatic drainage
Course—as indicated by monitoring patient closely	To place the patient in as many positions as possible; extreme positions (e.g., prone) are modified within the patient's limits of cardiopulmonary and hemodynamic responses and comfort
Increase duration in positions with favorable outcomes	
Decrease duration and minimize duration in positions with unfavorable outcomes	To change the patient's body position frequently with optimal assist from the patient (at least every 1-2 hr)
Avoid excessive duration in *any* single position	Even those positions with initially favorable outcomes will have an adverse effect after 1 to 2 hr as the dependent lung fields become compromised
Range-of-motion exercises (active and active assist) coordinated with breathing control and supported coughing maneuvers:	To exploit the cardiopulmonary effects of range-of-motion exercises primarily; secondarily their effects on joint range, muscle length, and stiffness
Upper extremities	To maintain optimal chest wall and upper extremity mobility immediately after surgery
Trunk	
Lower extremities especially hip and knee and foot and ankle exercises	
Continue hip and knee and foot and ankle exercises (hourly)	To maximize the effect of physical measures to control thrombi formation

Physical Therapy Diagnosis: Ineffective breathing pattern resulting from cardiovascular thoracic surgical procedure and median sternotomy, chest tubes, pain, recumbency, and restricted mobility

Signs and Symptoms: Reduced chest wall excursion, chest wall asymmetry, increased minute ventilation, atelectasis, absent sigh mechanism, suppressed cough, decreased lung compliance, increase airway resistance, monotonous tidal ventilation, and reluctance to change body position

INTERVENTIONS	RATIONALE
Monitor breathing pattern (tidal volume, respiratory rate, regularity, and work of breathing and of the heart)	To provide a baseline, ongoing assessment and measure of treatment response
Define outcome criteria: reversal or mitigation of the signs and symptoms	To provide a basis for defining treatment goals and criteria for discontinuing treatment
Mobilization, body positioning, and range-of-motion exercises coordinated with breathing control and supported coughing maneuvers	Normal breathing pattern will be restored with pain reduction, relaxation procedures coordinated with breathing control, and with the normal physiological stresses imposed by gravity and movement in the upright position
Pain control	To ensure that patient is adequately premedicated before treatment and maximally able to cooperate with treatment
Coordinate treatments with medication as required:	
Ensure that analgesics are at peak effectiveness during treatment	To ensure that patient's pain medication does not impair patient's arousal and ability to cooperate fully with treatment; provide input at rounds regarding the need for maximal patient arousal during treatment
Breathing control maneuvers	
Relaxation procedures	
Correct postural alignment:	To optimize breathing pattern, chest wall excursion, and distribution of ventilation; minimize compression atelectasis and suboptimal alveolar filling, gas mixing, and gas exchange
At rest	
In a chair	
Standing	
Walking	To relieve musculoskeletal rigidity and long-term cardiopulmonary sequelae of impaired postural alignment
Erect upright, and relaxed body posture	
Relaxed head and neck, upper extremities, chest wall, and abdominal muscles	To enhance breathing and movement efficiency and movement economy metabolically

Physical Therapy Diagnosis: Pain caused by incision, internal trauma, chest tube sites, posterior spinal pain from anterior chest wall retraction, persistent discomfort from artificial airway

Signs and Symptoms: Complaints of discomfort and pain, grimacing, guarding, splinting, holding body, rigid, moaning, reluctance to move and change body position, distracted, reduced ability to cooperate with treatment, fatigue and lethargy, disturbed rest and sleep, loss of sleep, and loss of appetite

INTERVENTIONS	RATIONALE
Monitor the quality, quantity, and location of patient's pain	To provide a baseline, ongoing assessment and measure of treatment response
Determine factors that increase and decrease pain and discomfort	
Define outcome criteria: reversal or mitigation of the signs and symptoms	To provide a basis for defining treatment goals and criteria for discontinuing treatment
Listen and attend to patient's complaints of discomfort	To minimize pain, suffering, and distress
Ensure that patient is appropriately medicated for treatments (preferably alternative agents to narcotics when possible) and medications are at peak efficacy	To promote pain self-management
Ice chips and mouth swabs to hydrate oral cavity and throat after extubation	
Teach relaxation procedures (e.g., breathing control, Jacobsen's relaxation procedure, Benson's relaxation method, autogenic training, biofeedback, visual imagery)	To minimize pain and discomfort by encouraging gentle movement and frequent body position changes, supported coughing, log rolling, and providing assistance when necessary
Coordinated treatments with breathing control and supported coughing maneuvers	To ensure that patient's pain medication does not impair patient's arousal and ability to cooperate fully with treatment; provide input at rounds regarding the need for maximal patient arousal during treatment (i.e., minimize narcotic analgesia when possible to enhance respiratory drive and arousal)
Pace each treatment and a series of treatments to permit optimal preparation and recovery from pain during uncomfortable maneuvers	To maximize tolerance of mobility exercises and body position changes with rest periods (i.e., these interventions are performed in stages and with optimal assistance such that the patient has the physiological benefits of actively, physically participating within his limits of pain and discomfort)
Intersperse rest periods within and between treatments	
Respond to patient's complaints of pain and make the patient as comfortable as possible at all times	Although weaning off pain medication is encouraged, the patient is encouraged to request analgesia before pain is excessive and unduly interferes with breathing, mobility, positioning, and ability to rest effectively
Promote good body alignment when sitting and standing, as well as when lying in bed	To ensure that alignment is optimal immediately after surgery to avoid long-term chest wall and postural deformity and associated residual discomfort and pain
Frequent body position changes	
Range-of-motion exercises: Upper extremities Trunk (forward flexion, extension, side flexion, rotation, and diagonal rotation) Lower extremities	Range-of-motion exercises maintain optimal joint range and muscle and connective tissue lengths of the chest wall; prevention of shortening and contracture minimizes long-term pain, discomfort, and stiffness

Physical Therapy Diagnosis: Decreased tolerance for physical activity and exercise resulting from surgery, surgical complications, pain, lack of sleep, and postsurgical fatigue

Signs and Symptoms: Physical activity restricted by complaints of pain, discomfort, apprehension about moving, fatigue, weakness, and loss of endurance

INTERVENTIONS	RATIONALE
Monitor tolerance for physical activity and exercise	To provide a baseline, ongoing assessment and measure of treatment response

Continued.

INTERVENTIONS	RATIONALE
Determine premorbid activity and aerobic conditioning level	To assist in prescribing exercise prescription
Determine optimal tolerance required by patient for his needs and optimal health	
Define outcome criteria: reversal or mitigation of the signs and symptoms	To provide a basis for defining treatment goals and criteria for discontinuing treatment
Mobilization and exercise prescription:	
Type—walking	To exploit the *long-term* effects of mobilization and exercise on cardiopulmonary function and oxygen transport (e.g., adaptation of lung parenchyma, pulmonary circulation, lymphatics; reduced minute ventilation and reduced perceived exertion and fatigue, rate pressure product, cardiac output at submaximal work rates, increased peripheral collateral circulation, and increased extraction and uptake of oxygen at the tissue level)
Intensity—low to moderate, pace within tolerance of strength, endurance, and pain, and cardiopulmonary and hemodynamic parameters; heart rate increase < 20-30 beats per minute; blood pressure increase < 30 mm Hg	
Duration—intersperse with sitting and standing rest periods; 5-30 minutes	To increase exercise stress and the volume of work the patient can perform; lower-intensity, shorter-duration exercise sessions are performed more frequently then higher-intensity, longer-duration exercise sessions
Monitor signs and symptoms of orthostatic intolerance with standing rests	
Frequency—throughout the day, activities of daily living (ADL) and bathroom, hallway walks—2-3 to several times daily	Initially the patient may be susceptible to postural hypotension; therefore a chair must be available initially when walking in case the patient becomes light-headed or fatigued
Course and progression—increase duration, speed; reduce rest periods; increase frequency	Monitor for signs and symptoms of postural hypotension; record heart rate and blood pressure before and after lying supine and assuming an upright seated or standing position
Prescriptive rest periods within treatments	The patient is in a hypermetabolic state caused by recovery from extensive surgery, anesthesia, sedation and narcotics, blood loss, anemia, healing and repair, and inadequate nutrition and fluid intake; mobilization/exercise stimuli are prescribed so that oxygen demand does not exceed the capacity for oxygen delivery
Prescriptive rest periods between treatments	Quality rest and sleep periods between treatments are essential to promote healing and repair, restore energy, and reduce fatigue, thereby enhancing functional activity and work output

Physical Therapy Diagnosis: Anxiety, reduced emotional and psychological well-being, and postsurgical depression

Signs and Symptoms: Emotional lability, being frightened, insecurity, frustration, fear, anger, increased arousal, restlessness, and tension

INTERVENTIONS	RATIONALE
To monitor anxiety	To provide a baseline and ongoing assessment
Comfort, reassurance, empathy	To improve psychological well-being
Caring	
Listen and be attentive to patient	
Be encouraging	
Make patient physically comfortable	
Involve patient in decision making	To promote patient's sense of control
	To promote self-responsibility
Support patient and family members	To help patient deal with coronary artery disease, surgery, and postsurgical lifestyle modifications

INTERVENTIONS	RATIONALE
Discuss transition to home, work, and performance of ADL	To facilitate rehabilitation planning when patient is discharged
Initiate discharge planning early (e.g., with other team members); prepare handouts of exercise regimens; communicate with home health care and physical therapist	To promote continuity of care and follow-up care, and referral to a physical therapist in the community or in a cardiac rehabilitation program

Physical Therapy Diagnosis: Threats to oxygen transport and gas exchange resulting from postsurgical status, type and duration of surgery, position during surgery, anesthesia and sedation, decreased arousal, fluid shifts and third spacing, infection, intubation, mechanical ventilation, extubation, recumbency, and restricted mobility

Signs and Symptoms: Hypoxemia, arterial desaturation, radiographic evidence of atelectasis, increased work of breathing, increased work of the heart, lethargy, fatigue, increased temperature, increased white blood cell count, age-related airway closure in sitting, age-related closure of dependent airways in recumbent positions, age-related inhomogeneity of ventilation, internal bleeding, cardiogenic pulmonary edema, blood transfusions (whole blood and blood products), circulatory stasis, venous thrombosis, fibrin and platelet microemboli, decreased clotting times caused by anticoagulant therapy, pulmonary embolism, age-related decrease of mucociliary clearance rate, age-related depression of cough, restricted mobility, recumbency, increased oxygen demands, and side effects of medications

INTERVENTIONS	RATIONALE
To monitor threats to oxygen transport and gas exchange	To provide a baseline and ongoing assessment
Define outcome criteria: prevention, reversal, or mitigation of the signs and symptoms	To provide a basis for defining treatment goals and criteria for discontinuing treatment
Preoperative and ongoing postoperative cardiopulmonary physical therapy assessments	The preoperative assessment includes a review of risk factors threatening cardiopulmonary and oxygen transport, lab tests and investigations, and the clinical examination
Preoperative teaching includes the disease pathology and surgery (type, body position, anesthesia and sedation, incision, duration, and dressings) and pain to be expected	Basic background regarding the disease and surgery provides a basis for understanding treatment, which enhances cooperation with treatment program when supervised and when not directly supervised
Preoperative teaching includes a description of when the patient will be seen by the physical therapist after surgery, the postoperative assessment and treatment interventions (including breathing control and supported coughing coordinated with positioning), frequent position changes and mobilization, and relaxation procedures	The patient is more cooperative and able to actively participate in treatment when exposed to the instructions before surgery
Teach preoperatively bed mobility exercises, transfers, changing body positions, mobilizing, and walking while supporting the incision site	
Teach the patient to coordinate the above activities with breathing control and coughing maneuvers	
Mobilization, walking; erect relaxed posture	To exploit the *preventive* effects of mobilization and exercise (i.e., to optimize alveolar volume and ventilation and minimize atelectasis, particularly of the dependent lung fields), to optimize mucociliary transport, to minimize secretion accumulation, to maximize functional residual capacity, to minimize airway closure, to minimize circulatory stasis, and to maximize circulatory blood volume
Intensity—within limits of hemodynamic stability, pain, endurance, and fatigue	
Frequency—as often as tolerated	
Course and progression—as tolerated	
Chair exercises (upright sitting position)	Avoid weight bearing on arms during dangling and transfers
Upper extremities	
Chest wall (without incision strain)	Avoid static postural stabilization, breath holding, Valsalva maneuver, and straining
Lower extremities (hip and knee and foot and ankle exercises hourly)	

Continued.

INTERVENTIONS	RATIONALE
Breathing control (relaxed deep inhalation, inspiratory hold, and exhalation to end-tidal volume) and supported coughing maneuvers Perform hourly Coordinate with position changes Coordinate with mobilization	To maximize alveolar ventilation, maximize functional residual capacity, maximize mucociliary transport, and reduce airway closure
Varied and extreme body positions when lying down Frequent body position changes (1-2 hr) Avoid excessive time in right side lying	Patients favor lying in restricted positions (e.g., the less painful side) for prolonged periods, thus are at risk of developing cardiopulmonary complications in the dependent lung fields
Optimize oxygen transport with cardiopulmonary physical therapy to reduce and then discontinue the need for supplemental oxygen	Oxygen increases the rate of airway collapse (denitrogen atelectasis), adversely affects surfactant composition, and contributes to ciliary dyskinesia
Monitor for signs of hemodynamic compromise Monitor for cardiogenic pulmonary edema Monitor for signs of deep vein thrombosis Monitor for signs of pulmonary emboli	To detect signs of impending cardiopulmonary dysfunction early and intervene accordingly

Physical Therapy Diagnosis: Risk of the negative sequelae of recumbency

Signs and Symptoms: Within 6 hours reduced circulating blood volume, decreased blood pressure on sitting and standing compared with supine, light-headedness, dizziness, syncope, increased hematocrit and blood viscosity, increased work of the heart, altered fluid balance in the lung, impaired pulmonary lymphatic drainage, decreased lung volumes and capacities, decreased functional residual capacity, increased closing volume, and decreased Pao_2 and Sao_2

INTERVENTIONS	RATIONALE
Monitor risks of the negative sequelae of recumbency Monitor responses to body position changes (e.g., supine to standing)	To provide a baseline and ongoing assessment
Define outcome criteria: prevention, reversal, or mitigation of the signs and symptoms	To provide a basis for defining treatment goals and criteria for discontinuing treatment
Frequent sitting upright position, standing and walking (every few hours)	The upright position is essential to shift fluid volume from central to peripheral circulation and maintain fluid volume regulating mechanisms and circulating blood volume
	The upright position maximizes lung volumes and capacities and functional residual capacity
	The upright position maximizes expiratory flow rates and cough effectiveness
	The upright position optimizes the length-tension relationship of the respiratory muscles and abdominal muscles, neural stimulation of the respiratory muscles, and cough effectiveness
	The upright position coupled with mobilization and breathing control and coughing maneuvers maximizes alveolar ventilation, ventilation and perfusion matching, and pulmonary lymphatic drainage

Physical Therapy Diagnosis: Risk of negative sequelae of restricted mobility	
Signs and Symptoms: Reduced activity and exercise tolerance, muscle atrophy and reduced muscle strength and tolerance, decreased oxygen transport efficiency at all steps in the pathway, increased heart rate, blood pressure, and minute ventilation at rest and submaximal work rates, reduced respiratory muscle strength and endurance, circulatory stasis, venous thrombosis, thromboemboli (e.g., pulmonary emboli), paralytic ileus, urinary stasis, pressure areas, skin redness, skin breakdown and ulceration, and cognitive dysfunction	

INTERVENTIONS	RATIONALE
Monitor the negative sequelae of restricted mobility	To provide a baseline and ongoing assessment
Define outcome criteria: prevention, reversal, or mitigation of the signs and symptoms	To provide a basis for defining treatment goals and criteria for discontinuing treatment
Mobilization and exercise prescription	Mobilization and exercise optimize circulating blood volume and enhance the efficiency of all steps in the oxygen transport pathway

Physical Therapy Diagnosis: Knowledge deficit	
Signs and Symptoms: Lack of information about coronary artery disease, risk factors, surgery, complications, and recovery	

INTERVENTIONS	RATIONALE
Assess patient's specific knowledge deficits related to coronary artery disease and cardiopulmonary physical therapy management	To address patient's specific knowledge deficits
Promote a caring and supportive patient-therapist relationship	To focus on treating the patient with coronary artery disease rather than coronary artery disease
Consider every patient interaction an opportunity for patient education	To promote patient's sense of responsibility for full recovery, health, and health promotion
Instruct the patient regarding avoidance of respiratory tract infections, nutrition, hydration and fluid balance, exercise, stress management, and quality sleep	To promote cooperation and active participation in treatment
Reinforce purposes of medication, their prescription parameters, and schedule	
Reinforce knowledge related to the roles of other health care team members	
Provide a personalized handout with a listing and description of exercises and their prescription parameters; precautions are emphasized	The patient can follow the handout instructions on his own between supervised treatments; he does not have to rely on memory, which will be impaired by the distractions of his postsurgical state and the hospital environment
Provide a handout of mobilization and exercise schedule, body positioning guidelines, and breathing control and supported coughing maneuvers	The content of the handout is reviewed with the patient
	On subsequent treatments, the physical therapist makes sure the patient can follow the handout and perform the exercises as prescribed
Teach, demonstrate, and provide feedback on interventions that can be self-administered	Between-treatment interventions are as important as treatment themselves to provide cumulative treatment effect
Teach patient regarding balance of activity and rest	Optimal balance between activity and rest is essential to exploit short-term, long-term, and preventive effects of mobilization and exercise
Prepare patient for functioning at home and work after discharge	To review home and work settings, such as stairs, walking distances, lifting, driving, ADL, and work, so patient is maximally prepared for discharge
Identify functional outcome goals with patient that should be achieved before discharge	

Continued.

INTERVENTIONS	RATIONALE
Provide written handouts that are specific to the patient regarding general and specific information and between-treatment prescriptions	To promote smooth transition to home, promote continuity of care with physical, a physical therapist in the community or cardiac rehabilitation program, and follow-up
Plan for discharge early; prepare handouts, including home exercise program, precautions	
Assess home and work physical environments to ensure that patient can function optimally	
Reinforce information on lifestyle modification, such as balanced healthy diet (low fat, low red meat, high complex carbohydrates), regular aerobic exercise, adequate sleep, stress management, assertiveness and coping training, and quality night's sleep	

PART IV

Special Case Studies

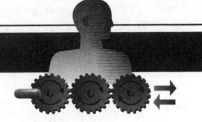

CHAPTER 15

Interstitial Pulmonary Fibrosis with Peripheral Vascular Disease

PATHOPHYSIOLOGY

Interstitial pulmonary fibrosis is an advanced stage of interstitial lung disease resulting from excessive deposition of connective tissue in the lung. It can be divided into granulomatous (secondary to pneumonia or sarcoidosis) and nongranulomatous (secondary to asbestosis, silicosis, and fibrosis alveolitis) types. Interstitial pulmonary fibrosis is associated with autoimmune and collagen diseases (e.g., rheumatoid arthritis, systemic lupus erythematosus), liver disorders, smoking, and genetic predisposition. The condition characterized by diffuse or localized inflammation leads to fibrosis of the alveolar walls and adjacent lung tissue. The thickened alveolar interstitium significantly reduces diffusing capacity, which results in mismatch in ventilation and perfusion, arterial hypoxemia, tachypnea at rest, cyanosis, and dyspnea on exertion. Right-sided heart failure occurs in the late stages of the disease. On auscultation, dry or coarse crackles on inspiration may be heard at the bases of the lungs.

Peripheral vascular insufficiency of the legs commonly results from atherosclerosis of the abdominal aorta, femoral arteries, and popliteal arteries. Other conditions associated with peripheral vascular complications include diabetes, thromboangiitis obliterans, vasospastic conditions such as Raynaud's phenomenon, and thromboemboli. Diabetes leads to microangiopathy and autonomic neuropathy, which affects vasomotor control, hence peripheral blood flow. In addition, compared with nondiabetic patients, the rate of atherosclerosis development is accelerated by a decade in patients with diabetes. The effects of these conditions are exacerbated with smoking because nicotine is a potent vasoconstrictor. Peripheral vascular insufficiency secondary to atherosclerosis and diabetes occurs most frequently in the lower extremities. Blood flow is chronically compromised, leading to poor limb nutrition, abnormal coloring, abnormal peripheral pulses and segmental blood pressures down the limb, reduced hair growth, thinning of the skin, scaliness and translucency, disappearance of skin ridges, heaping of nail growth, skin lesions, and ulcerations. Amputation of the limb is indicated in severe cases in which the skin lesions fail to heal, leading to infection, necrosis, and gangrene. Ischemic pain of the calf muscles (i.e., intermittent claudication), often exacerbated by exercise, which increases the metabolic demand of the muscles, is a common clinical symptom of peripheral vascular disease. In cases in which vessel stenosis develops slowly, collateral circulation may compensate for the compromised circulation. Although they may not have been symptomatic, patients with peripheral vascular insufficiency secondary to atherosclerosis have an increased incidence of coronary artery disease.

Case Study

The patient is a 55-year-old man. He is a grain farmer. He lives on the family farm with his wife and five children. His body mass index is 25. Since he was 36 years of age, he has developed increasing shortness of breath. His pulmonary function has been deteriorating steadily. He was diagnosed with interstitial pulmonary fibrosis related to having lived on a grain farm all his life. Three months ago, his forced expiratory volume in one second (FEV_1) was 2.8 L (60% of predicted), forced vital capacity (FVC) was 3.0 L (64% of predicted), and the FEV_1/FVC ratio was 93%. The diffusing capacity was 47% of predicted. In the middle of the harvest season he developed increasingly severe chest tightness and shortness of breath. He was admitted to hospital in acute distress. His arterial blood gases (ABGs) on room air were arterial oxygen pressure (Pao_2) 78 mm Hg, arterial carbon dioxide pressure ($Paco_2$) 37 mm Hg, and pH 7.39. His arterial oxygen saturation (Sao_2) decreased to 88% on exertion. He was put on a course of corticosteroids and immunosuppressive therapy. Oxygen and a pulmonary vasodilator were also administered. His medical history includes a prolonged history of respiratory allergies and moderately severe intermittent claudication in the right calf.

Oxygen Transport Deficits: Observed and Potential

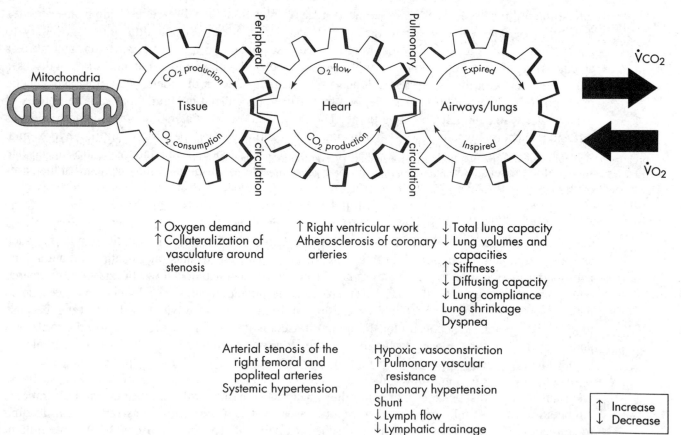

PHYSICAL THERAPY DIAGNOSES AND TREATMENT PRESCRIPTION

Physical Therapy Diagnosis: Altered cardiopulmonary function: alveolar hypoventilation and shunt

Signs and Symptoms: ABGs and pulmonary function tests consistent with hypoxemia and moderately severe interstitial lung disease, low lung volumes, ventilation-perfusion mismatch, decreased diffusing capacity, increased A − a oxygen gradient, decreased lung compliance, $Sao_2 < 90\%$ on exertion, increased pulmonary vascular resistance, pulmonary hypertension, increased work of the right side of the heart, increased work of breathing, increased respiratory rate, reduced tidal volume, increased resting heart rate; increased submaximal minute ventilation, heart rate, blood pressure, rate pressure product, breathlessness, and perceived exertion during exercise; age-related changes in the elastic recoil of the lung and age-related decrease in mucus clearance rate

INTERVENTIONS	RATIONALE
Monitor serial ABGs, pulmonary function tests, blood work, chest x-rays, and hemodynamic status	To provide a baseline, ongoing assessment and measure of treatment response
Monitor fluid and electrolyte balance	
Monitor subjective complaints of dyspnea	
Define outcome criteria: reversal or mitigation of the signs and symptoms	To provide a basis for defining treatment goals and criteria for discontinuing treatment
Supplemental oxygen	Supplemental oxygen is indicated to correct hypoxemia and reduce the work of breathing; ensure that oxygen delivery system (e.g., face mask and later nasal prongs) are fitted properly at all times
Teach breathing control and coughing maneuvers (maximal inhalation, 3-5 second hold, passive expiration to resting end-tidal volume)	To increase alveolar ventilation and breathing efficiency
Coordinate breathing control and coughing maneuvers with movement in upright sitting, standing and walking, and lying down resting	To exploit the *acute* effects of mobilization and exercise (i.e., maximize alveolar volume,, alveolar ventilation, lung volumes and capacities, functional residual capacity, ventilation and perfusion matching, mucociliary transport, lung motion, lymph flow, lymphatic drainage and reduce airway closure)
	To improve breathing efficiency during physical activity
	To reduce respiratory distress and the work of breathing and its energy cost
Teach body positions associated with the least work of breathing; upright (i.e., sitting and leaning forward, lean forward standing); head of bed up when recumbent	To reduce the work of the heart with body positioning to reduce dyspnea, reduce thoracic blood volume and displacement of the diaphragm by the abdominal viscera, and coordinate with rhythmic, self-paced breathing control maneuvers
Teach pacing of activities of daily living (ADL), physical activity, and exercise	
Exercise in upright body positions (e.g., walking, cycling ergometry)	
Teach chest wall stretching exercises	To optimize three-dimensional chest wall motion, including bucket handle and pump handle motion
Teach chest wall mobility exercises:	To minimize chest wall rigidity and deformity
Head and neck	
Upper extremity; flexion, extension, and rotation	
Thoracic forward flexion, back extension, side flexion, lateral rotation, and diagonal rotation	
Hip mobility and shifting of abdominal viscera	

Continued.

Physical Therapy Diagnosis: Inefficient breathing pattern due to restrictive lung pathology

Signs and Symptoms: Altered breathing pattern, ie, rapid shallow breathing, abnormal thoracoabdominal motion, rigid chest wall, restricted chest wall motion, low lung volumes, impaired distribution of ventilation, impaired ventilation perfusion matching, and impaired intrapulmonary gas mixing

INTERVENTIONS	RATIONALE
Monitor breathing pattern	To provide a baseline, ongoing assessment and measure of treatment response
Define outcome criteria: reversal or mitigation of the signs and symptoms	To provide a basis for defining treatment goals and criteria for discontinuing treatment
Teach breathing control and coughing maneuvers	To enhance efficiency of patient's breathing pattern at rest and during exercise and minimize the effects of relatively increased dead space ventilation
Teach relaxed breathing postures and positions	
Coordinate breathing control and coughing maneuvers with physical activity and exercise	To promote a more normal breathing pattern and optimize breathing efficiency
Identify which physical activities and exercise promote a more efficient breathing pattern (e.g., walking, cycle ergometer, swimming)	To minimize airflow obstruction
	To minimize the progression of restrictive pulmonary limitation
	To maximize ventilation and perfusion matching
Teach relaxation procedures: relaxed breathing, Jacobsen's relaxation procedure, Bensen's relaxation method, autogenic training, visual imagery, biofeedback	To reduce the undue energy cost of breathing and physical activity
Teach patient to coordinate breathing with exercise: in strengthening exercises, inspiration on extension movements, expiration on flexion movements; in aerobic exercise, establish breathing depth and rate that can be sustained comfortably for 10 to 40 minutes	

Physical Therapy Diagnosis: Intermittent claudication: ischemic leg pain caused by atherosclerosis in the right femoral and popliteal arteries

Signs and Symptoms: Complaints of right calf pain on walking, complaints of having to reduce pace or discontinue walking because of leg pain, motor and sensory deficits of the right leg

INTERVENTIONS	RATIONALE
Monitor leg pain	To provide a baseline, ongoing assessment and measure of treatment response
Teach patient to log triggers of leg pain, its severity, duration, and factors that relieve the pain	
Define outcome criteria: reversal or mitigation of the signs and symptoms	To provide a basis for defining treatment goals and criteria for discontinuing treatment
Teach patient a pain rating scale; for example, visual analog scale (mark pain severity on a 0 to 10 cm line with 0 no pain and 10 maximal, unbearable pain); monitor changes in pain with varying intensities of exercise	To promote patient's sense of control over ischemic pain and discomfort
Exercise prescription:	To exploit the *long-term* effects of exercise on the development of collateral circulation around the peripheral stenosis and alter rheology of the blood to promote improved perfusion and improve work performance
Medication: oxygen	
Type: walking	
Intensity: subclaudication threshold and breathlessness < 3-5 (0-10 scale)	To maximize central and peripheral adaptations to a prolonged aerobic stimulus
Duration: 20-60 minutes	To select subclaudication threshold to maximize walking duration
Frequency: several to 1 time daily	
Course and progression: as indicated	To avoid disabling pain that interferes with walking and promotes an abnormal gait and posture
Monitor arterial saturation continuously during exercise; maintain $SaO_2 > 90\%$	The duration is increased as the patient adapts to the exercise stimulus; as exercise duration increases, the intensity of the stimulus increases, and the frequency of the sessions correspondingly decreases

INTERVENTIONS	RATIONALE
Teach relaxation procedures (e.g., breathing control, pacing of activities, intermittent rest periods)	To integrate relaxation and pacing with activities to minimize metabolic demands on the affected leg; periodic rests permit the leg to reperfuse, eliminate metabolites, and reduce leg pain
Teach patient to examine right leg and foot daily for color, temperature, redness, abrasions, wounds, changes in muscle bulk, and motor and sensory deficits; notify health care professional of any changes	To protect the ischemic foot from prolonged impaired perfusion
	To seek attention if signs and symptoms of ischemia change
Reinforce foot and shoe hygiene	To minimize need for surgical intervention
Advise regarding appropriate footwear that minimizes the risk of foot abrasions	To minimize skin breakdown because the ischemic foot is slow to heal and has an increased risk of infection

Physical Therapy Diagnosis: Decreased physical activity and exercise tolerance resulting from dyspnea and intermittent claudication

Signs and Symptoms: Complaints of inability to perform ADL and exercise because of dyspnea and leg pain, claudication pain on walking short distances, and shortness of breath on exertion

INTERVENTIONS	RATIONALE
Monitor level of physical activity and exercise tolerance over past year	To provide a baseline, ongoing assessment and measure of treatment response
Define outcome criteria: reversal or mitigation of the signs and symptoms	To provide a basis for defining treatment goals and criteria for discontinuing treatment
Submaximal graded exercise tolerance test (GXTT) with ECG, Sao_2 monitoring, and monitoring of other exercise responses, including leg pain and breathlessness	To provide a baseline, ongoing assessment and treatment response
Medication: oxygen	A modified submaximal exercise can be safely performed with appropriate monitoring and predetermined end points of the exercise test; chest pain is an absolute criterion for termination of an exercise test in this patient (without a cardiologist present)
Type: treadmill walking	
Protocol: submaximal, symptom-limited	
Test termination: 75% age-predicted minimal heart rate, breathlessness 7-8 (0-10 scale), or leg pain 7 (0-10 scale); test terminated if angina reported or ECG changes	
Exercise prescription based on GXTT	To exploit the *long-term* effects of exercise on cardiopulmonary function and oxygen transport (i.e., optimize aerobic capacity, desensitization to dyspnea, maximize respiratory muscle strength, optimize movement efficiency and economy, and stimulate the development of collateral circulation around the stenosed artery in the right leg)
Interval training schedule: 5 minutes exercise–1 minute rest	
Type: walking	
Intensity: tolerable leg pain < 5, tolerable dyspnea < 5, Sao_2 > 90%	
Duration: 10-40 minutes	
Frequency: several to 2 times a day	
Course and progression: as indicated; several months	Interval training maximizes work output and is a primary training schedule for patients with significantly reduced functional work capacity
	As the patient adapts to chronic exercise stress, the interval schedule is progressed to bouts of high and low intensities and then to continuous training
	As the patient adapts to the chronic exercise stress, the intensity and duration of the sessions increase and the frequency of sessions decreases
	Focus on exercise-induced effects to minimize pain; as pain threshold increases, exercise intensity increases, which elicits effects that minimize breathlessness
	Several months of an exercise program are required to stimulate development of collateral circulation; with increased duration of sessions, frequency decreases

Continued.

INTERVENTIONS	RATIONALE

General strengthening program:
    Type—weights and pulleys for upper and lower extremities, thorax, and abdomen
    Intensity—low-medium intensity to keep breathlessness low, paced with patient's respiratory cycle (inhale on extension and exhale on flexion), avoid breath holding, straining, the Valsalva maneuver, and excessive static muscle contraction
    Duration—3 sets of 10 repetitions of each exercise with rests between sets and each exercise
    Frequency—daily to every other day
    Course and progression—as indicated
	To optimize patient's strength to enhance performance of ADL, physical activity and exercise, and oxygen transport overall
	As patient adapts to the exercise stimulus, resistance and duration of sessions increase and the frequency of sessions decreases

Supervised exercise program	To promote continuity and generalization to home setting; ensure that the exercise parameters are safe for the patient
Prepare home aerobic exercise program: stretching, warm-up, steady rate aerobic exercise, cool down, recovery	To wean patient from supervised to home program
Promote health promotion: exercise, fitness, nutrition, responsible use of medications, adequate and quality sleep and rest, relaxation, stress management	To reinforce self-responsibility and lifestyle changes for optimal health and well-being
Teach relaxation procedures, pacing, and energy conservation	Maximal work output is a function of both physical work output and optimal rest to promote restoration between physically demanding activities

Physical Therapy Diagnosis: Threats to oxygen transport and gas exchange related to progression of lung disease, age-related changes in the cardiopulmonary system, progression of peripheral vascular disease, increased risk of coronary artery disease in patients with ischemic limb pain, general deconditioning of the oxygen transport system, and restricted mobility

Signs and Symptoms: Fluid volume changes, impaired mucociliary transport, secretion accumulation, atelectasis, bronchospasm, inadequate tidal volume, increased pulmonary vascular resistance, pulmonry hypertension, thrombus formation, thromboemboli, diffusion defects, increased hematocrit and blood viscosity, impaired peripheral blood flow distal to site of vascular occlusion, impaired tissue perfusion with oxygenated blood and removal of CO_2 and metabolic wastes, motor and sensory deficits in the affected leg, skin breakdown, risk of infection, coronary artery occlusion, myocardial ischemia, angina, ECG irregularities, and systemic hypertension

INTERVENTIONS	RATIONALE
Monitor risks of impaired oxygen transport and gas exchange	To provide a baseline and ongoing assessment
Serial monitoring of ABGs, pulmonary function, ischemic leg pain, and exercise responses	To monitor and observe for changes in cardiopulmonary, cardiovascular, peripheral vascular, and systemic status
Serial cardiopulmonary clinical examinations	
Define outcome criteria: prevention, reversal, or mitigation of the signs and symptoms	To provide a basis for defining treatment goals and criteria for discontinuing treatment
Consider every patient interaction an opportunity for patient education	
Teach patient to monitor changes in cardiopulmonary cardiovascular and peripheral vascular status	To promote self-responsibility for health and wellness and management of lung disease and peripheral vascular disease
Reinforce lifestyle changes and healthy living	
Reinforce importance of daily exercise program	To exploit the *preventive* effects of exercise on oxygen transport and gas exchange
Reinforce active living	

Physical Therapy Diagnosis: Risk of negative sequelae of restricted mobility caused by cardiopulmonary pathophysiology and peripheral vascular disease

Signs and Symptoms: Reduced activity and exercise tolerance, muscle atrophy and reduced muscle strength, decreased oxygen transport efficiency, increased heart rate, blood pressure, and minute ventilation at submaximal work rates, reduced respiratory muscle strength and endurance, circulatory stasis, thromboemboli (e.g., pulmonary emboli), pressure areas, skin redness, skin breakdown and ulceration, weight gain, and reduced psychological well-being

INTERVENTIONS	RATIONALE
Monitor the negative sequelae of restricted mobility	To provide a baseline and ongoing assessment
Define outcome criteria: reversal or mitigation of the signs and symptoms	To provide a basis for defining treatment goals and criteria for discontinuing treatment
Mobilization and exercise prescriptions	To exploit the *preventive* effects of exercise on multisystem function; mobilization and exercise optimize circulating blood volume and enhance the efficiency of all steps in the oxygen transport pathway

Physical Therapy Diagnosis: Knowledge deficit

Signs and Symptoms: Lack of information about interstitial pulmonary fibrosis and peripheral vascular disease, their complications, and management

INTERVENTIONS	RATIONALE
Determine specific knowledge deficits related to interstitial pulmonary fibrosis and peripheral vascular disease and cardiopulmonary physical therapy management	To provide a baseline, ongoing assessment and measure of intervention response
Define outcome criteria: prevention, reversal, or mitigation of the signs and symptoms	To provide a basis for defining treatment goals and criteria for discontinuing treatment
Promote a caring and supportive patient-therapist relationship	To focus on treating the patient with interstitial lung disease and intermittent claudication rather than the conditions
Instruct regarding avoidance of respiratory tract infections, nutrition, weight control, hydration and fluid balance, rest and sleep, exercise	To promote patient's sense of responsibility for wellness and health promotion
	To promote cooperation and active participation in treatment
Teach, demonstrate, and provide feedback on interventions that can be self-administered	Between-treatment interventions are as important as treatments themselves to provide cumulative treatment effect
Teach patient to balance activity and rest	Optimal balance between activity and rest is essential to exploit acute, long-term, and preventive effects of mobilization and exercise
Patient is given a personalized handout with a listing and description of the exercises and their prescription parameters; precautions are emphasized	To maximize the cumulative effects of treatment
	To promote self-responsibility

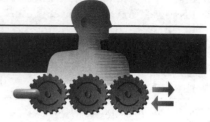

CHAPTER 16

Cystic Fibrosis

PATHOPHYSIOLOGY

Cystic fibrosis (CF) is an autosomal recessive disorder in which there is obstruction of the ducts of exocrine glands. Cystic fibrosis is a multisystem disorder involving the pulmonary, pancreatic, hepatic, gastrointestinal, and reproductive systems; it is characterized by altered electrolyte concentration in secretions (increased sweat electrolyte content), chronic airflow limitation, and pancreatic insufficiency. These signs and symptoms usually occur in childhood. Signs of pulmonary damage are mucus obstruction, inflammation and edema, decreased pulmonary compliance, and bronchospasm. Hemoptysis is caused by erosion of the bronchial vasculature from frequent and recurrent pulmonary infections. Pneumothorax occurs in 20% of adult CF cases and is due to rupture of cysts in the apices of the lung, which allows air from the lung to enter into the pleural space. Right-sided heart failure secondary to pulmonary hypertension develops in advanced stages of CF and is due to hypoxemia, which results from obstructed airways, atelectasis, and ventilation-perfusion mismatch. These changes in pulmonary function result in productive cough, recurrent bronchitis and pnuemonia, breathlessness and dyspnea on exertion, digital clubbing, and weight loss. Crackles and wheezes can be heard on auscultation. Chest x-rays may reveal hyperinflation of the lungs, small airway obstruction, bronchial cuffing, and bronchiectasis. The most severe changes are commonly displayed in the right upper lobe. Cardiopulmonary complications account for 95% of deaths in CF. Gastrointestinal and pancreatic involvement occurs in 20% of CF cases. Retention of enzymes in the pancreas eventually destroys the pancreatic tissue, resulting in malabsorption of fat and glucose intolerance. The inability of the gallbladder to secrete salt and water leads to biliary cirrhosis, bile duct proliferation, chronic cholecystitis, and cholelithiasis. Changes in gastrointestinal function result in weight loss; frequent, bulky, greasy stools; cramps; and abdominal pain. Children with CF have frequent absenteeism from school because of recurrent morbidity and hospitalization. Thus schooling and normal peer group and social interaction are disrupted.

Case Study

The patient is a 16-year-old girl. She is in the tenth grade. She lives with her parents and two brothers in an urban area. She is a high achiever and spends most of her time studying and practicing piano. The patient was diagnosed with cystic fibrosis at the age of 2. She developed a lower respiratory tract infection of sufficient severity to warrant hospitalization. She was productive for moderately large amounts of green foul-smelling sputum. Her breathing became labored, and she began showing signs of cyanosis. Her recent preadmission pulmonary function test results were forced expiratory volume in one second (FEV_1) 44% of predicted, forced vital capacity (FVC) 56% of predicted, and midexpiratory flow rate 54% of predicted. She is 5 feet 4.5 inches (164 cm) tall and weighs 101 pounds (46 kg); her body mass index is 17. She has had numerous exacerbations over the years, and in the past 2 years she has required hospitalization on three occasions. Her arterial blood gases (ABGs) on 2 L/min oxygen by nasal prongs were arterial oxygen pressure (Pao_2) 65 mm Hg, arterial carbon dioxide pressure ($Paco_2$) 50 mm Hg, bicarbonate (HCO_3) 30 mEq/L, and arterial oxygen saturation (Sao_2) 88%. During this acute period, she received broad-spectrum antibiotics, topical acetylcysteine, and aerosolized isoproterenol.

Oxygen Transport Deficits: Observed and Potential

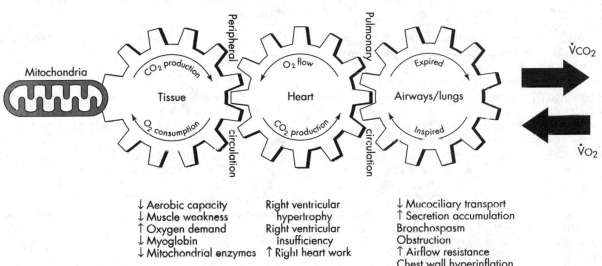

↓ Aerobic capacity
↓ Muscle weakness
↑ Oxygen demand
↓ Myoglobin
↓ Mitochondrial enzymes

Right ventricular hypertrophy
Right ventricular insufficiency
↑ Right heart work

↓ Mucociliary transport
↑ Secretion accumulation
Bronchospasm
Obstruction
↑ Airflow resistance
Chest wall hyperinflation
Flattened hemidiaphragms
Emphysematous changes
Impaired ventilation
Impaired ventilation=
   perfusion matching
Impaired gas mixing
Dyspnea
Use of accessory muscles
Inefficient respiratory
   muscle work
↑ Energy cost of breathing
↑ Work of breathing

↑ Central venous pressure
↑ Systemic blood
   pressure

↓ Diffusing capacity
Hypoxic vasoconstriction
↑ Pulmonary vascular
   resistance
Pulmonary hypertension
↑ Shunt
↓ Lymph motion
↓ Lymphatic
   drainage

Blood: ↑ Red blood cell count
   ↑ Hematocrit
   ↑ Viscosity
   Hypoxemia
   Hypercapnia
   Arterial desaturation at rest
      and in exercise

↑ Increase
↓ Decrease

PHYSICAL THERAPY DIAGNOSES AND TREATMENT PRESCRIPTION

Physical Therapy Diagnosis: Altered cardiopulmonary function: impaired gas exchange caused by alveolar hypoventilation and shunt

Signs and Symptoms: Decreased air entry, increased inhomogeneity of ventilation, ventilation and perfusion mismatch, increased mucus production, thick tenacious secretions, hypertrophy of mucus-producing glands, abnormal ciliary function, impaired mucociliary transport, secretion accumulation, airway obstruction, bacterial colonization and multiplication, decreased cough effectiveness, impaired airflow rate, hypoxemia, hypercapnia, signs of chronic airflow limitation (e.g., bronchiectatic changes), signs of restrictive lung disease (e.g., fibrosis secondary to chronic inflammation), diffusion defect, widening A − a oxygen gradient, breathlessness, right heart hypertrophy, hypoxic pulmonary vasoconstriction, pulmonary hypertension, crackles and wheezes on auscultation, bronchospasm, altered sputum characteristics, radiographic evidence of bronchial dilation and bronchiectasis, heart elongated and enlarged, and reduced mechanical efficiency of the myocardium

INTERVENTIONS	RATIONALE
Monitor ABGs, pulmonary function tests, Sao_2, hemodynamic status, fluid and electrolyte status, chest x-rays, sputum quantity and quality	To provide a baseline, ongoing assessment and measure of treatment response
Perform clinical cardiopulmonary assessment	
Define outcome criteria: reversal or mitigation of the signs and symptoms	To provide a basis for defining treatment goals and criteria for discontinuing treatment
Breathing control and coughing maneuvers (upright positions): breathing control maneuvers with maximal inspiration, 3-5 second hold, and passive expiration to resting end-tidal volume; pursed lips breathing	To minimize dynamic airway compression, alveolar collapse, and atelectasis
Coughing maneuvers: maneuvers with open glottis (e.g., huffing)	Open glottis coughing maneuvers reduce thoracic pressure, dynamic airway compression, and closure and minimize compromising venous return during coughing
	To enhance breathing efficiency
Mobilization coordinated with breathing control and coughing maneuvers (e.g., inspiration on extension movements and expiration on flexion movements): Upper extremities Trunk Lower extremities	To reduce myocardial stress by minimizing breath holding, straining, the Valsalva maneuver, and excessive static contractions
Exercise prescription based on response to physical challenges of activities of daily living (ADL) or modified exercise test (ensure that patient is adequately and appropriately premedicated and supplemental oxygen as indicated to maintain Sao_2)	To exploit the *acute* effects of exercise, including increased airway diameter, increased homogeneity of ventilation, increased area of ventilation and perfusion matching, increased mucociliary transport, reduced accumulation of secretions, increased peripheral to central movement of pulmonary secretions, increased cough effectiveness, increased lung movement, increased chest wall movement, increased alveolar ventilation, increased lymphatic drainage
Type—aerobic exercise coordinated with breathing control (pursed lips breathing) and coughing maneuvers (avoidance of heavy resistive exercise, exercise requiring excessive postural stabilization, and breath holding)	
Intensity—below breathlessness threshold and target heart rate based on the exercise challenge results	To maximize the efficacy of exercise stimulus in eliciting *acute* effects of exercise, medications must be administered so that they are at peak efficacy during treatment
Duration—10-40 minutes	
Frequency—several to 1 time daily	To stimulate surfactant production and distribution and thereby reduce alveolar surface tension and tendency toward alveolar collapse
Course and progression—as indicated	
	To avoid undue cardiac stress and myocardial work
Stretching and range-of-motion exercises for upper extremity and chest wall coordinated with breathing control and coughing maneuvers	To optimize chest wall configuration, mobility, and three-dimensional movement, including the bucket handle and pump handle movements
Intensity—no to minimal resistance	To minimize chest wall hyperinflation, need for accessory muscle
Duration—5-15 minutes	
Frequency—daily	To promote normal length of respiratory muscles and their length-tension relationships
Course and progression—as indicated	To promote normal posture and spinal alignment at rest and during physical activity and exercise

INTERVENTIONS	RATIONALE

Strengthening exercise:
  Upper extremity
  Chest wall
  Lower extremity
	To optimize muscle strength to facilitate ADL and perform physical activity

	To increase body mass, overall muscular strength, and endurance
Low to moderate intensity; breathlessness < 3-5 (0-10 scale); Sao$_2$ > 90%	To augment capacity for aerobic exercise
High repetitions (e.g., 3 sets of 10-25 repetitions)	As the patient responds to training, the intensity and duration of treatment sessions increases and the frequency decreases
Duration—15-30 minutes	
Frequency—1-2 times a day	
Course and progression—as indicated	
Ventilatory muscle training	To augment respiratory muscle strength and endurance
Intensity—progressive increase in resistance with gauge for rate of air flow	
Duration—5-10 minutes	
Frequency—2 times a day	
Course and progression—as indicated	

Relaxed breathing positions with controlled breathing, coughing maneuvers, and relaxation interventions:
  Sitting leaning forward with arms supported
  Lean forward standing with hands on knees
  Lean forward with back supported on wall
  Erect sitting
	Relaxed breathing positions to optimize accessory muscle use, stabilize upper chest wall, reduce abdominal encroachment, minimize the work of breathing and of the heart

Body positioning coordinated with breathing control (pursed lips breathing) and coughing maneuvers	Body positioning prescribed to optimize alveolar ventilation, ventilation and perfusion matching, surfactant production and distribution, and airway clearance
Postural drainage positions	Postural drainage positions when indicated in addition to mobilization for airway clearance and bronchial hygiene
Positions selected: most productive bronchopulmonary segments	To increase alveolar volume and ventilation and to drain pulmonary secretions
Postural drainage positions with percussion, shaking, and vibration	Postural drainage positions with manual techniques as indicated and appropriate monitoring to avoid arterial desaturation and other untoward effects
Positions selected: those that are most productive	Single-handed percussion at a frequency of 1 per second minimizes the risks associated with this intervention
Monitor breathing pattern, respiratory rate, heart rate, blood pressure, and Sao$_2$ before, during, and after treatment (immediately and 15 and 30 minutes after treatment)	Vigorous exhaustive coughing can contribute to arterial desaturation, dynamic airway compression, atelectasis, fatigue, nausea and vomiting, aspiration, increased myocardial work, and stress; thus coughing must be controlled as much as possible to minimize these untoward effects and maximize its beneficial effects as a primary airway clearance intervention
Autogenic drainage in the upright seated position	Autogenic drainage can be an alternative to postural drainage with manual techniques because it avoids their deleterious effects and the deleterious effects of uncontrolled coughing
	Controlled breathing intervention beginning at low tidal volume (unstick phase) and progressing to mid and high tidal volumes (clear phase); pulmonary secretions are believed to move from the peripheral to central airways, where they can be cleared
Flutter device	The patient exhales through the Flutter device until coughing is stimulated; sputum is expectorated
	Breathing through a Flutter device elicits fine chest wall vibrations that loosen and dislodge airway secretions
Ensure that aerosols and bronchodilators are being used appropriately as prescribed	To optimize the cardiopulmonary benefits of these interventions and minimize waste

Continued.

Physical Therapy Diagnosis: Abnormal breathing pattern

Signs and Symptoms: Air trapping, chest wall hyperinflation, abnormal chest wall configuration, decreased breath sounds, increased adventitious lung sounds, loss of normal bucket handle and pump handle movements, use of accessory muscles, dyspnea at rest and on minimal exertion, increased airway resistance, altered lung compliance, increased time constants, increased energy cost of breathing, increased work of breathing, increased work of the heart, abnormal thoracoabdominal motion, chest wall deformity, increased anteroposterior diameter, flattened hemidiaphragms, and poor posture

INTERVENTIONS	RATIONALE
Monitor breathing patterns (i.e., rate and depth during rest and activity/exercise, shortness of breath, use of accessory muscles of respiration, and abnormal thoracoabdominal motion)	To provide a baseline, ongoing assessment and measure of treatment response
Define outcome criteria: reversal or mitigation of the signs and symptoms	To provide a basis for defining treatment goals and criteria for discontinuing treatment
Body positioning to enhance efficiency of breathing pattern	To reduce the work and energy cost of breathing
Body positioning to reduce the work of breathing	To reduce the work of and stress on the heart
Body positioning to reduce the energy cost of breathing	To optimize functional work capacity
Breathing control and coughing maneuvers:	
Maximal inspiration with expiration to resting end tidal volume	To minimize dynamic airway compression, alveolar collapse, and atelectasis
Pursed lips breathing	To minimize work of the heart secondary to static exercise, breath holding, straining, and the Valsalva maneuver
Inhalation on extension movements and expiration on flexion movements	
Chest wall stretching and range-of-motion exercises	To promote normal chest wall shape and muscle and joint structure and function
Promote optimal posture and alignment	To promote optional chest wall configuration and respiratory mechanics

Physical Therapy Diagnosis: Decreased tolerance for physical activity and exercise

Signs and Symptoms: Shortness of breath at rest and during exercise, exercise-induced arterial desaturation, avoidance of physical activity and exercise, lethargy, social withdrawal and isolation, increased heart rate, blood pressure, rate pressure product, minute ventilation, and oxygen consumption at rest and during submaximal exercise, reduced functional work capacity, reduced respiratory muscle strength and endurance, and reduced movement efficiency and metabolic economy

INTERVENTIONS	RATIONALE
Monitor objective and subjective responses to a standardized clinical exercise test with patient appropriately premedicated	To provide a baseline, ongoing assessment and measure of treatment response
Define outcome criteria: reversal or mitigation of the signs and symptoms	To provide a basis for defining treatment goals and criteria for discontinuing treatment
Exercise prescription:	To exploit the *long-term* effects of exercise (i.e., increased efficiency of all steps of the oxygen transport pathway, including enhanced gas exchange and oxygen delivery, increased mobility of the chest wall, increased respiratory muscle strength and endurance, increased efficiency of the heart, increased collateral circulation, enhanced oxygen uptake and utilization at the cellular level; decreased minute ventilation, oxygen uptake, heart rate, blood pressure, rate pressure product at rest and submaximal work rates, hence decrease the work and energy cost of breathing, and the work of the heart at rest and submaximal work rates; increase immunity, increase psychological well-being; increase movement efficiency and metabolic economy, desensitization to dyspnea, and increased motivation)
Preconditions—45-60 minutes postprandial; patient appropriately and adequately premedicated; oxygen as required to maintain $Sao_2 > 90\%$	
Type—aerobic, rhythmic exercise, such as walking, running, cycling, swimming; interval training schedule	
Intensity—below breathlessness threshold; breathlessness < 3-5 (0-10 scale)	
Duration—20-40 minutes	
Frequency—1-2 times a day	
Course and progression—lifelong daily exercise	

INTERVENTIONS	RATIONALE
	Daily exercise between exacerbations is essential for optional management of cystic fibrosis and for bronchial hygiene
	To optimize absorption of food, the patient delays exercising after eating for 45-60 minutes
	During exacerbations, mobilization is essential to exploit the *acute* effects of exercise on cardiopulmonary function and bronchopulmonary hygiene in addition to maintaining long-term conditioning effects
	During exacerbations, exercise intensity is reduced, duration of the sessions is reduced, and frequency of sessions may be increased
	Exercise intensity set such that oxygen demand is within patient's capacity for oxygen delivery
Prescriptive pacing of physical activity	Maximize work output of training with interval schedule (e.g., work-rest intervals or high-low intensity intervals)
Interval training schedule	
Prescriptive pacing of each exercise session	Maximize ADL performance with interspersed rest periods, high demand–low demand pacing, adequate sleep, and energy conservation interventions (e.g., performing ADL as mechanically efficiently as possible, using alternate means of performing ADL, and using aids and devices)
Monitor adequacy of rest and sleep	Optimal rest and sleep are essential for physiological restoration; physical activity and exercise should be followed by a rest period
Teach relaxation procedures	To minimize systemic oxygen demands
Coordinate breathing control with relaxation procedures	

Physical Therapy Diagnosis: Anxiety: shortness of breath

Signs and Symptoms: Shortness of breath at rest and during exercise, panicked appearance, verbalization of anxiety and air hunger, arterial desaturation, increased respiratory rate, reduced tidal volume, increased heart rate and blood pressure, and fear of triggering uncontrolled bouts of exhaustive coughing

INTERVENTIONS	RATIONALE
Monitor anxiety and shortness of breath	To provide a baseline, ongoing assessment and measure of treatment response
Define outcome criteria: reversal or mitigation of the signs and symptoms	To provide a basis for defining treatment goals and criteria for discontinuing treatment
Teach patient to identify specific triggers of increased shortness of breath	To minimize anxiety associated with shortness of breath
Teach patient to remain below a shortness of breath threshold (on 0-10 scale)	To reduce autonomic arousal
Teach patient to identify factors that improve and worsen shortness of breath	To minimize the energy cost associated with anxiety
	To enable the patient to control shortness of breath as much as possible
Coordinate physical activity, breathing control, and coughing maneuvers	To minimize the increased energy expenditure associated with the work of breathing; increased oxygen demand further increases the work of breathing and anxiety
Teach pacing and energy conservation	
Reinforce the importance of daily physical exercise as per the exercise prescription parameters	Regular physical activity maintains optimal work performance and desensitizes patient to dyspnea
Relaxed breathing positions coordinated with breathing control maneuvers	Optimize coughing effort (i.e., promote coughing when needed to clear airways or shift secretions) and minimize exhausting, uncontrolled bouts of coughing; such coughing contributes to dynamic airway compression, airway closure, arterial desaturation, vomiting, risk of aspiration, and significantly increased energy expenditure
Relaxation procedures (e.g., Jacobsen's relaxation technique, Benson's relaxation method, autogenic training, biofeedback, visual imagery)	
Supplemental oxygen	Pharmacological support may be indicated if other methods do not relieve shortness of breath related to anxiety

Continued.

Physical Therapy Diagnosis: Reduced emotional and psychological well-being

Signs and Symptoms: Verbalization of not fitting into peer group; lack of friends, alienation, time out of school and away from peer group when ill or hospitalized, cystic fibrosis support group for the patient and family, and worsening of posture and self image

INTERVENTIONS	RATIONALE
Monitor emotional and psychological well-being	To provide a baseline and ongoing assessment
Define outcome criteria: reversal or mitigation of the signs and symptoms	To provide a basis for defining treatment goals and criteria for discontinuing treatment
Training exercise program, including aerobic exercise, stretching and range-of-motion exercises, and general strengthening exercises	To promote the *preventive* and health benefits of exercise on psychological well-being To maintain the highest possible degree of oxygen transport efficiency and aerobic capacity
Postural correction exercises	To help improve physical self-image
A variety of physical activities and games enjoyed by patient and her peer group	To foster physical activity and active living consistent with patient's peer group To promote physical activities that foster social interaction and integration with others
Encourage recreational activities and laughter	Recreational activities that promote diverse body positions and movement in different planes elicit many *acute* benefits of exercise and elicit gravitational stress on the cardiopulmonary system Laughter promotes deep breaths and mucociliary transport
Provide emotional support for patient and her family	Median survival is improving: up to 30 years

Physical Therapy Diagnosis: Threats to oxygen transport and gas exchange: disease progression, recurrent infections, hospitalization, blood sugar abnormalities, intercurrent illness, arthritis or hypertrophic osteopathy, anemia

Signs and Symptoms: Gastroesophageal reflux, small intestinal obstruction with abdominal distention, increased intraabdominal pressure, discomfort, encroachment of the diaphragm, hemoptysis, bronchopulmonary infection, increased work of breathing, increased work of the heart, reduced functional capacity, decreased appetite, increased energy cost of eating, fatigue, and immunosuppression

INTERVENTIONS	RATIONALE
Monitor ABGs, Sao_2, pulmonary function tests, breathlessness, aerobic capacity, performance of ADL	To provide a baseline and ongoing assessment
Define actions criteria: prevention, reversal, or mitigation of the signs and symptoms	To provide a basis for defining treatment goals and criteria for discontinuing treatment
Teach patient to self-monitor cardiopulmonary status	To detect changes in cardiopulmonary status early, hasten intervention, and minimize morbidity and deterioration
Teach pacing of physical activity, interspersing rest periods, and optimizing sleep and nutrition	To exploit the *preventive* effects of exercise on cardiopulmonary function and oxygen transport Optimal performance reflects a balance among physical activity, rest, sleep, and nutrition
Teach energy conservation (i.e., how to perform ADL and recreational activities such that excessive energy expenditure is minimized)	To minimize undue energy expenditure to minimize excessive demands on oxygen transport
Teach stress management and coping skills	To reduce anxiety, stress, and undue physiological arousal

Physical Therapy Diagnosis: Risk of negative sequelae of restricted mobility

Signs and Symptoms: Reduced activity and exercise tolerance, muscle atrophy and reduced muscle strength, decreased oxygen transport efficiency, increased heart rate, blood pressure, and minute ventilation at submaximal work rates, reduced respiratory muscle strength and endurance, circulatory stasis, thromboemboli (e.g., pulmonary emboli), pressure areas, skin redness, skin breakdown, and ulceration

INTERVENTIONS	RATIONALE
To monitor the negative sequelae of restricted mobility	To provide a baseline and ongoing assessment
Define outcome criteria: prevention, reversal, or mitigation of the signs and symptoms	To provide a basis for defining treatment goals and criteria for discontinuing treatment
Mobilization and exercise prescription	To exploit the *preventive* effects of exercise on the cardiopulmonary system and oxygen transport in addition to its multisystemic effects; mobilization and exercise optimize circulating blood volume, enhance the efficiency of all steps in the oxygen transport pathway

Physical Therapy Diagnosis: Knowledge deficit

Signs and Symptoms: Lack of information about cystic fibrosis, acute exacerbations, and complications

INTERVENTIONS	RATIONALE
To determine specific knowledge deficits of child and caregivers	To provide a baseline and ongoing assessment
Define outcome criteria: reversal or mitigation of the signs and symptoms	To provide a basis for treatment goals and criteria for discontinuing interventions
Promote a caring and supportive patient-therapist relationship	To focus on treating the patient with cystic fibrosis rather than the cystic fibrosis
Consider every patient interaction an opportunity for patient education	To promote cooperation and active participation in treatment
Instruct regarding avoidance of respiratory tract infections, nutrition, weight control, hydration and fluid balance, and stress management	To promote patient's sense of responsibility for wellness and health promotion
Reinforce the purpose of medication, its prescription parameters, and medication schedule	To ensure that aerosols and bronchodilators are used effectively to maximize treatment effects
	To encourage the patient to balance sedentary interests (i.e., studying and piano with regular physical exercise)
Teach, demonstrate, and provide feedback on interventions that can be self-administered	Between-treatment interventions are as important as treatments themselves to provide cumulative treatment effect
Teach patient to balance activity and rest	Optimal balance between activity and rest is essential to exploit short-term, long-term, and preventive effects of mobilization and exercise
Promote active living	To incorporate the acute, long-term, and preventive effects of physical activity and regular exercise into the patient's daily life
Promote optimal rest and sleep	To optimize the patient's functional capacity by optimizing her needs for rest and sleep

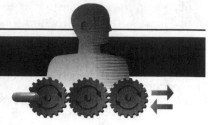

CHAPTER 17

Rheumatoid Arthritis

PATHOPHYSIOLOGY

Rheumatoid arthritis (RA) is a chronic inflammatory condition that is more prevalent in women than men. The condition is multisystemic and is characterized by persistent inflammation of the synovial joints. The cause of RA remains unknown, although several areas are being investigated. They include immune mechanisms (the interaction of the IgG immunoglobins with the rheumatoid factor), genetic and metabolic factors, and viral infections. Joints that are most commonly affected are those of the hands, wrists, elbows, feet, ankles, and knees. The inflammation occurs in a bilaterally symmetric pattern, involving the same joints on both sides of the body. At onset, there is synovitis with edema, vascular congestion, fibrin exudate, and cellular infiltration. This triggers migration of white blood cells into the affected region, releasing various enzymes. The enzyme collagenase is especially damaging to the joint because it breaks down collagen. Synovial thickening occurs at the articular junctions with continued inflammation, and granulation tissue forms a pannus (mantle) over the cartilage surface. The pannus impedes normal nutrition to the cartilage, causing it to become necrotic. The pannus eventually invades underlying bone, tendons, and ligaments and destroys them. Erosion of the articular cartilage, bone, and surrounding soft tissue may lead to subluxation or dislocation of the joints and osteoporosis. Nerve entrapments and neuropathies are common. Inflammation of tendon sheaths, muscle spasm and guarding, and formation of subcutaneous nodules near the affected joints contribute to joint deformity, restriction of range-of-motion, and muscle weakness and atrophy. Early signs and symptoms of RA include fever, weight loss, fatigue, and generalized aching and morning stiffness. As the condition progresses, these symptoms are replaced by localized joint swelling, pain, warmth, redness, and tenderness. Excerbations of RA are triggered by either an irritation or damage to the joint. There are periods of exacerbation and remission during the course of the disease. The clinical presentation of RA is associated with reduced activity and exercise, which contributes to deconditioning, reduced functional work capacity, decreased strength, impaired movement efficiency and economy, and inefficiency of oxygen transport overall. RA affects other organs in the body, such as the heart, lungs, and spleen. Multisystemic manifestations of RA include pleuritis, pulmonary fibrosis, pericarditis, cardiac valve dysfunction, lymphadenopathy, and splenomegaly.

Case Study

The patient is a 67-year-old woman. She continues to work part time as a librarian. She lives alone in a one-bedroom, second-floor apartment. The patient has a close relationship with her sister and family, who live in the neighborhood. Her body mass index is 15; she has never smoked. She was diagnosed with rheumatoid arthritis 27 years ago. Her condition is moderately severe and has necessitated hospitalization previously. She was admitted to a rehabilitation hospital for an acute exacerbation, which included fever of 102.2°F (39°C), fatigue, anorexia, generalized weakness, severe shortness of breath, coughing, joint swelling, and pain in her arms and legs. The chest x-ray showed infiltrates over the lingula and left lower lobe and a small left pleural effusion. She has signs of vasculitis, impaired diffusing capacity, and pericarditis. The patient is known to have moderately severe osteoporosis aggravated by prolonged corticosteroid therapy and restricted mobility.

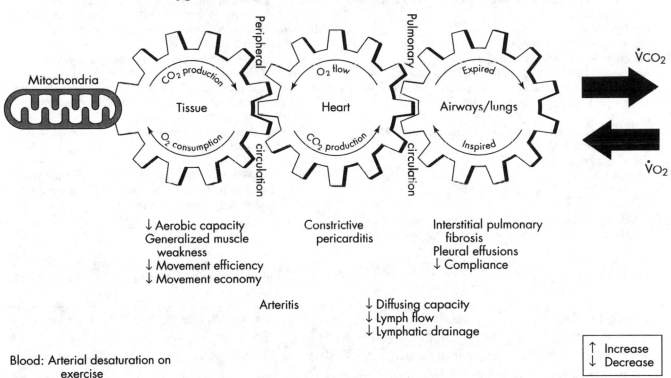

Oxygen Transport Deficits: Observed and Potential

↓ Aerobic capacity
Generalized muscle weakness
↓ Movement efficiency
↓ Movement economy

Constrictive pericarditis

Interstitial pulmonary fibrosis
Pleural effusions
↓ Compliance

Arteritis

↓ Diffusing capacity
↓ Lymph flow
↓ Lymphatic drainage

Blood: Arterial desaturation on exercise

↑ Increase
↓ Decrease

PHYSICAL THERAPY DIAGNOSES AND TREATMENT PRESCRIPTION

Physical Therapy Diagnosis: Altered cardiopulmonary function: alveolar hypoventilation and pleuropulmonary manifestations of rheumatoid arthritis, including pleural disease, interstitial pulmonary fibrosis, pleuropulmonary nodules, pneumonitis, and arteritis; cardiopulmonary dysfunction secondary to deformity and osteoporosis, age-related decreases in velocity of mucociliary clearance and cough reflex

Signs and Symptoms: Pleural effusions, pulmonary fibrosis, impaired diffusing capacity, radiographic evidence of atelectasis, pleural effusion, and chest wall distortion and deformity

INTERVENTIONS	RATIONALE
Monitor cardiopulmonary, musculoskeletal, and neuromuscular status Perform a clinical cardiopulmonary physical therapy assessment	To provide a baseline, ongoing assessment and measure of treatment response
Define outcome criteria: reversal or mitigation of the signs and symptoms	To provide a basis for defining treatment goals and criteria for discontinuing treatment
Mobilization coordinated with breathing control and coughing maneuvers	To exploit the *acute* effects of active living and mobilization on cardiopulmonary function and gas exchange
Intensity—low Duration—10-30 minutes	Mobilization is prescribed at very low intensity while patient is acute
Frequency—several to 2 times a day	When the patient is subacute, the intensity and duration are increased and the frequency of sessions is decreased
Course and progression—as indicated; the mobilization sessions are coordinated with medications and the patient's peak energy periods as much as possible	Because of the presence of osteoporosis secondary to long-term corticosteroid use, straining and forced coughing maneuvers are contraindicated
Stretching and range-of-motion exercises (gentle, rhythmic, paced movements): Head and neck Upper extremity Chest wall Lower extremity	To optimize chest wall excursion and three-dimensional movement, including bucket handle and pump handle motions
Coordinate stretching, chest wall mobility exercises, and range-of-motion exercises with breathing control maneuvers	Because of joint laxity and instability, stretching and range-of-motion exercises are performed gently and within the limits of joint deformity and comfort
Reinforce patient's medication schedule to optimize comfort and work performance	The patient can cooperate and actively participate with treatment more effectively if pain is optimally controlled

---

Physical Therapy Diagnosis: Fatigue: constitutional effect of rheumatoid arthritis, deconditioning, weakness, overuse, impaired movement economy, anemia, and anorexia

Signs and Symptoms: Complaints of excessive fatigue, decreased capacity to perform ADL, reduced functional work capacity, and nonrestorative sleep and rests

INTERVENTIONS	RATIONALE
Monitor pattern of fatigue and relationship to exercise, sleep/rest, diet, medications, and stress management Monitor patient's fatigue using a semiquantitative scale (0-10 scale with descriptors or an analog scale)	To provide a baseline, ongoing assessment and measure of treatment response
Define outcome criteria: reversal or mitigation of the signs and symptoms	To provide a basis for defining treatment goals and criteria for discontinuing treatment
Teach patient to monitor fatigue patterns and events around periods of fatigue	To enable patient to control fatigue and its impact on function rather than be victimized by it
Review patient's activity-fatigue log so she can understand the relationship between activity, fatigue, and other factors that contribute to fatigue	To provide guidance to patient to manage fatigue after discharge and thus optimize functional work capacity

INTERVENTIONS	RATIONALE
Prescribe rests based on the patient's fatigue logs Coordinate physical activity with fluctuations in fatigue Exercise regularly and at the best times of day Coordinate physical activity/exercise with medication schedule Pace physical activities and exercise Teach energy conservation strategies Perform ergonomic assessment of home and work to enhance body position, body alignment, biomechanical stresses, and movement efficiency Review patient's sleeping patterns, pillows, and mattress Teach patient to modify her activity and exercise program based on fatigue levels and general well-being	Timing of exercise sessions is critical to ensure that energy stores are optimal and that the patient has a good sense of well-being

Physical Therapy Diagnosis: Discomfort and pain

Signs and Symptoms: Verbalization of discomfort/pain, physical expression of discomfort/pain, reduced physical activity, reduced participation in cross-training exercise program, withdrawal from social activity, and lethargy

INTERVENTIONS	RATIONALE
Monitor discomfort/pain (0-10 scale or a visual analog scale) Define outcome criteria: reversal or mitigation of the signs and symptoms Teach patient to log discomfort/pain and its relationship to activity and other factors and diurnal variations Teach patient to modify physical activity and the exercise program with fluctuations in discomfort/pain Reinforce medication schedule Ensure that medications agree with the patient Review patient's rest periods Teach patient to perform activities of daily living (ADL), physical activity, and exercise within prescribed discomfort/pain threshold Review orthotics, shoes, and walking aids Reinforce pacing of activities Reinforce avoidance of precipitating factors and teach alternative activities	To provide a baseline, ongoing assessment and measure of treatment response To provide a basis for defining treatment goals and criteria for discontinuing treatment To teach patient to manage discomfort/pain rather than being victimized by it To optimize function, minimize suffering, and minimize the rate of deterioration To promote active living and aerobic exercise

Physical Therapy Diagnosis: Decreased physical activity and exercise tolerance because of pain, inflammation, deformity, abnormal gait, fatigue, muscle atrophy, weakness, postural deviations, chest wall abnormalities, limb length discrepancy, hip and knee deformity, foot deformity, curvature of the spine, and osteoporosis

Signs and Symptoms: Verbalization of pain, physical expression of pain, inflamed swollen joints, chronic deformities of the affected hands, hips, knees, and feet, excessive fatigue, constitutional complaints, inefficient gait (e.g., wide base), nonerect posture, use of walking aid, genu valgum, asymmetric disease severity in the legs

INTERVENTIONS	RATIONALE
Monitor physical activity and exercise performance Monitor activity-to-rest patterns Monitor fatigue profile	To provide a baseline, ongoing assessment and measure of treatment response To establish the limits to activity and exercise performance

Continued.

INTERVENTIONS	RATIONALE
Monitor deformity of limbs and compensatory changes in gait	To establish treatment goals and to modify treatment prescription with changes in the patient's condition
Monitor analgesic and antiinflammatory medication schedule	
Monitor orthosis and effectiveness	
Perform a modified exercise test or assess exercise responses to an ADL challenge	
Monitor constitutional complaints and rule out other contributing factors *not* amenable to physical therapy	
Establish preadmission level of activity and conditioning	
Define outcome criteria: reversal or mitigation of the signs and symptoms	To provide a basis for defining treatment goals and criteria for discontinuing treatment
Teach patient criteria for exercising at any given session (e.g., generally feels well, no acute inflammation, baseline discomfort acceptable, best time of day)	Patients with progressive conditions or with conditions that have fluctuations must learn how to modify their activity and exercise on a day-to-day basis to optimize work output and minimize strain and overuse
Prescribe a modified cross-training exercise program	To exploit the *long-term* effects of exercise on functional capacity in a patient with rheumatoid arthritis, including reduced resting and submaximal heart rate, blood pressure, rate pressure product, improved cardiac output, coronary perfusion, perceived exertion, breathlessness, fatigue, and discomfort/pain; increase alveolar ventilation, diffusing capacity, gas exchange, increased peripheral collateral circulation, oxygen delivery and extraction at the muscle level, improved removal of metabolites
All exercises are rhythmic, nonstraining, and exclude heavy resistive exercise	
All exercise is performed within limits of comfort, fatigue, and exertion	
All physical activity and exercise are coordinated with breathing control maneuvers	
Interval training schedule: 3-5 minutes exercise to 30-60 second rest for all types of prescribed exercise	
Type—modified aerobic exercise, such as walking	
Intensity—perceived exertion 3-5 (0-10 scale); minimal discomfort/pain < 3 (0-10 scale); fatigue < 3-5 (0-10 scale)	To exploit weight-bearing effects of walking to decelerate rate of bone demineralization, bone loss and related morbidity, deformity, and loss of function
Duration—10-30 minutes	
Frequency—several to 2 times a day	
Course and progression—as indicated	
Type—modified aerobic exercise, such as hydrotherapy (e.g., walking in pool, swimming, chair exercises in water, range of motion all joints, strengthening exercises)	Establish optimal water depth for hydrotherapy; increased depth of water up to the chest increases resistance to ventilation and chest expansion and increases the work of breathing
Intensity—perceived exertion 3-5 (0-10 scale); discomfort/pain < 3 (0-10 scale); fatigue < 3-5 (0-10 scale)	As the patient's condition fluctuates or exercise tolerance improves, the intensity and duration vary inversely with the frequency of the sessions
Duration—10-30 minutes	
Frequency—2 times a week	
Course and progression—as indicated	
Type—cycle ergometer	
Intensity—comfortable pedaling cadence	
Duration—10-20 minutes	
Frequency—2-3 times on alternate days or once daily	
Course and progression—as indicated	
Type—range-of-motion exercises; head and neck, upper extremities, chest wall (three planes), lower extremities	
Intensity—no resistance; within minimal pain range	
Duration—20-30 minutes	
Frequency—daily	
Course and progression—as indicated	

INTERVENTIONS	RATIONALE
Type—postural correction exercises, including spinal alignment, level of shoulders and pelvis, leg length, juxtaposition of musculoskeletal structures in the legs, chest wall mobility and capacity for normal three-dimensional movement (including bucket handle and pump handle motions), stretching of neck muscles, upper extremities, chest wall (forward flexion, extension, side flexion, rotation, and diagonal rotation)	To optomize alignment, chest wall excursion and symmetry, breathing patterns and efficiency, and movement economy
Intensity—low	
Duration—10-30 minutes	
Frequency—daily	
Course and progression—as indicated	
Type—general strengthening program with wrist and ankle weights for arms and legs; modified sit-ups and bridging	A requisite degree of strength is required to perform ADL and perform aerobic, endurance activity (e.g., walking)
Positions—standing, sitting, and lying down	A requisite degree of muscle strength enhances aerobic metabolism and functional capacity
Intensity—0.5-1 lb weights on arms; 1-2 lb weights on legs	
Duration—3 sets of 5-10 repetitions	
Frequency—daily	
Course and progression—as indicated	
Promote active living	Whenever possible and commensurate with the patient's status on any given day, the patient is encouraged to be as active as possible provided that preset discomfort/pain and fatigue thresholds are not exceeded

Physical Therapy Diagnosis: Risk of negative sequelae of restricted mobility

Signs and Symptoms: Reduced activity and exercise tolerance, muscle atrophy and reduced muscle strength, increased stiffness, decreased oxygen transport efficiency, increased heart rate, blood pressure, and minute ventilation at rest and submaximal work rates, reduced respiratory muscle strength and endurance, circulatory stasis, thromboemboli (e.g., pulmonary emboli), pressure areas, skin redness, skin breakdown and ulceration, and increased deformity

INTERVENTIONS	RATIONALE
Monitor the negative sequelae of restricted mobility	To provide a baseline and ongoing assessment
Define outcome criteria: prevention, reversal, or mitigation of the signs and symptoms	To provide a basis for defining treatment goals and criteria for discontinuing treatment
Mobilization and exercise prescription	Mobilization and exercise optimize circulating blood volume and enhance the efficiency of all steps in the oxygen transport pathway
	To exploit the *preventive* effects of mobilization and exercise

Continued.

Physical Therapy Diagnosis: Threats to oxygen transport: pleural effusion, pneumothorax, bronchopleural fistula, obliteration of the pulmonary vasculature, pulmonary hypertension, upper airway obstruction, pericarditis, pericardial effusion, tamponade, chronic constrictive pericarditis, anemia, arrhythmias, thrombocytopenia, increased intraabdominal pressure secondary to splenomegaly, leukopenia, increased frequency of infection, gastrointestinal bleeding, discomfort/pain, fatigue, weakness, deformity, reduced functional work capacity and deconditioning, osteoporosis, deformity, and decreased functional capacity caused by long-term steroid use

Signs and Symptoms: Clinical signs of cardiopulmonary pathophysiology, signs of constitutional problems, abnormal laboratory tests and clinical investigations consistent with impaired oxygen transport, signs and symptoms of discomfort/pain, fatigue, weakness, deformity, and clinical signs of gastrointestinal dysfunction

INTERVENTIONS	RATIONALE
Serial monitoring of oxygen transport variables and the function of multiple organ systems	Rheumatoid arthritis is a multisystemic condition with cardiopulmonary manifestations
	To provide a baseline, ongoing assessment and measure of treatment response
Define outcome criteria: prevention, reversal, or mitigation of the signs and symptoms	To provide a basis for defining treatment goals and criteria for discontinuing treatment
Teach patient to monitor changes in multiorgan status	Involvement of other organs can produce cardiopulmonary effects (e.g., gastrointestinal dysfunction)
	Rheumatoid arthritis is associated with iatrogenic complications (e.g., osteoporosis, deformity, and loss of functional capacity) as a result of long-term use of corticosteroids
Teach patient to modify physical activity and the cross-training program according to changes in health status	Impaired cardiopulmonary function and oxygen transport result from reduced physical activity, weakness, pain, deformity, and reduced aerobic exercise
Reinforce when changes in status require medical attention	To promote self-management of rheumatoid arthritis

Physical Therapy Diagnosis: Knowledge deficit

Signs and Symptoms: Lack of information about rheumatoid arthritis, preventive measures, relapses, or complications

INTERVENTIONS	RATIONALE
Assess specific knowledge deficits related to rheumatoid arthritis, cardiopulmonary manifestations, and physical therapy management	To provide a baseline, ongoing assessment and response to interventions
Define outcome criteria: reversal or mitigation of the signs and symptoms	To provide a basis for defining treatment goals and criteria for discontinuing treatment
Promote a caring, supportive patient-therapist relationship	To focus on treating the patient with rheumatoid arthritis rather than the rheumatoid arthritis
Consider every patient interaction an opportunity for education	To promote patient's sense of responsibility for wellness and health promotion
Instruct regarding avoidance of respiratory infections, nutrition, hydration and fluid balance, exercise, stress management, quality rest and sleep, joint protection, and movement efficiency	To promote cooperation and active participation in treatment
Reinforce medication schedule	
Teach, demonstrate, and provide feedback on interventions that can be self-administered	Between-treatment interventions are as important as treatments themselves to provide cumulative treatment effect
Teach patient to balance activity and rest	Optimal balance between activity and rest is essential to exploit short-term, long-term, and preventive effects of mobilization and exercise
Prepare a personalized handout with a listing and description of the exercises and their prescription parameters; precautions are emphasized	The patient can follow the handout on her own between supervised treatments to maximize the cumulative benefits of the treatments

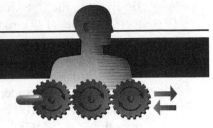

CHAPTER 18

Stroke with Sleep Apnea

PATHOPHYSIOLOGY

Stroke is an acute neurologic injury involving the blood vessels of the brain. It is manifested as cerebral ischemia and infarction or cerebral hemorrhage. The arteries most commonly affected are the middle cerebral artery and the internal carotid artery. Cerebral ischemia results from thrombosis or embolism. Thrombosis accounts for about 90% of all stroke cases. It usually occurs in older individuals (60 to 90 years old) and is characterized by atherosclerosis in the cerebral arteries. Embolism tends to occur in younger individuals. Hemorrhage results from rupture of an aneurysm, arteriovenous malformation, trauma, or hypertension. The extent of deficits caused by a stroke depends on the area of the brain that is affected. Thrombotic strokes cause transient symptoms whereas embolic strokes occur abruptly with fluctuating symptoms. The most common signs and symptoms of stroke are contralateral paralysis; contralateral sensory loss; sensory and motor loss in the face, neck, and upper extremity; dysphagia or aphagia with involvement of the dominant hemisphere; spatial and perceptual problems, such as neglect of the affected side; deterioration in judgment; behavioral change; anosognosia; and contralateral hemianopia. The pathogenesis of stroke includes atherosclerosis, lipohyalinosis, dilation of an aneurysm, venous thrombosis, emboli from the heart, decreased perfusion pressure, increased blood viscosity with inadequate cerebral blood flow, and rupture of a blood vessel in the subarachnoid space or intracerebral tissue. Cardiopulmonary manifestations of stroke include breathing irregularities, hypotonia of the respiratory muscles, chest wall asymmetry, impaired saliva control, weak ineffective cough, movement inefficiency, impaired movement economy, and cardiac dysrhythmias.

Sleep apnea is a condition characterized by collapse of the pharyngeal structures in the upper airway during sleep. The condition is caused by an anatomic abnormality, an abnormality of the protective mechanisms during swallowing, or reduced tone of the upper airway musculature. This leads to significant fluctuations in arterial oxygen levels during sleep. Large negative intrathoracic pressures are generated to overcome the resistance of the occluded upper airway. Venous return and systemic blood pressure are increased. Patients may have 60 to 120 apneic episodes a night, which can significantly compromise their daytime function. The clinical presentation includes reports of chronically disrupted night's sleep, waking in the night gasping for air, fatigue and somnolence during the day, and complaints by the patient's partner of periods of loud snoring.

Case Study

The patient is a 73-year-old man. He is a retired plumber who enjoys traveling, golf, and swimming. He lives on the outskirts of a large metropolitan area in a single-story home with his wife. He is 5 feet 9.5 inches (177 cm) tall and weighs 198 pounds (90 kg); his body mass index is 29. He had smoked socially in the past but not for many years. Six months ago, his pulmonary function test results were at the low end of the normal range. He collapsed at home. He was found 12 hours later when his wife returned from a weekend trip. On admission to the emergency room, he was diagnosed with a right cerebral vascular accident and left side paralysis. His heart rate was 118 beats per minute and his blood pressure was 163/100 mm Hg. He had a rapid shallow breathing pattern, and crackles were audible in both bases. Within a few days he developed moderately severe spasticity in the left arm and left shoulder pain. His past medical history included sleep apnea, which was diagnosed 6 months ago. His symptoms included loud snoring and significant apneic episodes at night that caused him to waken and gasp for air. A trial of nighttime ventilation (continuous positive airway pressure [CPAP]) was not successful because he had difficulty adjusting to the face mask. The patient is also edentulous and has poorly fitting dentures.

Oxygen Transport Deficits: Observed and Potential

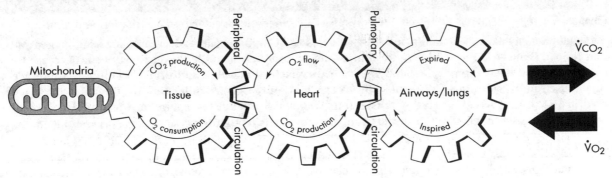

↓ Aerobic capacity
↑ Muscle weakness
Unilateral paresis
Movement inefficiency
↓ Movement economy
↑ Oxygen consumption of
    spastic muscles
↓ Oxygen consumption of
    flaccid muscles
Fatigue
Sleep deprivation

Compression of heart due
    to postural list to left
↑ Myocardial work

↓ Airway diameter
↑ Airway resistance
Mucus retention
↓ Saliva control
Aspiration
Hypotonia of pharyngeal
    structures
Upper airway obstruction
Age-related decrease in rate of
    mucociliary transport
Age-related depression of
    cough reflex
Lung compression on
    paralyzed side
↓ Volumes on paralyzed
    side
Age-related increase in airway
    closure
↑ Closing volumes on
    affected side
↓ Chest wall excursion
Chest wall asymmetry
    (leans to paralyzed side)
Abnormal hemidiaphragm
    excursion on the
    paralyzed side
↓ Cough reflex
↓ Cough effectiveness
Abnormal breathing
    pattern
Nocturnal breathing
    disturbance
↓ Respiratory muscle
    strength
↓ Chest wall motion
↓ Volumes and capacities
↓ Forced expiratory flow
    rates
Nocturnal hypoxemia and
    desaturation
Shortness of breath
↑ Use of accessory
    respiratory muscles
↓ Myoelectric activity of
    respiratory muscles on
    paralyzed side

Systemic hypertension
Atherosclerosis

↓ Lymph flow
↓ Lymphatic drainage

Blood:
    ↓ Viscosity due to
        medications

↑ Increase
↓ Decrease

Physical Therapy Diagnosis: Altered cardiorespiratory function: alveolar hypoventilation and shunt

Signs and Symptoms: Abnormal arterial blood gases (ABGs), hypoxemia, decreased arterial oxygen saturation (Sao_2), reduced arousal, shortness of breath, decreased left hemidiaphragm excursion, decreased muscle activity of the left intercostals, abdominals, paravertebral muscles, and pectoral muscles, use of accessory muscles of respiration on exertion, electrocardiogram (ECG) irregularities, hypertension, increased myocardial work, increased oxygen demand at submaximal work rates, age-related loss of elastic recoil of the lungs, reduced mucociliary transport rate, and decreased cough reflex and effectiveness

INTERVENTIONS	RATIONALE
Monitor vital signs, ABGs, ECG, Sao_2 and signs of cardiopulmonary respiratory insufficiency before, during, after, and between treatments	To provide a baseline, ongoing assessment and measure of treatment response
Define outcome criteria: reversal or mitigation of the signs and symptoms	To provide a basis for defining treatment goals and criteria for discontinuing treatment
Maximize duration in erect, relaxed, upright positions	To optimize alveolar ventilation and the distributions of ventilation, perfusion, and ventilation and perfusion matching, lung volumes and capacity, and reduce airway closure
Maximize duration in the upright position and moving	
Monitor vital signs and Sao_2 during treatments	
Ensure that patient's blood pressure is within acceptable limits before, during, and after treatment	To exploit the *acute* effects of mobilization/exercise on cardiopulmonary function and gas exchanges (i.e., maximize alveolar ventilations, optimize the distributions of ventilation, perfusion, and ventilation and perfusion matching, increase functional residual capacity, decrease airway closure, decrease airway resistance, increase lung compliance, increase mucociliary transport, decrease secretion accumulation, promote pulmonary lymph flow and lymphatic drainage)
	To ensure that patient is not exposed to further risk of stroke, vital signs are recorded before, during, and after treatment; blood pressure must be maintained within acceptable limits
	To facilitate coughing and airway clearance by optimizing the length-tension relationships of the respiratory muscles in the erect, upright positions and of the abdominal muscles
	To facilitate normal thoracoabdominal motion
	To mobilize secretions from the peripheral to central airways for clearance with exercise-induced deep breaths and spontaneous coughing
	To stimulate exercise-induced cardiopulmonary responses to optimize alveolar ventilation and airway clearance
When in bed, promote frequent body position changes coordinated with breathing control and coughing maneuvers; change position every 1-2 hr	To promote physiological "stir-up" to increase alveolar volume and ventilation, reduce airway closure, reduce compression atelectasis
Frequent body position changes with least time in left side lying	To enhance mucociliary transport and minimize bacterial colonization, multiplication, and infection
Minimize duration in supine; avoid supine for sleeping	To avoid apneic episodes and apneic hypoxemia in supine; tongue falls back and apposes the lateral and posterior walls of the pharyngeal lumen
	To minimize positional hypoxemia caused by weight of abdomen and restriction of descent of the diaphragm in supine
	To promote quality sleep; optimize physiological effects of sleep

INTERVENTIONS	RATIONALE
Minimize neck flexion	Neck flexion is minimized by using a soft, nonrestrictive cervical collar

360 degree positional rotation side to side
  ¾ supine to either side
  ¾ prone to either side
  Supine, head of bed up
	To optimize cardiopulmonary function and gas exchange

Maximize patient's comfort in each position with optimal support for left shoulder, arm, and leg in all body positions	To reduce suffering, maximize the therapeutic benefits of each position, and maximize patient's ability to cooperate with treatment
Promote adequate rest and sleep; minimize effects of sleep apnea	To maximize physiological benefits of sleep, minimize hypersomnalence during waking hours, and increase arousal

Physical Therapy Diagnosis: Altered cardiopulmonary function: altered breathing pattern caused by hypotonia of chest wall muscles, residual chest wall asymmetry and deformity of thoracic cavity, and sleep apnea

Signs and Symptoms: Increased respiratory insufficiency, shortness of breath, and use of the accessory muscles of respiration; loss of normal chest wall motion, abnormal thoracoabdominal motion, classic hemiplegic posture (uneven shoulders, lean to affected side, affected arm in sling support for pain), circumduction of affected leg, and reduced electrical activity of inspiratory muscles on the involved side

INTERVENTIONS	RATIONALE
Monitor breathing patterns (tidal volume and respiratory rate, chest wall excursion, and symmetry)	To provide a baseline, ongoing assessment and measure of treatment response
Define outcome criteria: reversal or mitigation of the signs and symptoms	To provide a basis for defining treatment goals and criteria for discontinuing treatment
Manual stretching and mobilization of the chest wall coordinated with body positioning and breathing control maneuvers	To stimulate normal varied breathing pattern (i.e., changes in rate and depth) and minimize monotonous tidal ventilation

Range-of-motion exercises:
  Head and neck
  Upper extremities
  Chest wall
  Lower extremities
	To stimulate a ventilatory response
	To stimulate recruitment of paralyzed muscles
	To reduce spasticity

Apply sling to left arm when mobilizing patient	To maximize comfort and stability
Promote upright position (i.e., erect sitting; standing and walking)	To mobilize the chest wall and promote improved alveolar ventilation, improved distributions of ventilation, perfusion, and ventilation and perfusion metching, and symmetric breathing pattern

Postural correction:
  Head and neck alignment
  Sitting (upright, erect)
  Standing
  Walking with an ankle foot orthosis and tripod
	To optimize alveolar ventilation, mucociliary transport, airway clearance, three-dimensional chest wall movement; minimize accessory muscle use
	Upright position facilitates nerve impulse transmission to inspiratory muscles
	To optimize postural alignment and its effects on cardiopulmonary function, minimize residual musculoskeletal dysfunction, and minimize the risk of falling and its sequelac
	To reduce thoracic blood volume and closure of the dependent airways and minimize airway closure
	To optimize fluid pressure and volume regulating mechanisms in the systemic circulation

Continued.

INTERVENTIONS	RATIONALE
Promote side lying positions for sleeping and avoidance of neck flexion	Episodes of sleep apnea increase in the supine position; neck flexion further narrows the pharyngeal lumen Sleep apnea is associated with abnormal breathing patterns during sleep, which contributes to apneic hypoxemia; sleep is nonrestorative To minimize effects of apneic hypoxemia, which could contribute to further cerebral dysfunction

Physical Therapy Diagnosis: Risk of pulmonary aspiration and impaired airway protection resulting from neuromuscular weakness, hypotonia of the posterior pharyngeal structures, sleep apnea, and improperly fitting false teeth

Signs and Symptoms: Increased cardiorespiratory insufficiency, asymmetric breathing pattern, aberrant postural alignment, snoring, sleep disturbance, waking unrested in the morning, upper airway obstruction, depressed cough, depressed cough effectiveness, decreased Pao_2 and Sao_2, complaints about fit of false teeth, inability to chew food thoroughly, choking and discomfort, increased heart rate and blood pressure, atelectasis, intrapulmonary shunt, spasticity of the muscles of respiration, chest wall, upper airway, mouth and face, abdomen and limbs, abnormal gag and cough reflex, age-related decrease in rate of mucociliary transport, age-related depression of cough reflex and effectiveness, increased pulmonary secretions, recumbency, and restricted mobility

INTERVENTIONS	RATIONALE
Assess risks and incidence of pulmonary aspiration	To provide a baseline and ongoing assessment
Define outcome criteria: prevention, reversal, or mitigation of the signs and symptoms	To provide a basis for defining treatment goals and criteria for discontinuing treatment
At rest, place patient in bed with head of bed up (minimally 10-30 degrees) and in side lying	To minimize the risk of oral and gastric secretions entering the upper airway
Place in high Fowler's position	
Recommend dental review	To ensure that false teeth fit well, are comfortable; maximize chewing ability, minimize risk of aspiration, maximize nutrition
Work with speech pathologist regarding swallowing difficulty	To reinforce recommendations of speech pathologist regarding aspiration avoidance and facilitating swallowing
Patient exercises 45-60 minutes after feeds	To ensure that food is further down gastrointestinal tract after meals and has the least risk of being regurgitated with exercise
Recommend side lying positions for sleeping and when lying down	Avoid aspiration associated with the supine position Avoid obstruction of the upper airway with lax oropharyngeal structures; minimize snoring and sleep disruption
Review with team if patient is a candidate for sleep apnea studies	Sleep apnea is a serious disorder and may require medical or surgical interventions if refractory to conservative management Risk of pulmonary aspiration may be increased if the patient is fatigued through sleep deprivation

Physical Therapy Diagnosis: Decreased activity and exercise tolerance

Signs and Symptoms: Aerobic deconditioning and low maximal functional work capacity, increased heart rate, blood pressure, rate pressure product, and minute ventilation at rest and submaximal work rates, impaired recovery from exercise, disproportionate exertion, breathlessness, and fatigue during and after exercise, neuromuscular deficits (including upper extremity flaccidity and lower extremity spasticity), pain in affected shoulder, and musculoskeletal deficits (including postural malalignment, chest wall asymmetry, unequal shoulder and pelvis level, drop foot, upper extremity in a sling, lean forward and to the affected side gait)

INTERVENTIONS	RATIONALE
Assess physical activity and exercise tolerance	To provide a baseline, ongoing assessment and measure of treatment response
Determine premorbid conditioning level	
Identify factors that interfere with mobilization and exercise	All factors that can affect oxygen transport must be considered and integrated into the exercise prescription
Define outcome criteria: reversal or mitigation of the signs and symptoms	To provide a basis for defining treatment goals and criteria for discontinuing treatment
Modified submaximal exercise test, such as exercise challenge of activities of daily living (ADL) or short walk	Exercise test is modified and submaximal to avoid negative effects of a maximal test, which is invalid in patients whose maximal capacity is limited by neuromuscular or musculoskeletal dysfunction
Monitor heart rate, blood pressure, rate pressure product, ECG, Sao_2, breathing pattern, and subjective responses of exertion and fatigue	To prescribe exercise within limits of that determined to be optimally therapeutic and safe by modified exercise test
	To ensure that blood pressure is within therapeutic and safe limits
Modified exercise training program	To exploit the *long-term* effects of mobilization/exercise on cardiopulmonary, oxygen transport and functional capacity (i.e., increase activity and exercise tolerance while minimizing fatigue and exhaustion and maximizing safety)
Type—walking, ergometry, aquatic exercise, swimming	
Interval training: several bouts of work and rest cycles	To optimize cardiopulmonary reserve capacity
Intensity—low-moderate, heart rate < 75% age-predicted maximum, blood pressure < 160 mm Hg, perceived exertion rating 3-5 (0-10 scale), fatigue < 3-4 (0-10 scale)	When patient's functional return has been maximized the exercise test is repeated, and the exercise prescription parameters are designed to maintain that level of function
Duration—20-40 minutes	
Frequency—3-1 times a day	As the patient's tolerance increases, the intensity and duration of the sessions increase and the frequency decreases
Course and progression—when plateau in functional improvement prescribe a maintenance program	
Reduce spasticity; normalize muscle tone	To promote normal cardiopulmonary function, normal biomechanics during gait, minimize undue oxygen demand, and minimize gait abnormalities and risk of falling
Reduce shoulder pain (e.g., heat, ice, range of motion, sling)	To reduce pain, minimize distraction, and maximize tolerance to physical activity
Orthotic fitting	Aids are fitted to optimize patient's body alignment, comfort, and safety
Cane	
Shoulder sling	Optimal body alignment and reduced sway from midline reduces excessive energy cost of ambulation and oxygen demand
Gait reeducation	
Lightweight, well-supported shoes	
General strengthening exercises (erect starting position) coordinated with breathing control (i.e., inspiration on extension, expiration on flexion)	Optimize coordination of breathing with physical activity and exercise
Optimize muscle strength and endurance where possible, particularly in postural muscles	Avoid isometric contractions, exercises requiring undue postural stabilization, Valsalva maneuver, straining, or breath holding
	To optimize respiratory muscle strength and endurance

Continued.

INTERVENTIONS	RATIONALE
Outcome measures: pulmonary function (i.e., maximal inspiratory and expiratory pressures, Sao$_2$, shortness of breath, perceived exertion, fatigue, and serial exercise tests) and functional outcomes, such as the ability to move or wheel purposefully in physical environment, bed mobility, transfers, ambulation, bathroom and kitchen skills	Outcome measures include physiological indices of cardiopulmonary function and oxygen transport, which are correlated with functional outcomes such as walking and propelling a wheel chair
Increased use of aids and devices (e.g., orthoses, ambulation aids, and selective use of a wheelchair)	To reduce undue oxygen demands and cardiopulmonary stress
	To preserve physiological reserve for worthwhile activities by using a wheelchair on excursions rather than expending energy in ambulation
Prescriptive rest within and between activities and exercise sessions	To optimize energy stores and avoid energy depletion
Optimize quality of patient's night sleep	To ensure that patient is receiving full physiological benefits of sleep; review use of noctural ventilation, sleeping positions, mattress quality, and bedtime environment and activities

Physical Therapy Diagnosis: Threats to oxygen transport and gas exchange, including pulmonary aspiration, chest wall asymmetry, increased energy and oxygen demands, depressed mucociliary transport and cough reflexes, reduced ventilatory capacity, reduced functional work capacity, morbidity associated with falls, restricted mobility, atherosclerosis, hypertension, dysrhythmias, and disturbed sleep

Signs and Symptoms: Abnormal breathing pattern, chest wall deformity, reduced chest wall expansion, asymmetric chest wall expansion, hypotonia of chest wall muscles, abnormal breathing coordination, altered cough and gag reflexes, decreased air entry, hypoxemia, decreased cough effectiveness, poorly protected upper airway, impaired saliva control, cardiopulmonary deconditioning, impaired movement efficiency and metabolic economy, and increased oxygen demands resulting from spasticity

INTERVENTIONS	RATIONALE
Monitor oxygen transport and gas exchange	To provide a baseline and ongoing assessment
Define outcome criteria: prevention, reversal, or mitigation of the signs and symptoms	To provide a basis for defining treatment goals and criteria for discontinuing treatment
Promote active living	To exploit the "stir-up" principle in this patient (i.e., maximize alveolar ventilation, ventilation and perfusion matching, facilitate mucociliary transport, promote airway clearance, facilitate spontaneous coughing, minimize bacterial colonization and multiplication, and facilitate lymphatic drainage)
Frequent mobilization during the day	
Body positioning	
Frequent changes in body positions	
	To maximize cardiopulmonary protection associated with an optimal conditioning level
Reduce spasticity with body positioning and neurological techniques	Spasticity compromises oxygen transport and gas exchange via several mechanisms: it affects the respiratory muscles, the accessory muscles, the abdominal muscles, and the limbs, which impedes range-of-motion and mobilizing and positioning the patient; it restricts chest wall movement; it impedes airway clearance via cough or suctioning; and it significantly increases oxygen demand and the demands on the oxygen transport system
Minimize postures and activity that facilitate spasticity	
Maximize postures and activity that inhibit spasticity	
	Determine whether spasticity reduction with body positioning could be augmented with antispasticity medication; consult with team if indicated

INTERVENTIONS	RATIONALE
Promote relaxation	Handle patient gently and with appropriate support and assist from others as necessary
	Speak to patient in calm, reassuring manner
	Observe what factors in the social and physical environment stimulate or reduce spasticity and incorporate this information during treatment

Physical Therapy Diagnosis: Risk of negative sequelae of restricted mobility

Signs and Symptoms: Reduced activity and exercise tolerance, muscle atrophy, flaccidity, reduced muscle strength and endurance, decreased oxygen transport efficiency, increased heart rate, blood pressure, and minute ventilation at submaximal work rates, reduced respiratory muscle strength and endurance, circulatory stasis, thromboemboli (e.g., pulmonary emboli), pressure areas, skin breakdown and ulceration

INTERVENTIONS	RATIONALE
Monitor negative sequelae of restricted mobility	To promote a baseline and ongoing assessment
Define outcome criteria: prevention, avoidance, reversal, or mitigation of the signs and symptoms	To provide a basis for defining treatment goals and criteria for discontinuing treatment
Mobilization and exercise prescription	To exploit the *preventive* effects of mobilization and exercise (i.e., mobilization and exercise enhance the efficiency of all steps in the oxygen transport pathway)

Physical Therapy Diagnosis: Knowledge deficit

Signs and Symptoms: Lack of information about hemiplegia, sleep apnea, relationship to heart disease, nocturnal ventilation, preventive measures, and complications

INTERVENTIONS	RATIONALE
Determine specific knowledge deficits related to pathology and physical therapy management	To provide a baseline and ongoing assessment
Define outcome criteria: reversal or mitigation of the signs and symptoms	To provide a basis for defining treatment goals and criteria for discontinuing treatment
Promote a caring, supportive patient-therapist relationship	To focus on treating the patient with a stroke rather than the stroke
Consider every patient interaction an opportunity for patient education	To promote patient's sense of responsibility for wellness, health promotion, and prevention
Instruct regarding optimal functional work capacity, including avoidance of respiratory tract infections, nutrition, weight control, hydration and fluid balance, sleep, and exercise	To promote cooperation and participation in treatment
	To promote weight control through proper diet and exercise to improve general health and help reduce blood pressure and severity of sleep apnea
Reinforce purpose of medication and its prescription parameters and schedule	To ensure that patient understands the importance of taking hypertension medications and taking them on schedule
Teach, demonstrate, and provide feedback on interventions that can be self-administered	Between-treatment interventions are as important as treatments themselves to provide cumulative treatment effect
Teach patient to balance activity and rest	Optimal balance between activity and rest is essential to exploit acute, long-term, and preventive effects of mobilization and exercise
Review with the patient nocturnal ventilation, its indications, and benefits	To encourage the patient to reconsider CPAP at night to maximize the benefits of a night's sleep
Suggest use of nasal CPAP rather than face mask	Many patients find the nasal CPAP more comfortable than the face mask
Prepare a personalized handout with a listing and description of the exercises and their prescription parameters; precautions are emphasized	The patient can follow the handout instructions on his own between supervised treatments
	The content of the handout is reviewed with the patient and modified as the patient's functional capacity improves

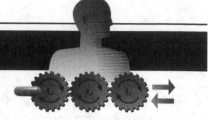

CHAPTER 19

Late Sequelae of Poliomyelitis

PATHOPHYSIOLOGY

The last poliomyelitis epidemic in the Western world was in the 1950s and early 1960s. The incidence of poliomyelitis dramatically decreased with the advent of the Salk and Sabin vaccines. Poliomyelitis continues to be endemic, however, throughout most developing nations. The disease is caused by a virus that attacks the anterior horn cells of the spinal cord. Although spinal poliomyelitis was the most common form, bulbar and encephalatic forms also occurred. Involvement of the respiratory muscles necessitated mechanical ventilation. At that time use of the iron lung, a body tank that inflated the lungs using negative pressure, was prevalent. The disease was formerly known as infantile paralysis because children under the age of 10 years were primarily affected. Symptoms at onset included fever, chills, nuchal stiffness, and paresis. Of those patients who developed paralytic poliomyelitis, 50% made significant functional recovery. The remaining 50% had significant residual weakness, spinal and limb deformity, and functional loss. Most poliomyelitis survivors returned to school and carried on with their lives.

Some 30 to 35 years after onset, a significant proportion of survivors are experiencing new problems. These are termed the *late sequelae,* or the late effects, of poliomyelitis and include fatigue, weakness, pain, reduced endurance, shortness of breath, swallowing and choking difficulty, sleep disturbance, increased sensitivity to cold, and psychological problems. The cause of these problems has been attributed to overwork of both affected and unaffected musculature, biomechanical inefficiency, abnormal wear patterns through joints, terminal axon degeneration, impaired impulse transmission, and the confounding effect of aging. The incidence of late-onset problems is increased in individuals who had paralysis of all four limbs at onset, who had ventilatory complications, and who contracted the disease after the age of 10 years.

Case Study

The patient is a 55-year-old man. He is a lawyer who lives with his wife and two children in a small town. He is 22 pounds (10 kg) overweight. He has never smoked. He referred himself to a private physical therapy clinic for increased weakness and reduced endurance. His medical history includes poliomyelitis, which he contracted when he was 7 years old. He had generalized paralysis with ventilatory compromise; however, he was able to return to school within 8 months. He had residual left leg weakness, 3 cm limb length discrepancy, and moderately severe scoliosis. He walks with a long leg brace on the left leg and a cane. He has always pushed himself physically but had pushed himself harder over the past few years because he believed that he was deconditioning because his work is sedentary. He had been experiencing increased fatigue, pain, and muscle weakness in both legs and in his right arm. He has difficulty getting up in the morning and is extremely tired by midafternoon. In addition, he becomes short of breath at intensities of exercise that he previously tolerated. He can now walk only one block.

Oxygen Transport Deficits: Observed and Potential

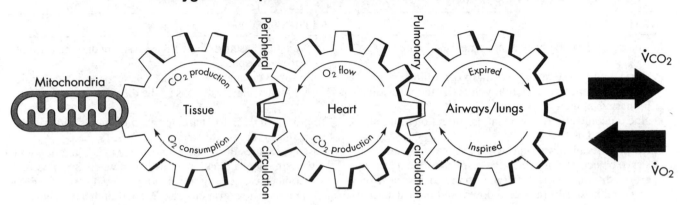

↓ Aerobic capacity	Distortion due to postural asymmetry	Hypotonia of pharyngeal structures
Muscle weakness	Axis deviation	Hypotonia of laryngeal structures
Muscle fatigue	Displacement	Dysphagia
Overuse/abuse of affected and nonaffected muscles	Age-related atherosclerosis	Choking problems
↓ Movement efficiency		Mucus retention
↓ Movement economy		Respiratory muscle weakness
		Abdominal muscle weakness
		↓ Maximal inspiratory pressure
		↓ Maximal expiratory pressure
		Ineffective cough
		↓ Chest wall excursion
		Chest wall asymmetry
		Distortion due to postural asymmetry
		↓ Volumes and capacities
		↓ Forced expiratory flow rates
		Impaired gas mixing

Systemic hypertension	Impaired gas exchange	↑ Increase
	↓ Lymph flow	↓ Decrease
	↓ Lymphatic drainage	

PHYSICAL THERAPY DIAGNOSES AND TREATMENT PRESCRIPTION

Physical Therapy Diagnosis: Decreased physical activity and exercise tolerance

Signs and Symptoms: Reduced pulmonary function (including maximal inspiratory and expiratory pressures), decreased functional work capacity, decreased aerobic capacity, decreased mechanical efficiency, decreased metabolic economy, abnormal pulmonary function (e.g., restrictive lung dysfunction secondary to chest wall deformity and respiratory muscle weakness), complaints of reduced endurance and dyspnea, complaints of disproportionate fatigue, complaints of joint and muscle pain, complaints of disrupted and nonrestorative sleep, complaints of being unable to perform activities of daily living (ADL), complaints of being unable to perform a full day's work

INTERVENTIONS	RATIONALE
Monitor response to physical activities and exercise	To provide a baseline, ongoing assessment and measure of treatment response
Perform a multisystem assessment to determine the effects of the late sequelae of poliomyelitis, including cardiopulmonary dysfunction	Polio survivors may have primary or secondary late cardiopulmonary manifestations of the disease
Define outcome criteria: reversal or mitigation of the signs and symptoms	To provide a basis for defining treatment goals and criteria for discontinuing treatment
Perform a modified walking steady-rate exercise test	Based on the results of the exercise test in conjunction with the clinical examination, to establish whether a modified aerobic exercise program is indicated and if so its parameters; or an exercise program is contraindicated because it contributes to overuse abuse and if so to establish the parameters to maximize functional capacity
Observe objective and subjective responses (perceived exertion, discomfort/pain, fatigue) to increasing intensity of exercise, steady-rate, cool down, and immediate and long-term (day or two) recovery	

Exercise prescription:
  Type—walking with optimal orthotic fitting and footwear (optimally fitted, supporting, cushioned, and lightweight)
  Intensity—within the limits of discomfort/pain, such as <3 (0-10 scale); within the limits of fatigue, such as < 3 (0-10 scale)
  Select smooth, paved surfaces; avoid hills
  Duration—10-30 minutes with rests
  Frequency—daily
  Course and progression—as indicated; maintain intensity within specified limits
  Type—water exercises
  Intensity—within the limits of discomfort/pain, such as < 3 (0-10 scale); within the limits of fatigue, such as < 3 (0-10 scale)
  Duration—10-30 minutes with rests
  Frequency—1-2 times a week
  Course and progression—as indicated; maintain intensity within specified limits
	To exploit the *long-term* effects of exercise in a polio survivor with requisite physiological reserve capacity (i.e., optimize aerobic capacity and efficiency of oxygen transport at all steps of the pathway within the restrictions of the modified exercise prescription, increase respiratory muscle strength and endurance, reduce dyspnea, enhance biomechanical efficiency and movement economy, and improve motivation)
	Age-related decrease in motor units in polio survivors contributes to a disproportionate decrease in function, which predisposes the patient to overuse of the affected muscles
	Patients with no demonstrable physiological reserve capacity will deteriorate given a conventional exercise program; functional work capacity in these patients is enhanced with judicious activity and exercise reduction, pacing, energy conservation, prescriptive rest periods, and major changes in lifestyle and employment and the use of walking/locomotion aids

Assess muscle strength of all muscle groups (polio affected and nonaffected)	To provide a baseline, ongoing assessment and measure of treatment response To discriminate weak versus fatigued polio-affected muscles To identify all muscle groups affected by polio; frequently muscles other than those identified by the patient are affected

INTERVENTIONS	RATIONALE

Muscle strengthening prescription for weak polio-affected muscle groups:
  Type—nonfatiguing strengthening exercises
  Intensity—low resistance exercise (i.e., below the fatigue threshold for each muscle group)
  Duration—3 sets of 10 repetitions
  Frequency—daily to 3 times a week
  Course and progression—as indicated by increase in muscle strength or decreased rate of deterioration and loss of strength
	To strengthen *weak* polio-affected and overused polio-unaffected muscles
	Avoid exposing fatigued polio-affected muscles to strengthening exercises; *fatigued* muscles deteriorate further with use and require rest (either locally or generally)
	To provide a basic strength for ADL and ambulation and efficient postural support and stability
	To optimize alignment, enhance mechanical efficiency, and minimize the metabolic cost of activity and ambulation; hence optimize oxygen transport
	To maximize functional capacity without undue strain on the musculature

Prescriptive rests:
  Within an exercise session
  Regular rest periods
  Reduced exercise intensity
  Between exercise sessions
Pacing
Energy conservation
	To optimize physiological recovery of muscle energy stores and energy transfer systems with prescriptive rests interspersed within and between exercise sessions

Optimize postural alignment:
  Postural correction in various postures
  Postural correction exercises
  Orthoses and walking aids
	To maximize biomechanical efficiency and minimize metabolic energy cost of physical activity, particularly walking
	Minimizing the energy cost of walking maximizes the energy available for ADL and increases overall endurance

Physical Therapy Diagnosis: Discomfort and pain: muscle aches, cramps, twitching, joint pain, deformity, biomechanical stress in affected and unaffected (compensating) limbs, spinal curvature and deformity, muscle weakness, muscle imbalance

Signs and Symptoms: Complaints of discomfort and pain in polio-affected or unaffected muscles and joints at rest or on exertion, reduced ability to perform ADL, altered gait, musculoskeletal discomfort/pain secondary to compensatory biomechanical changes for muscle paresis, limb length discrepancy, or deformity, and musculoskeletal discomfort/pain from repetitive strain (e.g., crutch or cane walking)

INTERVENTIONS	RATIONALE
Monitor pain; type, triggers, intensity, duration and course (what makes it better) Define outcome criteria: reversal or mitigation of the signs and symptoms	To provide a baseline, ongoing assessment and measure of treatment response To provide a basis for defining treatment goals and criteria for discontinuing treatment

Correct postural alignment deficits
  Postural correction in different positions (e.g., sitting, standing, walking, and lying down)
  Postural correction exercises
  Pelvic tilt
  Stretching exercises
	To analyze contributing causes of pain; prioritize these and treat
	Pain management is a priority because pain compromises function and functional work capacity

Select appropriate walking aids and devices; types:
  Long leg brace—review fit, its weight
  Shoe raise—for limb length discrepancy
  Cane—review use and efficiency
  Electric wheelchair/scooter—review potential use
Parameters:
  Intermittent or continuous use of aids depending on the activity and its physical demands on the patient
	Walking aids and devices maintain alignment and conserve energy
	Work with the patient and orthotist to achieve optimal orthotic fitting; patient's input is essential to ensure that the devices are acceptable, fit comfortably, enhance function, and increase the frequency with which they are worn
	Excessive weight of a brace, orthosis, or shoe significantly increases the energy cost of walking

Continued.

INTERVENTIONS	RATIONALE
	Muscles of polio survivors atrophy readily; intermittent use of orthoses and aids may initially be preferable to continuous use of these aids to provide specific muscles with some rest but not impose relative disuse
	Electric wheelchairs/scooters increase functional capacity by conserving energy for specific activities rather than expending excessive energy during ambulation
	This patient walks at significantly increased energy cost because of muscle weakness, muscle imbalance, limb length discrepancy, use of cane, and postural deformity
	A treatment goal is to minimize the energy cost of walking by normalizing biomechanics wherever feasible

Physical Therapy Diagnosis: Fatigue: reduced physiological muscle reserve, impaired neuromuscular transmission, deconditioning, reduced movement efficiency and metabolic economy, disturbed nonrestorative sleep, cardiopulmonary dysfunction

Signs and Symptoms: Inability to perform ADL, inability to complete a day's work without excessive fatigue, loss of function, reduced walking capacity, inability to participate in social and recreational activities, nonrestorative sleep; waking up fatigued, cycle of fatigue, reduced activity and greater fatigue, patient reports hitting the "polio wall" at a comparable time each day, dyspnea, reduced endurance, need to rest frequently, and need for increased sleep

INTERVENTIONS	RATIONALE
Monitor fatigue and its relationship to work, exercise, stress, and diet	To provide a baseline, ongoing assessment and measure of treatment response
Define outcome criteria: reversal or mitigation of the signs and symptoms	To provide a basis for defining treatment goals and criteria for discontinuing treatment
Patient completes an activity-rest log	Patient completes a log of activity and rest patterns and the associated level of fatigue during activities and before and after rests and a night's sleep
	Based on the log, the patient is advised to maintain fatigue (in addition to discomfort/pain) at a subthreshold level (the level at which a disproportionate amount of time is required to recover)
	The term *polio wall* describes a "point of no return fatigue," which occurs for many patients at the same time of day
Monitor quality of rest and patient's night sleep	Break negative cycle of overtiring, which compromises ability to restore from rest and sleep
Teach patient to anticipate fatigue triggers (e.g., type of activity, intensity or duration of that activity), to maintain fatigue below a predetermined threshold (e.g., 3 on a 0-10 scale), and rest until fatigue is down to a predetermined lower limit (e.g., 1 on the 0-10 scale)	To determine the balance between activity and level of exertion and an acceptable fatigue level or threshold that the patient can adequately recover from physiologically
Pace activity	Rest is prescribed as objectively as exercise in that injudicious rest and restricted activity are deleterious to health, well-being, and function; excessive muscle work in poliomyelitis survivors contributes to further muscle deterioration and loss of function
Teach energy conservation strategies	The fatigue threshold is set from an analysis of the activity-rest log and represents the highest level of fatigue from which the patient can readily recover
Review orthoses and walking aids, refer to orthotist for orthoses as indicated	To optimize patient's alignment, and minimize biomechanical stresses (hence muscle and joint pain) and optimize movement efficiency and metabolic economy of movement (hence reduce fatigue)

INTERVENTIONS	RATIONALE
Review work, home, and leisure activities and make recommendations	Recommend working part-time or flexihours to work within limits of physiological capacity
Ergonomic assessment of work and home settings	To minimize undue biomechanical strain, fatigue, undue energy expenditure
	Drastic recommendations may need to be made (e.g., change work hours, change living accommodation, reduce commute time, change habitual activities such as sports and exercise, and learn how to be assertive to modify others' expectations)
Weight control and optimal nutrition	Weight control and optimal nutrition are priorities for patients with chronic disabilities, including the late sequelae of poliomyelitis; in addition to increasing fatigue, excess weight contributes to increased muscle and joint strain and overuse, altered biomechanics and alignment, and reduced endurance and strength; optimal nutrition is essential to maximize muscle fuels for optimal functional work performance
Promote optimal rest periods and a good night's sleep	To exploit those aspects of rest that are optimally recuperative for the patient and integrate these into his ADL as much as possible
	To review the patient's sleep habits, the quality and quantity of his night's sleep, and his mattress to ensure that he is maximally restored in the morning

Physical Therapy Diagnosis: Threats to oxygen transport and gas exchange

Signs and Symptoms: Further reduction in exercise tolerance, increasing fatigue, shortness of breath on exertion, worsening endurance, increasing incapacity to perform ADL, work, and leisure activities, increasing choking and swallowing problems, deterioration in pulmonary function, increasing weight, hypertension, restricted mobility, weak cough, ineffective cough, weak abdominal muscles, increasing chest wall deformity, increasing postural deformity, impaired sleep, hypertension, increased risk of infections, increasing respiratory muscle weakness, sleep apnea, musculoskeletal deformity, inefficient, metabolically costly gait, obesity, pain, generalized weakness, and risk of choking and aspiration

INTERVENTIONS	RATIONALE
Monitor threats to oxygen transport and gas exchange	To provide a baseline and ongoing assessment
Define outcome criteria: prevention, reversal, or mitigation of the signs and symptoms	To provide a basis for defining treatment goals and criteria for discontinuing treatment
Maintain optimal functional work capacity	To exploit *preventive* effects of exercise; exercise prescribed specifically to optimize function and conditioning level while minimizing the risk of further overuse
Maintain ideal body weight
Reinforce optimal nutrition and balanced diet	Depending on the severity of muscle wasting and paralysis and abnormalities of growth and development, body mass index should be at the low to mid portion of the normal range (20-25)
Reinforce optimal hydration	Patients with loss of muscle mass should have body mass indices below normal proportional to reduced muscle mass
Promote a good night's sleep	To promote good general health and maintain optimal immunity

Continued.

INTERVENTIONS	RATIONALE
Teach Heimlich maneuver; self-application and with assist by family member or others	To ensure that patient is protected in the event of an airway obstruction
Reinforce avoiding troublesome foods; avoidance of eating and talking, eat slowly; have head up if lying down after meals	
Avoid exercise for 45-60 minutes after meals	
Reinforce eating small, frequent meals	
Pace activities; discontinue activity when predetermined fatigue or pain thresholds are reached; rest until fatigue and pain have subsided to lower acceptable limits	

Physical Therapy Diagnosis: Risk of negative sequelae of restricted mobility

Signs and Symptoms: Reduced activity and exercise tolerance, muscle atrophy and reduced muscle strength, decreased oxygen transport efficiency, increased heart rate, blood pressure, and minute ventilation at submaximal work rates, reduced respiratory muscle strength and endurance, circulatory stasis, thromboemboli (e.g., pulmonary emboli), pressure areas, skin redness, skin breakdown and ulceration

INTERVENTIONS	RATIONALE
Monitor the negative sequelae of restricted mobility	To provide a baseline and ongoing assessment
Define outcome criteria: prevention, reversal, or mitigation of the signs and symptoms	To provide a basis for defining treatment goals and criteria for discontinuing treatment
Mobilization and exercise prescription	To exploit the *preventive* effects of mobilization and exercise
	Mobilization and exercise optimize circulating blood volume and enhance the efficiency of all steps in the oxygen transport pathway

Physical Therapy Diagnosis: Knowledge deficit

Signs and Symptoms: Lack of information about the late sequelae of poliomyelitis, its management, and prognosis

INTERVENTIONS	RATIONALE
Determine specific knowledge deficits related to late sequelae of poliomyelitis, its cardiopulmonary manifestations, and physical therapy management	To promote patient's sense of responsibility for wellness, health promotion, and prevention
Define outcome criteria: reversal or mitigation of the signs and symptoms	To provide a basis for defining treatment goals and criteria for discontinuing treatment
Promote a caring and supportive patient-therapist relationship	To treat the patient with the late sequelae of poliomyelitis rather than the late sequelae of poliomyelitis
Consider every patient interaction an opportunity for patient education	To promote cooperation and active participation of the patient in treatment
Instruct regarding maximizing function, rest and sleep, nutrition, weight control, hydration and fluid balance, exercise, activity pacing, activity-rest pacing, orthoses and mobility aids, and flu prophylaxis	To promote patient's sense of responsibility for health, wellness, and health promotion
Teach, demonstrate, and provide feedback on interventions that can be self-administered	Between-treatment interventions are as important as treatments themselves to provide cumulative treatment effect
Teach patient to balance activity and rest	Optimal balance between activity and rest is essential to exploit acute, long-term, and preventive effects of mobilization and exercise
Provide individualized written handout on general information, treatment, and treatment prescription	To promote cumulative benefits of the treatment

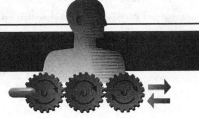

CHAPTER 20

Chronic Renal Failure

PATHOPHYSIOLOGY

Chronic renal failure (CRF) is a progressive condition in which there is scarring of the kidneys and loss of function. The causes of CRF are recurrent infections and exacerbations of nephritis, obstruction of the urinary tract, destruction of blood vessels from diabetes, long-term hypertension, and use of nephrotoxic drugs. Chronic renal failure has multisystemic manifestations. It affects the neuromuscular, cardiovascular, pulmonary, gastrointestinal, endocrine, hematologic, immunologic, and integumentary systems. It is characterized by four stages of kidney damage: decreased renal reserve, renal insufficiency, renal failure, and end-stage renal disease. Some nephrons remain intact and others are destroyed. The functioning nephrons hypertrophy and produce an increased volume of filtrate with increased tubular reabsorption. These changes cause fluid and electrolyte imbalance, leading to an increase or decrease in urinary output, solute retention, an increase in nitrogenous products in the blood, impaired potassium and hydrogen ion excretion, and acidosis. Anemia occurs because there is a decrease in the secretion of erythropoeitin by the kidney, which results in a decrease in red blood cell production. Hyperuricemia, hypertension, and glucose intolerance are common signs of end-stage renal disease. In severe cases of renal failure, anorexia, persistant nausea, vomiting, dyspnea on minimal exertion, pitting edema, and pruritis are evident. Other changes include increase in skin pigmentation, muscular twitching, numbness of feet and legs, pericarditis, and pleuritis. Dialysis is indicated to replace kidney function with significant renal impairment. In severe cases, renal transplantation is indicated.

Case Study

The patient is a 32-year-old man. He is a graphic designer. He lives with his girlfriend in a downtown apartment. His body mass index is 18.5. He does not smoke. He had chronic renal failure secondary to recurrent bouts of nephritis. Over the past month he has become increasingly lethargic, irritable, fatigued, and short of breath on minimal exertion. He was admitted to hospital in renal failure. His glomerular filtration rate was 25% of normal; blood urea nitrogen and serum creatinine were significantly elevated. He had mild anemia and azotemia, which worsened with stress. He was in a state of metabolic acidosis. He had developed increasing problems with nocturia and polyuria. Clinical examination revealed pericarditis and pleuritis. He also experienced moderately severe muscle cramping and pain in his legs. He responded well to medical management aimed at normalizing fluid and electrolyte balance with dialysis, optimizing nutrition and caloric intake, minimizing secondary gastrointestinal complications and bleeding, and promoting comfort and rest.

Oxygen Transport Deficits: Observed and Potential

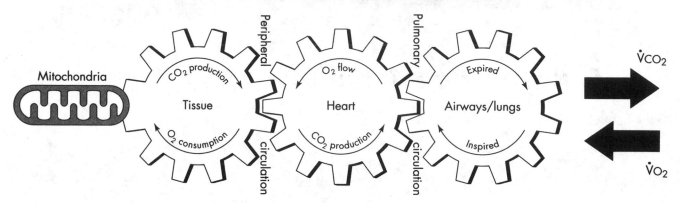

↓ Aerobic capacity
↓ Muscle strength
Edema
Impaired muscle blood
    flow
Muscle irritability
Oliguria
↓ Glomerular filtration
    rate
Abdominal distension
↑ Intraabdominal
    pressure

Tachycardia
Dysrhythmias
↑ Work of the heart
Congestive
    heart failure
Pericarditis

Airway obstruction
Airway closure
↑ Airflow resistance
Alveolar hemorrhage
↓ Compliance
↓ Vital capacity
↓ Residual volume
↓ Forced expiratory flow
    rates
Alveolar inflammation
Atelectasis
Pleuritis

Systemic hypertension

↑ Diffusing capacity
Shunt
Pulmonary hypertension
↓ Lymph flow
↓ Lymphatic drainage

Blood: ↓ Red blood production
Leukocytosis
↓ Hormone production of
    the kidneys (renin and
    angiotensin)
↑ Fluid retention
Hypervolemia
Hemodilution
Abnormal electrolyte
    balance
Anemia
↑ Serum creatinine
↑ Blood urea nitrogen
Azotemia
Thrombocytopenia
Altered platelet function

↑ Increase
↓ Decrease

PHYSICAL THERAPY DIAGNOSES AND TREATMENT PRESCRIPTION

Physical Therapy Diagnosis: Altered cardiopulmonary function caused by chronic renal failure (i.e., alveolar hypoventilation, pleuritis, pericarditis, and inefficient oxygen transport)

Signs and Symptoms: Reduced lung volumes, fluid accumulation, edema, accumulation of crystalloid solutes and waste products, altered electrolyte balance, altered acid-base balance, gastrointestinal distress, severe anemia, impaired efficiency of oxygen uptake and extraction at the tissue level, increased heart rate, increased blood pressure, decreased urine output, and electrolyte imbalance

INTERVENTIONS	RATIONALE
Serial monitoring of chronic renal insufficiency	To provide a baseline, ongoing assessment and measure of treatment response
Serial monitoring of cardiopulmonary manifestations of chronic renal failure	To provide an indication of how the exercise program should be modified with fluctuations in the patient's condition
Define outcome criteria: reversal or mitigation of the signs and symptoms	To provide a basis for defining treatment goals and criteria for discontinuing treatment
Mobilization coordinated with breathing control and coughing maneuvers	To exploit the *acute* effects of mobilization (i.e., increased alveolar volume, alveolar ventilation, functional residual capacity, ventilation-perfusion matching, decreased airway closure, increased mucociliary transport, increased airway clearance, increased lymph flow, increased diaphragmatic excursion)
Type—dangling over bed, transfer to chair, ambulating	
Intensity—exertion < 4 (0-10 scale) and within limits of comfort	
Duration—5-20 minutes	
Frequency—several times daily	
Cause and progression—as indicated	
Type: range-of-motion exercises coordinated with breathing control and coughing maneuvers	To exploit the cardiopulmonary benefits of range-of-motion exercises (i.e., ventilatory and cardiopulmonary effects)
Intensity—low resistance	
Duration—10-20 minutes	
Frequency—daily	
Course and progression—as indicated; discontinue when walking regularly	
360 degree positional rotation when resting in bed	To promote physiologic "stir-up" until fully ambulating
Frequent position changes (every 1-2 hr)	
Coordinate mobilization and body positioning with rest periods	To minimize undue fatigue and maximize patient's energy to optimize treatment effect

Physical Therapy Diagnosis: Decreased physical activity and exercise tolerance

Signs and Symptoms: Reduced capacity to perform ADL, increased heart rate, blood pressure, rate pressure product, minute ventilation, cardiac output, and perceived exertion at rest and during exercise, reduced maximal oxygen consumption, fatigue, generalized weakness, inability to produce erythropoietin, anemia, shortness of breath, defect in platelet function, osteodystrophy, renal rickets, joint pain, muscle cramping, and impaired blood flow to muscle

INTERVENTIONS	RATIONALE
Serial monitoring of blood work, including hemoglobin	To provide a baseline, ongoing assessment and measure of treatment response
Serial monitoring of nutritional status	
Serial monitoring of fluid and electrolyte status	
Serial monitoring of responses to a modified graded exercise tolerance test (GXTT)	
Define outcome criteria: reversal or mitigation of the signs and symptoms	To provide a basis for defining treatment goals and criteria for discontinuing treatment
Prescribe a comprehensive exercise program including aerobic exercise, strengthening exercises, and range-of-motion exercises	To exploit the combined effects of a comprehensive exercise program

Continued.

INTERVENTIONS	RATIONALE
Prescribe an exercise program based on the GXTT	To exploit the *long-term* effects of aerobic exercise and maximize patient's functional capacity; patient is a potential renal transplant candidate
Serial monitoring of fluid and electrolyte balance and general systemic status; modify the parameters of the exercise prescription as indicated	The fluid and electrolyte status of patients with chronic renal failure fluctuate daily, thus the exercise prescribed is precisely modified to maximize the benefit-to-risk ratio of each session
Serial monitoring of hemoglobin and adequacy of muscle blood flow	To prescribe exercise when anemia and nutrition are controlled and significant muscle blood flow abnormality is ruled out
Treat pain (e.g., heat, massage)	To minimize discomfort/pain and maximize treatment effect
Exercise prescription	To exploit the *long-term* effects of aerobic exercise when patient's status stabilizes
Type—walking	
Intensity—within limits of comfort, tolerance; exertion < 5 (0-10 scale)	To enhance walking endurance for functional activities
Duration—20-60 minutes	To maximize health benefits to optimize patient's cardiopulmonary capacity should he be slated for renal transplant
Frequency—several to 2 times a day	
Course and progression—as indicated; commensurate with physical status and well-being in any given day	As patient adapts to exercise stress, intensity and duration of sessions increase and frequency decreases.
Type—ergometer, cadence that is comfortably maintained	To enhance aerobic capacity with non–weight bearing exercise
Intensity—low; exertion < 5 (0-10 scale), discomfort/pain < 3 (0-10 scale)	
Frequency—1-2 times a day	
Duration—10-30 minutes	
Course and progression—as indicated	
Type—muscle strengthening exercises; arms and legs	Chronic renal failure can contribute to impaired muscle blood flow and nutrition; muscle does not have the normal capacity to adapt to exercise and is prone to injury
Intensity—low; light resistance, 3 sets of 10 repetitions	
Duration—20-30 minutes	
Frequency—alternate days	
Course and progression—as indicated	
Type—range-of-motion exercises	To maintain muscle at optimal length and joint flexibility
Upper extremity	
Trunk	
Lower extremity	
Intensity—minimal resistance	
Duration—10-20 minutes	
Frequency—daily	
Course and progression—as indicated	
Activity and exercise pacing	Physical activity and endurance can be augmented by judiciously reducing energy demands
Energy conservation techniques	
Prescriptive rest periods	
Restorative sleep	

Physical Therapy Diagnosis: Threats to oxygen transport: sequelae of chronic renal failure, deconditioning, continual constitutional debility and lethargy, iatrogenic effects of hemodialysis (bleeding, coagulopathies, pericarditis, hypotension, vascular access infections, hypoxemia) and medications, increased risk of infection, renal osteodystrophy, anemia, thromboses, pericarditis, pericardial effusion, cardiac tamponade, ascites, hypertension, atherosclerosis, congestive heart failure, arrhythmias, hyperlipidemia, fluid excess, hypoalbuminemia, capillary damage, pulmonary edema, pulmonary calcification, reduced diffusing capacity, azotemia, acidosis, suppression of red blood cell production, decreased survival time of red blood cells, bleeding, loss of blood through dialysis, thrombocytopenia, decreased platelet activity, decreased cardiac output, drug toxicity, and decreased renal perfusion

Signs and Symptoms: Hypoxemia, arterial desaturation, altered arterial blood gases (ABGs), arrhythmias, input > output, edema, weight gain, electrolyte imbalance, radiographic evidence of pleural effusions and pericardial fluid, increased work of breathing, increased work of the heart, malaise and lethargy, increased heart rate and blood pressure, decreased specific gravity, increased blood urea nitrogen, increased creatinine, fluid losses with nausea and vomiting, anorexia, drowsiness, inability to concentrate, memory deficits, high levels of nitrogenous wastes, decreased breath sounds, crackles/wheezes, chest pain, pallor, easy bruising and bleeding, and insomnia

INTERVENTIONS	RATIONALE
Serial monitoring of the signs and symptoms related to the cardiopulmonary manifestations of systemic dysfunction	To provide a baseline and follow systemic effects of chronic renal insufficiency
Define outcome criteria: reversal or mitigation of the signs and symptoms	To provide a basis for defining treatment goals and criteria for discontinuing treatment
Promote active living	To exploit the *preventive* effects of physical activity and exercise
Promote regular physical exercise	
Promote adherence to an exercise prescription	
Teach patient to balance activity and rest	

Physical Therapy Diagnosis: Fatigue

Signs and Symptoms: Verbalization of fatigue, physical expressions of fatigue, reduced activity, reduced exercise, and withdrawal from social and recreational activities

INTERVENTIONS	RATIONALE
Assess pathophysiological factors contributing to fatigue (e.g., anemia, poor nutrition, fluid imbalance, muscle weakness, cardiopulmonary deconditioning)	To discriminate the contribution of various factors to overall experience of fatigue in order to determine the degree to which fatigue is amenable to physical therapy management; and to modify treatments accordingly
Monitor fatigue using a semiquantitative or analog scale	To provide a baseline, ongoing assessment and index of treatment response
Define outcome criteria: prevention, reversal, or mitigation of the signs and symptoms	To provide a basis for defining treatment goals and criteria for discontinuing treatment
Teach the patient to log fatigue	Logging fatigue identifies its precipitating and mitigating factors; thus information is used by the patient to maintain low levels of fatigue, exercise at subthreshold levels, and to avoid exceeding fatigue levels, which do not respond as readily to rest periods
Teach activity pacing	Controlling fatigue improves functional capacity and minimizes the risk of chronic excessive fatigue
Teach energy conservation procedures	
Integrate rest periods within and between treatments	To prescribe rest periods objectively based on the quality and quantity of rest that has the optimal effect on the patient (i.e., maximally restorative)
Reinforce patient's nutritional plan	To promote good nutrition for optional performance, health, and well-being and minimize overworking the kidneys

Continued.

INTERVENTIONS	RATIONALE
Reinforce medication schedule	To reinforce medication schedule to maximize function and minimize suffering
Review the quality and quantity of patient's sleep and make recommendations	To review sleep pattern (i.e., quality and quantity, including presleep activities, mattress, pillows, noise, ventilation, warmth, eating, drinking, hours of sleep, number and duration of wakeful periods, what patient does when awake)

Physical Therapy Diagnosis: Risk of the negative sequelae of recumbency

Signs and Symptoms: Within 6 hours reduced circulating blood volume, decreased blood pressure on sitting and standing compared with supine, light-headedness, dizziness, syncope, increased hematocrit and blood viscosity, increased work of the heart, altered fluid balance in the lung, impaired pulmonary lymphatic drainage, decreased lung volumes and capacities, decreased functional residual capacity, increased closing volume, decreased arterial oxygen pressure (Pao_2) and arterial oxygen saturation (Sao_2)

INTERVENTIONS	RATIONALE
Monitor the signs and symptoms of the negative sequelae of recumbency	To provide a baseline, ongoing assessment and measure of treatment response
Define outcome criteria: prevention, reversal, or mitigation of the signs and symptoms	To provide a basis for defining treatment goals and criteria for discontinuing treatment
Sitting upright position, standing and walking	The upright position is essential to shift fluid volume from central to peripheral circulation and maintain fluid volume regulating mechanisms and circulating blood volume
	The upright position is essential to maximize lung volumes and capacities and functional residual capacity
	The upright position is essential to maximize expiratory flow rate and cough effectiveness
	The upright position is essential to optimize the length-tension relationship of the respiratory muscles and abdominal muscles and to optimize cough effectiveness
	The upright position coupled with mobilization and breathing control and coughing maneuvers maximizes alveolar ventilation, ventilation and perfusion matching, and pulmonary lymphatic drainage

Physical Therapy Diagnosis: Risk of negative sequelae of restricted mobility

Signs and Symptoms: Reduced activity and exercise tolerance, muscle atrophy and reduced muscle strength, decreased oxygen transport efficiency, increased heart rate, blood pressure, and minute ventilation at submaximal work rates, reduced respiratory muscle strength and endurance, circulatory stasis, thromboemboli (e.g., pulmonary emboli), pressure areas, skin redness, skin breakdown and ulceration

INTERVENTIONS	RATIONALE
Monitor the signs and symptoms of the negative sequelae of restricted mobility	To provide a baseline, ongoing assessment and measure of treatment response
Define outcome criteria: prevention, reversal, or mitigation of the signs and symptoms	To provide a basis for defining treatment goals and criteria for discontinuing treatment
Mobilization and exercise prescription	To exploit the *preventive* effects of mobilization/exercise; mobilization and exercise optimize circulating blood volume and enhance the efficiency of all steps in the oxygen transport pathway

Physical Therapy Diagnosis: Knowledge deficit

Signs and Symptoms: Lack of information about chronic renal failure, preventive measures, relapse, or complications

INTERVENTIONS	RATIONALE
Monitor knowledge deficits with respect to chronic renal failure, its cardiopulmonary consequences, and physical therapy management	To provide a baseline, ongoing assessment and measure of response to interventions
Define outcome criteria: reversal or mitigation of the signs and symptoms	To provide a basis for defining treatment goals and criteria for discontinuing treatment
Promote a caring and supportive patient-therapist relationship	To focus on treating the patient with chronic renal failure rather than the chronic renal failure
Consider every patient interaction an opportunity for patient education	To promote cooperation and active participation in treatment
Instruct regarding avoidance of infections, nutrition, weight control, hydration and fluid balance, and exercise	To promote patient's sense of responsibility for wellness and prevention
Reinforce patient monitoring himself at home (e.g., vital signs, edema, input and output)	
Reinforce restriction of dietary sodium and potassium sources	
Reinforce seeking medical attention with increased weight, decreased urinary output, or increased blood pressure	
Reinforce medication schedule (e.g., diuretics and antihypertension medications)	
Teach the patient fatigue-control strategies and self-management	
Teach, demonstrate, and provide feedback on interventions that can be self-administered	Between-treatment interventions are as important as treatments themselves to provide cumulative treatment effect
Teach patient regarding balance of activity and rest	Optimal balance between activity and rest is essential to exploit short-term, long-term, and preventive effects of mobilization and exercise
Prepare an individualized information handout and exercise prescription; precautions are emphasized	To augment the cumulative effects of treatment

PART V

Critical Care Case Studies

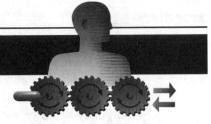

CHAPTER 21

Adult Respiratory Distress Syndrome

PATHOPHYSIOLOGY

Adult respiratory distress syndrome (ARDS) is a rapidly progressive syndrome that can follow any medical or surgical condition without underlying cardiopulmonary pathology. The initial defect results in damage to the pulmonary capillary endothelium and increased microvascular permeability. This may result from direct lung injury, such as aspiration of gastric contents, inhalation of toxins, oxygen toxicity, or pulmonary contusion. Another mechanism involves the neutrophils, which are attracted to the interstitium and release oxygen free radicals, proteases, platelet-activity factor, and arachidonic acid metabolites. These substances damage the pulmonary capillary endothelium, causing fluid and proteins to leak into the interstitium and then into the alveoli. Various other cells and debris also leak into the interstitium. Enzymes such as elastase and collagenase disrupt the elastic and collagen fibers in the interstitium. The plasma proteins and protein by-products released by this breakdown increase oncotic pressure, drawing more water into the interstitium. Fluid pours into the alveoli from the interstitium, causing alveolar collapse. Loss of surfactant production leads to an increase in surface tension, which worsens the alveolar collapse and decreases the functional work capacity. A right-to-left intrapulmonary shunt develops, leading to refractory hypoxemia. Various pulmonary perfusion defects also occur, leading to increased pulmonary vascular resistance and dead space. Symptoms develop 1 to 7 days after the initial injury or insult. Most patients develop symptoms within the first 3 days. Capillary leak syndrome from disruption of the capillary endothelium results in leaking and accumulation of fluid, protein, and cellular material in the interstitium, causing noncardiogenic pulmonary edema. Decreased surfactant activity allows fluid to enter the alveoli, resulting in alveolar collapse (atelectasis). This increases shunting and worsens hypoxemia. Hyaline membrane is formed and causes stiffening of the lungs, which decreases compliance, increases shunting, and increases hypoxemia. Mortality rates exceed 50%. Associated organ failure increases mortality significantly.

Four stages of ARDS have been described. The least severe stage involves acute lung injury that occurs with 24 hours of the initial insult and is associated with clear lungs, normal chest x-ray, tachycardia, hyperventilation, and respiratory alkalosis. The most severe stage involves severe respiratory failure with severe refractory hypoxemia, acidosis with severe hypoxemia, acute respiratory distress, and acute pulmonary edema and decreased sensorium. Neuromuscular blockade therapy is indicated in the presence of low pulmonary compliance and high peak airway pressures. Muscular relaxation or induced paralysis can facilitate mechanical ventilation and reduce systemic and cardiac oxygen demand. A peripheral nerve stimulator is used to stimulate a twitch response of the ulnar nerve, specifically finger flexion, to regulate the level of neuromuscular blackade (every 15 minutes initially to every 1 to 4 hours over the long term).

Case Study

The patient is a 19-year-old man. He is a student at a technical school and lives in an apartment with a roommate near campus. He has a normal body mass index, does not smoke, and drinks socially. On his way to visit his parents for the weekend, he failed to negotiate a curve on his motorcycle, plunged into a river, and nearly drowned. He was quickly resuscitated by passersby. On arrival at the emergency room of a nearby hospital he was found to be oriented; however, he was belligerant and anxious. His heart rate was 113 beats per minute, blood pressure was 143/95 mm Hg, and respiratory rate was 29 breaths per minute. On auscultation, breath sounds were diminished throughout, and diffuse fine crackles and inspiratory wheezes were heard bilaterally. On a fractional inspired oxygen concentration (Fio_2) of 0.40 by mask, his arterial blood gases (ABGs) were pH 7.45, oxygen pressure (Po_2) 65 mm Hg, carbon dioxide pressure (Pco_2) 35 mm Hg, and bicarbonate (HCO_3) 26. Over the next 48 hours, his condition deteriorated. He became increasingly tachycardic, hypertensive, dyspneic, and hypoxemic. His Fio_2 was increased to 1.00 and his gases were pH 7.45, Po_2 50 mm Hg, Pco_2 33 mm Hg, and HCO_3 26. His chest x-ray showed bilateral, diffuse patchy infiltrates. He was mechanically ventilated on assist control: tidal volume 750 ml and respiratory rate 14 breaths per minute. Positive end-expiratory pressure (PEEP) was set at 10 mm Hg. His static effective compliance was 37 ml/cm H_2O. His peak inspiratory pressures were 35 cm H_2O. A pulmonary artery catheter was inserted and the following hemodynamic profile was recorded: pulmonary artery pressure (PAP) 30/12 mm Hg, pulmonary artery wedge pressure (PAWP) 10 mm Hg, central venous pressure (CVP) 10 cm H_2O, cardiac arrest (CI) 4.2, arterial oxygen saturation (Sao_2) 88%, and mixed venous oxygen saturation (Svo_2) 74%. The patient was diagnosed with ARDS. Pulmonary lung compliance was significantly reduced and peak airway pressure increased. Paralysis was induced with neuromuscular blocking agents to facilitate mechanical ventilation and reduce metabolic demands. A trial of PEEP at 15 mm Hg caused deterioration and was returned to 10 mm Hg. Clinical signs of elevated intracranial pressure were absent. Spinal cord involvement was ruled out.

Oxygen Transport Deficits: Observed and Potential

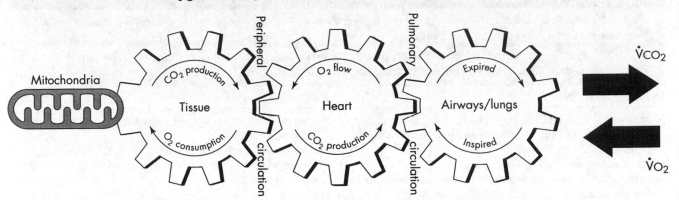

↑ Anaerobic metabolism
↑ Tissue oxygen demand

↑ Heart rate
Dysrhythmias
↑ Pulmonary artery
   pressure
↑ Pulmonary artery
   capillary wedge
   pressure

Bilateral infiltrates
Inflammation
↓ Volumes and capacities
↑ Closing volume
Atelectasis
↑ Work of breathing
Monotonous ventilation
   on ventilator
↓ Cough reflex
↓ Compliance
Ventilation-perfusion
   mismatch
Crackles
↑ Bibasilar breath sounds
Alveolar capillary
   membrane leak
Pulmonary edema
Acute lung injury
↓ Mucociliary transport
↑ Mucus retention
Tenacious secretions
Bronchial irritation
Bronchospasm

↑ Systemic blood pressure

Pulmonary vascular
   congestion
Shunt
↓ Lymph flow
↓ Lymphatic drainage

Blood: Hypoxemia
   ↓ pH
   Arterial desaturation
   ↑ Serum lactate levels
   Cyanosis
   Respiratory alkalosis
   Metabolic acidosis
   ↑ White blood cell counts
   ↑ Temperature

↑ Increase
↓ Decrease

PHYSICAL THERAPY DIAGNOSES AND TREATMENT PRESCRIPTION

Physical Therapy Diagnosis: Decreased oxygen delivery caused by decreased level of consciousness, cardiopulmonary arrest, myocardial ischemia, and impaired hemodynamics; acute lung injury

Signs and Symptoms: Increased intracardiac pressures, increased shunt, tachycardia, hypertension, dyspnea, hypoxemia, $Sao_2 < 98\%$, and diffuse bilateral crackles

INTERVENTIONS	RATIONALE
Monitor vital signs, ABGs, blood work, Sao_2, electrocardiogram (ECG), hemodynamics and peripheral tissue perfusion, urinary output	To provide a baseline, ongoing assessment and measure of treatment response
Monitor serum lactate levels	Serum lactate levels reflect anaerobic metabolism (i.e., increase when oxygen demand exceeds delivery)
Assess patient's capacity to supply oxygen in relation to oxygen demands	
Monitor changes in mechanical ventilation mode and parameters and Fio_2	These factors have significant effects on oxygen supply (i.e., delivery)
Monitor administration of muscle relaxants and neuromuscular blockade	These factors have significant effects on oxygen demand (i.e., consumption)
Monitor stressors of and factors that affect the oxygen transport system, such as routine intensive care unit (ICU) procedures, body positioning, lab tests and procedures, cardiopulmonary physical therapy, and visitors	All physical and psychological stressors increase or decrease oxygen demands; factors that reduce oxygen demands can be integrated into management
	Cardiopulmonary physical therapy interventions affect cardiac output, hence oxygen delivery and tissue oxygenation
To assess oxygen delivery (Do_2) with changes in the patient's management, such as changes in PEEP: $Do_2 = $ cardiac output (CO) $\times$ arterial O_2 content (Cao_2) $\times$ 10, where $Cao_2 = $ (hemoglobin $\times 1.39 \times Sao_2$) + (0.003 $\times Pao_2$)	To determine the effect of interventions on Do_2; Do_2 was reduced at PEEP of 15 mm Hg compared with 10 mm Hg; normally PEEP is set to maintain $Pao_2 > 60$ mm Hg, $Sao_2 > 90\%$ at an $Fio_2 < 0.60$, but the effect on Do_2 must also be considered
	PEEP reduced cardiac output, which significantly reduced Do_2
To assess oxygen consumption (Vo_2): $Vo_2 = CO \times (Cao_2 - Cvo_2) \times 10$, where $Cvo_2 = $ (hemoglobin $\times 1.39 \times Svo_2$) + (0.003 $\times Pvo_2$)	The oxygen extraction ratio (i.e., the ratio of oxygen consumption to oxygen delivery) is increased in critically ill patients because oxygen demands increase and oxygen delivery decreases (normal $Vo_2/Do_2 = 23\%$)
Define outcome criteria: reversal or mitigation of the signs and symptoms	To provide a basis for defining treatment goals and criteria for discontinuing treatment
	To integrate hemodynamic data and degree of stability into treatment prescriptions and define prescription parameters
Minimize use of those interventions or specific parameters of a given prescription that impair venous return, cardiac output, and oxygen delivery to the tissues	To ensure that treatments produce optimal effects on oxygen transport (i.e., maximum benefit with the least risk
	Impaired cardiac output results in impaired oxygen delivery to vital organs and other tissues; peripheral tissue oxygen extraction is increased to compensate; arterial hypoxemia is associated with tissue hypoxia and cardiac dysrhythmias
Monitor the effects of mobilization, body positioning, and range-of-motion exercises on hemodynamic status	To ensure that oxygen demand (Vo_2) does not exceed oxygen delivery (Do_2)
	Kinetic beds are indicated for patients who are extremely hemodynamically unstable, who tolerate positioning poorly, and whose capacity to deliver oxygen cannot meet the demand for oxygen

INTERVENTIONS	RATIONALE
Monitor mechanical ventilation parameter and PEEP	To establish the extent to which mechanical ventilation affects hemodynamics (i.e., venous return, stroke volume, and cardiac output), increases pulmonary vascular resistance, reduces left ventricular afterload, alters left and right venticular geometry and compliance, elevates peak geometry and compliance, elevates peak airway pressure, and impairs lymph flow

Physical Therapy Diagnosis: Cardiopulmonary dysfunction: impaired gas exchange caused by alveolar hypoventilation, shunt, and collapse

Signs and Symptoms: Dyspnea, tachypnea, tachycardia, decreased breath sounds, ventilation and perfusion mismatch, decreased lung volumes and capacities, bilateral, diffuse patchy infiltrates on chest x-ray, diffuse crackles, $Pao_2 < 60$ mm Hg, $Sao_2 < 98\%$, cyanosis, decreased level of consciousness, Fio_2 0.40, shunt > 20%, static effective compliance < 50 ml/cm H_2O, pulmonary capillary wedge pressure (PCWP) < 18 mm Hg

INTERVENTIONS	RATIONALE
Monitor vital signs, ABGs, chest x-rays, ECG, intracardiac pressures, pulmonary function, airflow resistance, lung compliance	To provide a baseline, ongoing assessment and measure of treatment response
Monitor mechanical ventilator parameters and response to PEEP	To augment the benefits of mechanical ventilation and particularly PEEP on maximizing functional residual capacity and minimizing airway closure
Monitor supplemental oxygen requirements and responses	To establish whether hypoxemia is responsive to supplemental oxygen; True shunts are refractory to increases in Fio_2
Closely monitor patient's cardiopulmonary status and fluid and electrolyte balance	Adult respiratory distress syndrome severely compromises cardiopulmonary status; frequent ongoing assessment is essential to determine progression of syndrome in order to plan, implement, and evaluate treatment
	Loss of fluid into the pulmonary interstitium and alveoli contributes to fluid deficits, resulting in further intrapulmonary shunting
Monitor ABGs and pulse oximetry after ventilator and Fio_2 changes	Refractory hypoxemia is a hallmark of adult respiratory distress syndrome; respiratory alkalosis is seen in early stages
Ensure that bronchodilators are administered as indicated, particularly before treatment; ensure that peak effect occurs during treatment	To promote adequate oxygenation and correct hypoxemia
	To reduce shunting and improve gas exchange
Monitor mechanical ventilation settings, PEEP level, and Fio_2 before each treatment	To determine the effects of cardiopulmonary physical therapy interventions on oxygen transport versus changes in ventilatory support
Monitor fatigue in addition to oxygen transport variables before, during, and after treatment	To avoid undue oxygen demands and fatigue
Monitor extent of neuromuscular blockade	To determine patient's oxygen demands during induced paralysis and the implications for treatment
Monitor patient's requirements for analgesia and sedation	The need for analgesia and sedation warrant particular attention because neuromuscular blockade masks the patient's need for these; the patient feels pain and anxiety, but the clinical indicators are masked
Define outcome criteria: reversal or mitigation of the signs and symptoms	To provide a basis for defining treatment goals and criteria for discontinuing treatment

Continued.

INTERVENTIONS	RATIONALE
Ensure that patient is premedicated before treatment (i.e., bronchodilators) and medication is at peak potency during treatment	To maximally dilate airways to optimize treatment response

Body positioning:
  High Fowler's position
  Reverse-Trendelenburg position (head up and feet down)
  Side lying
  ¾ supine to each side
  ¾ prone to each side
  Supine; head of bed > 10-30 degrees
	To maximize alveolar volume, alveolar ventilation, ventilation and perfusion matching, reduce airway resistance, increase pulmonary compliance, induce vigorous stimulation of mucociliary transport, minimize intrapulmonary shunting, increase chest wall excursion, stimulate surfactant production and distribution, promote lymphatic drainage

	To minimize FiO_2 required and facilitate patient's readiness for spontaneous breathing
	To reduce the work of the heart
Monitor closely hemodynamic responses to all interventions	To modify treatment prescription parameters accordingly to maximize their benefit and minimize their risks
Protect patient during positioning and provide supports once in position	Neuromuscular blockade exposes the patient to musculoskeletal and neuromuscular injury
Variants of body positions with varying degrees of head up and down and feet up and down	Change body positions frequently to simulate gravitational and exercise stimuli associated with being upright and moving
Change body positon every 1 to 2 hr; change from one extreme position to another as tolerated	To maximize alveolar ventilation and induce vigorous stimulation of mucociliary transport to prevent further airflow obstruction, atelectasis, and inrrapulmonary shunting
Suction before and after body positon changes as indicated	To remove secretions that have been mobilized by having assumed a given position for a period of time or by the effect of changing body position
Suction judiciously; hyperventilate and hyperoxygenate	Critically ill patients readily desaturate with suctioning unless hyperoxygenated beforehand
Optimize duration in physiologically favorable body positions; monitor ongoing responses	Favorable positions can have adverse effects if assumed for longer than 1 to 2 hr
When the patient is stable, promote extubation as soon as possible by maximizing cardiopulmonary function and gas exchange and decreasing work of breathing	To assist patient to return to spontaneous breathing as soon as possible and to prevent atelectasis and secondary infection

Range-of-motion exercises:
  Upper extremities
  Trunk
  Lower extremities (hip and knee and foot and ankle)
Intensity—active-assisted or passive
Duration—10-15 minutes
Frequency—2-3 times a day
Course and progression—as indicated; commensurate with changes in patient's status
	To exploit the cardiopulmonary effects of range-of-motion exercises (i.e., ventilatory and circulatory effects)

Minimize undue oxygen demands by monitoring factors that contribute to increased oxygen demand (i.e., pathology, physical demands of interventions, increased temperature, stress of illness, impaired thermoregulation, routine procedures, handling, and suctioning)	To ensure that oxygen demands do not exceed oxygen supply
Optimize oxygen transport efficiency	To minimize FiO_2 required and facilitate patient's readiness for spontaneous breathing

INTERVENTIONS	RATIONALE
Prescribe mobilization/exercise when the patient's hemodynamic status can support requisite oxygen delivery and the patient is weaned off neuromuscular blockade Type—dangling, transfer to chair; walking, when extubated Intensity—low; heart rate increase < 20 beats per minute, blood pressure increase < 30 mm Hg, SaO_2 > 95% Duration—10-30 minutes Frequency — several to 2 times a day Course and progression—as indicated Coordinate breathing control and coughing maneuvers with mobilization and body position changes when the patient is extubated	After neuromuscular blockade and its associated effects on muscular aerobic deconditioning, mobilization can be aggressive provided the patient remains hemodynamically stable; he is young, in good health with no underlying cardiopulmonary pathology, and encountered no significant complications To exploit the *acute* effects of mobilization/exercise and maximize the efficiency of the oxygen transport system overall

Physical Therapy Diagnosis: Impaired mucociliary transport and airway clearance caused by mechanical ventilation, monotonous tidal ventilation, loss of normal lung movement, and impaired ability to cough

Signs and Symptoms: Distant breath sounds, crackles, and wheezes on auscultation, increased secretions, increased airflow obstruction, and resistance

INTERVENTIONS	RATIONALE
Monitor mucociliary transport, lung motion, secretion accumulation, and secretions suctioned (quantity and quality) Define outcome criteria: reversal or mitigation of the signs and symptoms Place patient in high Fowler's position Place patient in variants of high Fowler's position Ensure that patient is well supported	To provide a baseline, ongoing assessment and measure of treatment response To provide a basis for defining treatment goals and criteria for discontinuing treatment The upright position maximizes lung volumes and capacities, maximizes descent and expansion of the diaphragm, maximizes expiratory flow rates, facilitates mucociliary transport, facilitates airway clearance of specific lung fields, and minimizes aspiration
Monitor for absent or decreased breath sounds	Early indications of respiratory compromise or complications

Turn patient at least every 2 hr
Suction as indicated using hyperventilation with 100% oxygen before and after suctioning
Lavage using 1-3 cc sterile normal saline directly into endotracheal tube before mechanically hyperventilating
Body positioning:
    360 degrees positional rotation
    Erect high or semi-Fowler's position
    Reverse-Trendelenburg position (head up and feet down)
    ¾ supine to both sides
    ¾ prone to both sides
    Side lying on both sides
    Supine, head of bed up > 10-30 degrees
	To facilitate ciliary action and prevent pooling of secretions
	
	To mechanically promote loosening of secretions and ensure adequate oxygenation before and after suctioning
	To elicit physiological "stir-up"
	To elicit the cardiopulmonary benefits of the position change and the specific benefits associated with each position

Incorporate postural drainage positions into the 360 degrees positional rotation regimen Attempt to position patient in as many extreme positions as possible Duration—1-2 hr Frequency—every 1-2 hr Course and progression—as indicated	The patient has impaired mucociliary transport so he can benefit from postural drainage positioning to promote mucociliary transport Single-handed percussion, if indicated, at a frequency of 1 per second minimizes the adverse effects of this intervention (particularly on hemodynamics in this patient)

Continued.

Physical Therapy Diagnosis: Ineffective breathing pattern caused by acute lung injury

Signs and Symptoms: Mechanical hyperventilation, increased pulmonary artery pressure, hypoxemia, dyspnea, fighting the ventilator, changes in mental status, radiographic atelectasis, use of accessory muscles, decreased bibasilar breath sounds, and decreased chest wall movement

INTERVENTIONS	RATIONALE
Monitor respiratory pattern; absent, unequal, or decreased breath sounds; wheezes and crackles; tidal volume, respiratory rate, airflow resistance, asymmetric chest wall expansion, and pulmonary compliance	To provide a baseline, ongoing assessment and measure of treatment response
	Increased edema and fibrosis causes lungs to become stiff and decrease compliance, resulting in increased work of breathing
Monitor pulmonary function, ABGs, gas exchange, and hemodynamic status	To assess efficiency of breathing pattern, airflow resistance, lung compliance, and work of breathing
Monitor neuromuscular blockade and sedation	Patient may fight mechanical ventilation, has sensation of being unable to breathe; neuromuscular blockade allows for complete mechanical control of ventilation; sedation allows patient more comfort and reduced panic
Monitor for adverse effects of mechanical ventilation	Decreased venous return, stroke volume, cardiac output, and barotrauma are common adverse effects of mechanical ventilation
Define outcome criteria: reversal or mitigation of the signs and symptoms	To provide a basis for defining treatment goals and criteria for discontinuing treatment
Body positions:	Positions are selected that promote respiratory efficiency and gas exchange at reduced work and energy cost
Type—those positions that optimize breathing efficiency and gas exchange	
Duration—1-2 hr	
Frequency—every 1-2 hr	
Course and progression—as indicated	
Base duration in any body position on assessment of outcome variables	Even beneficial positions become deleterious over time
Allow for periods of rest within and between treatments; treatment sessions are short and frequent	To allow the patient to rest and regain strength and endurance for breathing and to maximize treatment effects
	To minimize the risk of oxygen demand exceeding oxygen supply and metabolic acidosis

Physical Therapy Diagnosis: Decreased capacity to accommodate to physical stress because of neuromuscular blockade (e.g., gravitational stress from body position changes, ICU interventions, range-of-motion exercises, and activity)

Signs and Symptoms: Dyspnea, fatigue, and exaggerated increase in heart rate and blood pressure in response to physical stressors

INTERVENTIONS	RATIONALE
Assess hemodynamic, respiratory, and gas exchange variables in response to physical stressors (e.g., body position changes, routine ICU care and procedures, range-of-motion exercises, suctioning, assessments)	To provide a baseline, ongoing assessment and measure of treatment response
Define outcome criteria: reversal or mitigation of the signs and symptoms	To provide a basis for defining treatment goals and criteria for discontinuing treatment
360 degree positional rotation	
Erect high or semi-Fowler's positions	
Horizontal positions with head of bed up > 10-30 degrees	To optimize responses to gravitational stress on hemodynamics and gas exchange
Frequent body position changes at least every 1-2 hr if tolerated	To reduce the risks associated with maintaining a given body position for more than 1-2 hr
	To decrease risk of complications and promote venous return

INTERVENTIONS	RATIONALE
Check heart rate and blood pressure in high and semi-Fowler's positions and in the reverse-Trendelenburg position (head up and feet down)	To monitor for orthostatic hypotension and capacity for fluid pressure and volume regulation
Monitor heart rate, blood pressure, and Sao₂ during exposure to physical stress	To maintain heart rate within 10-20 beats per minute of baseline and maintain blood pressure within 20-30 mm Hg; if a drop occurs it may indicate decreased cardiac output
Intersperse frequent rest periods within and between interventions	To prevent oxygen demand exceeding oxygen supply To prevent excessive fatigue
As the patient's oxygen reserve capacity improves and the patient is weaned from neuromuscular blockade, prescribe mobilization initially for its *acute* effects on oxygen transport and then for its *long-term* effects	To exploit the *long-term* effects of mobilization/exercise and maximize the efficiency of the oxygen transport system overall
Coordinate breathing control and coughing maneuvers with mobilization and body position changes when the patient is extubated	Breathing control and coughing maneuvers are coordinated with treatments after extubation and until normal functional capacity is attained
Type—strengthening exercises	To increase strength (muscles atrophy from neuromuscular blockade and restricted mobility)
Coordinate breathing control and coughing maneuvers	To promote sufficient strength needed for aerobic exercise stimulation
Intensity—low; rhythmic; avoid high-resistance exercise	
Duration—10-30 minutes	As the patient's functional capacity improves, the intensity and duration of treatment sessions increase and the frequency decreases
Frequency—several to 2 times a day	
Course and progression—as indicated	

Physical Therapy Diagnosis: Anxiety caused by respiratory distress, neuromuscular blockade, and hospitalization

Signs and Symptoms: Agitation, restlessness, confusion, impaired concentration, hyperventilation, diaphoresis, tachycardia, tension, lethargy, and fatigue

INTERVENTIONS	RATIONALE
Monitor anxiety and its effects on hemodynamics and gas exchange	To provide a baseline, ongoing assessment and measure of response to interventions Adult respiratory distress syndrome is characterized by severe refractory hypoxemia; factors that threaten oxygenation are minimized
Monitor anxiolytic medications being administered	To ensure that medication does not adversely affect oxygen transport
Define outcome criteria: reversal or mitigation of the signs and symptoms	To provide a basis for defining treatment goals and criteria for discontinuing treatment
Place patient in relaxation positions when resting	Dyspnea, shortness of breath, and hyperventilation are early signs of impending respiratory failure and cause high anxiety, which worsens cardiopulmonary status Upright positions decrease compression of diaphragm by the abdomen, maximize ventilation and perfusion, and decrease sensation of inability to breathe
Prepare patient for interventions and expected sensations	To minimize anxiety and maximize cooperation
Provide emotional support	To help patient and family deal with patient's illness
Ensure that patient is appropriately medicated before treatment	To maximize comfort, reduce suffering, promote maximal cooperation with treatments
Scheduled treatments between interventions	To optimize oxygen transport To optimize the effect of sleep To minimize undue oxygen demand
Promote optimal rest and sleep	To offset sleep deprivation common in hospitalized patients; if possible allow for 60-90 minute sleep segments to optimize sleep cycle patterns

Continued.

Physical Therapy Diagnosis: Threats to cardiopulmonary function and gas exchange

Signs and Symptoms: Pulmonary fibrosis and worsening compliance, alteration in fluid status (e.g., overload), refractory hypoxemia, inadequate tissue oxygenation, multiorgan system failure, oxygen toxicity, risk of infection, edema, weight gain, fluid overload, increased central venous pressure, increased pulmonary capillary wedge pressure, electrolyte abnormalities, noncardiogenic pulmonary edema, sequelae of neuromuscular paralysis, recumbency, and restricted mobility

INTERVENTIONS	RATIONALE
Monitor threats to cardiopulmonary function and gas exchange	To provide a baseline, ongoing assessment and measure of treatment response
Monitor fluid inputs and outputs, weight, pulmonary artery pressure, pulmonary capillary wedge pressure, cardiac output, and mean arterial pressure	Loss of fluid to the pulmonary interstitium and alveoli leads to intravascular depletion, further exacerbating pulmonary shunting
Monitor electrolytes	Intravascular overload leads to decreased Hb/Hct and alters electrolytes
Define outcome criteria; prevention, reversal, or mitigation of the signs and symptoms	To provide a basis for defining treatment goals and criteria for discontinuing treatment
Promote treatments to enhance efficiency of oxygen transport and minimize Fio_2	To reduce risks associated with high oxygen tensions (e.g., denitrogen atelectasis, ciliary dykinesis, impaired migration of alveolar macrophages, and increased adherence of gram-negative organisms to lower respiratory tract epithelium)
Approximate upright sitting positions	To exploit the *preventive* effects of body positioning and mobilization on cardiopulmonary function and gas exchange
	To decrease pulmonary pressures and further pulmonary capillary leaks
	To promote renal drainage and decrease renal stasis
Place in high and semi-Fowler's positions	To promote optimal lung expansion and diaphragmatic descent
Turn patient every 1-2 hr as tolerated	To elicit physiological "stir-up"
Integrate active and active-assist mobilization and range of motion when neuromuscular blockade is discontinued	To optimally stress cardiopulmonary and cardiovascular systems as soon as possible to minimize effects of restricted mobility
Promote breathing control and coughing maneuvers and coordinate with mobilization and body positioning when extubated	To prevent atelectasis
	To prevent circulatory stasis
Monitor temperature every 4 hr and changes in white blood cell count	Increased temperature and increased white blood cell count are signs of infection
Maintain scrupulous cleanliness in handling patient	To decrease risk of infection

Physical Therapy Diagnosis: Risk of the negative sequelae of recumbency

Signs and Symptoms: Within 6 hours reduced circulating blood volume, decreased blood pressure on sitting and standing compared with supine, light-headedness, dizziness, syncope, increased hematocrit and blood viscosity, increased work of the heart, altered pulmonary fluid balance, impaired pulmonary lymphatic drainage, decreased lung volumes and capacities, decreased forced expiratory flow rates, decreased functional residual capacity, decreased pulmonary compliance, increased closing volume, increased airflow resistance, and decreased Pao_2 and Sao_2

INTERVENTIONS	RATIONALE
Monitor the negative sequelae of recumbency	To provide a baseline and ongoing assessment
Define outcome criteria: prevention, reversal, or mitigation of the signs and symptoms	To provide a basis for defining treatment goals and criteria for discontinuing treatment

INTERVENTIONS	RATIONALE
Sitting upright position is the most physiological position that can be assumed by this patient with neuromuscular blockade Ensure that patient is well supported Sitting upright position with feet dependent Coordinate physical activity and mobilization with breathing control and coughing maneuvers when the patient is extubated	To exploit the benefits of the upright position on hemodynamics and plasma volume regulation The upright position is essential to shift fluid volume from central to peripheral circulation and maintain fluid volume regulating mechanisms and circulating blood volume The upright position maximizes lung volumes and capacities, especially functional residual capacity, and minimizes airway closure The upright position maximizes expiratory flow rates and cough effectiveness The upright position optimizes the length-tension relationship of the respiratory muscles and abdominal muscles, neural stimulation of the respiratory muscles, and cough effectiveness The upright position coupled with mobilization and breathing control and coughing maneuvers maximizes alveolar ventilation, ventilation and perfusion matching; optimizes respiratory mechanics, mucociliary transport, and pulmonary lymphatic drainage

Physical Therapy Diagnosis: Risk of negative sequelae of restricted mobility

Signs and Symptoms: Reduced activity and exercise tolerance, muscle atrophy and reduced muscle strength, decreased oxygen transport efficiency, increased heart rate, blood pressure, and minute ventilation at rest and submaximal work rates, neuromuscular blockade, reduced respiratory muscle strength and endurance, circulatory stasis, thromboemboli, pulmonary emboli, pressure areas, skin redness, skin breakdown and ulceration, and cognitive dysfunction

INTERVENTIONS	RATIONALE
Monitor the negative sequelae of restricted mobility Determine premorbid cardiopulmonary status Define outcome criteria: prevention, reversal, or mitigation of the signs and symptoms Mobilization and exercise prescription is limited to passive range of motion until neuromuscular blockade is discontinued Mobilization and exercise are prescribed when neuromuscular blockade is discontinued, commensurate with hemodynamic stability Base mobilization parameters on the hemodynamic responses to routine ICU and nursing procedures	To provide a baseline and ongoing assessment To provide a basis for defining treatment goals and criteria for discontinuing treatment To exploit the ventilatory and cardiovascular effects of range-of-motion exercises To exploit the *preventive* effects of mobilization and exercise (e.g., optimize circulating blood volume and enhance the efficiency of all steps in the oxygen transport pathway) To minimize the untoward effects of mobilization on hemodynamics by prescribing the parameters judiciously based on the hemodynamic responses

Physical Therapy Diagnosis: Knowledge deficit

Signs and Symptoms: Lack of knowledge related to adult respiratory distress syndrome and cardiopulmonary physical therapy management

INTERVENTIONS	RATIONALE
Monitor specific knowledge deficits related to near drowning, adult respiratory distress syndrome, and cardiopulmonary physical therapy and management	To provide a baseline, ongoing assessment and response to interventions To address specific knowledge deficits

Continued.

INTERVENTIONS	RATIONALE
Monitor patient's cognitive and physical capacity to understand these conditions and related cardiopulmonary physical therapy management	Although patient is under neuromuscular blockade and sedation, the patient hears, sees (vision somewhat impaired by ocular muscle weakness), and feels pain
Define outcome criteria: reversal or mitigation of signs and symptoms	To provide a basis for defining treatment goals and criteria for discontinuing treatment
Promote a caring and supportive patient-therapist relationship	To focus on treating the patient with adult respiratory syndrome rather than the syndrome
	To promote trust and confidence
Consider every patient interaction as an opportunity for education	To promote patient's sense of responsibility for recovery
Impart knowledge and information commensurate with the patient's capacity to receive and respond to the information on a day-to-day basis	To maximize patient's active cooperation with treatment

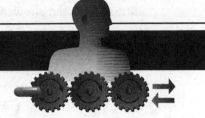

CHAPTER 22

Infant Respiratory Distress Syndrome

PATHOPHYSIOLOGY

Infant respiratory distress syndrome (IRDS), or hyaline membrane disease, is a direct result of premature birth. Type II alveolar cells, which produce surfactant, are not mature until 35 weeks of gestation; thus children delivered before this critical period are at risk of developing IRDS. A reduction in pulmonary surfactant results in increased surface tension. The immature respiratory system is incapable of generating the large intrapleural pressures needed to counter the increased surface tension, hence airway closure and atelectasis result. Reduced surfactant results in alveolar collapse with each breath so that a normal functional residual capacity is not established. Respiratory insufficiency and failure ensue. Respiratory function and gas exchange are further compromised by poorly developed elastic properties of the lungs, weak ventilatory muscles, fewer collateral ventilatory channels, and poorly developed cilia.

Case Study

The patient is a 2-day-old boy. He is the second child in the family. He was admitted to the neonatal intensive care unit within 1 hour of birth. His gestational age was 29 weeks. The patient's mother is a 27-year-old woman who has miscarried twice before. There is no evidence of substance abuse. Labor was precipitated by premature rupture of the membranes. Apgar scores were 4 after 1 minute and 7 after 5 minutes. The patient breathed spontaneously once his mouth and nose were suctioned and almost immediately showed signs of respiratory distress manifested by intercostal and subcostal retractions, expiratory grunts, and nasal flaring. The patient's condition deteriorated rapidly. When his arterial blood gases (ABGs) indicated an arterial oxygen pressure (Pa_{O_2}) of 30 mm Hg and arterial carbon dioxide pressure (Pa_{CO_2}) 70 mm Hg, he was intubated and placed on continuous positive airway pressure (CPAP) with an Fi_{O_2} of 0.40. At 48 hours, a ductal murmur, secondary to patent ductus arteriosus (PDA), was detected on auscultation. The patient underwent a left thoracotomy incision and PDA ligation. He was intubated with an orotracheal tube and received 28% oxygen and intermittent mandatory ventilation of 12 breaths per minute. Positive end-expiratory pressure (PEEP) was +2 cm H_2O. His ABGs were pH 7.41, Pa_{CO_2} 36 mm Hg, Pa_{O_2} 68 mm Hg, and transcutaneous arterial oxygen tension (Tc_{PO_2}) 64 mm Hg. Vital signs were heart rate 140 beats per minute, blood pressure 150 mm Hg, and temperature 101.8°F (38.8°C). Chest x-ray showed reticulogranular pattern of infiltrate and air bronchogram consistent with IRDS. Right upper lobe and left lower lobe atelectasis were apparent.

The patient had a transpyloric tube in place and received continuous infusion of formula. An umbilical arterial catheter was inserted. The patient was placed on a radiant warmer. He had electrocardiogram (ECG) leads, a temperature probe, and a TcPo₂ sensor attached to his chest, back, and abdomen. An ultrasound scan showed a grade II subependymal hemorrhage.

Oxygen Transport Deficits: Observed and Potential

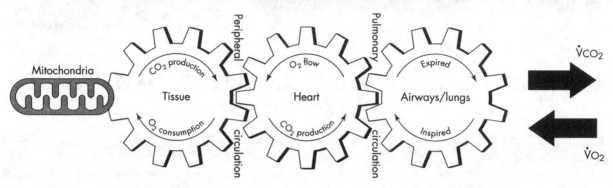

Hypoxia
Hypermetabolic
Hypothermia
↑ Oxygen demand

↑ Work of the heart
↑ Heart rate
↓ Cardiac output

Narrowed airways
↓ Mucociliary transport
Airflow obstruction
↑ Airway resistance
Airway closure
↑ Airway compression
Ciliary dyskinesis
Bronchospasm
Low lung volumes
Dyspnea
↑ Work of breathing
↓ Collateral channels
↓ Functional residual capacity
↓ Surfactant production
↓ Surfactant distribution
Unstable alveoli
Subcostal, intercostal, and
    epigastric retraction
Atelectasis
↑ Circumferential diameter
    of chest wall
Horizontal position of ribs
↑ Diaphragm level
↓ Cough reflex
↓ Cough effectiveness
Inefficient length-tension
    relationship of
    respiratory muscles
Weak respiratory muscles
Diaphragmatic fatigue
↑ Abdominal size and
    encroachment under
    diaphragm
Ventilation-perfusion
    mismatch
Abnormal breathing pattern

↑ Systemic blood pressure

Fluid imbalance
Shunt
Diffusion defect
↑ Vascular resistance
↓ Lymph flow
↓ Lymphatic drainage

Blood: Hypoxemia
        Arterial desaturation
        Fever
        Electrolyte imbalance
        Metabolic acidosis

↑ Increase
↓ Decrease

PHYSICAL THERAPY DIAGNOSES AND TREATMENT PRESCRIPTION

Physical Therapy Diagnosis: Abnormal hemodynamic status and increased metabolic demands

Signs and Symptoms: Pao_2 < predicted for a neonate (< 55-65 mm Hg on room air), Sao_2 < 90%, hypermetabolic, impaired thermoregulaton, surgical repair of PDA, mechanical ventilation

INTERVENTIONS	RATIONALE
Monitor vital signs, ABGs, $TcPo_2$, blood work, hemodynamics, peripheral perfusion, urinary output	To provide a baseline, ongoing assessment and measure of treatment response
Define outcome criteria: reversal or mitigation of signs and symptoms	To provide a basis for defining treatment goals and criteria for discontinuing treatment
Body positioning: in upright position head of bed up > 30 degrees and right side lying	To reduce hemodynamic stress and work of the heart
Minimize undue physical stress (positions that increase the work of the heart, excessive handling, noises, temperature changes, and suctioning)	To minimize intracerebral pressure (ICP)

Physical Therapy Diagnosis: Impaired gas exchange caused by alveolar hypoventilation and shunt

Signs and Symptoms: Pao_2 < predicted for neonate (< 55-65 mm Hg on room air) Sao_2 < 90%, hypermetabolic, fever, increased resistance to air flow, decreased lung compliance, increased airway compression and alveolar collapse, radiographic evidence of infant respiratory distress syndrome, atelectasis in the right upper lobe and left lower lobe, increased work of breathing, weak respiratory muscles, inefficient circumferential configuration of the chest wall, compliant chest wall, subcostal and intercostal retraction, diffusion defect, ventilation and perfusion mismatch, left-to-right pulmonary shunt, and fluid and electrolyte imbalance

INTERVENTIONS	RATIONALE
Monitor vital signs, ABGs, $TcPo_2$, blood work, chest x-rays, heart rate, blood pressure, peripheral perfusion, ECG, Sao_2, urinary output, signs of altered intracerebral pressure	To provide a baseline, ongoing assessment and measure of treatment outcome
Monitor oxygen transport variables, i.e., delivery, uptake, and extraction	
Ongoing clinical cardiopulmonary assessment	
Define outcome criteria: reversal or mitigation of the signs and symptoms	To provide a basis for defining treatment goals and criteria for discontinuing treatment
Body positioning prescription in conjunction with ongoing monitoring of oxygen transport variables (i.e., respiratory, hemodynamic and gas exchange variables)	To exploit the *acute* effects of gravity via frequent body position changes (e.g., optimize alveolar volume, ventilation, and ventilation and perfusion matching; minimize compression alelectasis and airway closure, optimize mucociliary transport, minimize secretion retention and bacterial colonization; minimize the work of breathing and of the heart; promote chest tube drainage and lymphatic drainage)
Type: high supported sitting (e.g., in Tumbleform chair)	Upright positions relieve compression on dependent lung fields in the neonate and elicit normal gravitational stimulation on cardiopulmonary function
	Because neonates are incapable of supporting themselves, they must be well supported in upright positions
	To reduce thoracic blood volume, work of the heart, visceral compression on the underside of the diaphragm, and compression of lower lobes; maximize lung volumes and capacities, reduce the work of breathing
	Minimize weight and compression on the chest wall to allow for normal excursion and thoracoabdominal motion
	To maximize duration in erect upright (nonslumped) body positions and thereby maximize normal chest wall excursion and minimize chest wall and parenchymal compression

Continued.

INTERVENTIONS	RATIONALE

Postural drainage positions—right upper lobe:
   Apical segment—high Fowler's position
   Anterior segment—head of bed 45 degrees
   Posterior segment—¾ prone to left with head of bed 30 degrees
Left lower lobe:
   Anterior segment—supine with head of bed down 30-45 degrees
   Lateral segment—right side lying with head of bed down 30-45 degrees
   Posterior segment—prone with head of bed down 30-45 degrees
Duration—maintain those positions that are most efficacious in clearing secretions for as long as possible within the patient's tolerance, in the presence of beneficial outcome and absence of deleterious outcome
360 degrees position rotational schedule (within limits of catheters, lines, and chest tubes)
Side lying on either side
¼ side lying on either side
¾ prone to either side
Prone with abdomen free
Supine
Variants of the head up and head down positions at various angles
Frequency—1-2 hr
Duration—1-2 hr
Course and progression—as indicated
	Positions are selected to maximize alveolar volume and ventilation and minimize airway closure, particularly in the right upper lobe and left lower lobe
	To exploit the secretion clearance benefits of the most effective positions
	To exploit the benefits of specific postural drainage positions, minimize the effect of diminishing returns with excessive duration in a given position, and deleterious outcome
	Modify head down position because of subependymal hemorrhage and possibly increased intracerebral pressure; a grade II is not an absolute contraindication to the head down position, but the patient requires close monitoring
	To minimize compression of abdominal viscera on the underside of the diaphragm and closure of the dependent airways
	Patient should be positioned from one extreme position to another (i.e., dependent compressed areas should be moved to nondependent positions)
	The prone abdomen free position displaces the viscera downward and promotes diaphragmatic excursion, tidal volume, and lung compliance and enhances Pao_2 and Sao_2

Frequent body position changes Maximize duration in body positions with a favorable effect on oxygen transport Minimize duration in body positions with a deleterious effect on oxygen transport Avoid excessive time (1-2 hr) in any single static position, even one with favorable effects	To elicit physiological "stir-up" To avoid deleterious hydrostatic effects on cardiopulmonary function
Monitor the patient's response to handling and other potentially adverse stimuli	Frequent handling can contribute to respiratory distress in the neonate; thus the maximal frequency of positioning is based on close monitoring of the patient's responses (i.e., the maximal frequency that is tolerated without cardiorespiratory compromise and deterioration of oxygen transport variables)

Physical Therapy Diagnosis: Impaired mucociliary transport and secretion accumulation

Signs and Symptoms: Crackles on auscultation, airflow obstruction and resistance, increased system pressure, increased work of breathing, decreased $TcPo_2$ and Sao_2

INTERVENTIONS	RATIONALE
Monitor gas exchange, airflow resistance, airway obstruction, and bronchospasm Monitor quantity and quality of sputum suctioned Define outcome criteria: reversal or mitigation of the signs and symptoms Body positioning for postural drainage of the right upper lobe and the left lower lobe	To provide a baseline, ongoing assessment and measure of treatment response To provide a basis for defining treatment goals and criteria for discontinuing treatment To drain pulmonary secretions to reduce airflow resistance, airway irritation, and bronchospasm

INTERVENTIONS	RATIONALE
Postural drainage positions with manual techniques as indicated for airway clearance of the right upper lobe and left lower lobe	Relative contraindications to manual percussion in this patient: low birth weight, compliant chest wall, intraventricular hemorrhage, and healing thoracic incision
	Manual percussion, if indicated, performed with a couple of fingers at a frequency of 1 per second minimizes the risks associated with this intervention
	Chest wall vibration may have some additional benefit to postural drainage in the presence of retained airway secretions
	Chest wall percussion has been associated with deleterious effects on oxygen transport; if indicated (given hemorrhage grade II), the patient requires close monitoring before, during, and after treatment
Suctioning when indicated with hyperoxygenation and rests between catheter passes	Patient should be hyperoxygenated to minimize arterial desaturation and atelectasis
Observe for adverse effects of suctioning (e.g., bleeding, cyanosis, bradycardia)	Suctioning is performed only when indicated, rather than routinely, to minimize the trauma and adverse effects associated with this procedure
Instillation with hypertonic saline before suctioning	Instillation with hypertonic saline can assist secretion removal
Mobilization	Because the patient cannot cooperate with treatment, spontaneous movement, although apparently minimal, constitutes a mobilization stimulus capable of eliciting the *acute* effects beneficial to oxygen transport
Type—spontaneous movement of arms, legs, and trunk	
Intensity—low intensity	
Duration—5-10 minutes	
Frequency—several times a day	
Course and progression—as indicated; within limits of hemodynamic stability and optimal gas exchange	
Body positions to stimulate spontaneous movements in a variety of body positions	To exploit gravitational effects in facilitating and resisting spontaneous movement
Monitor hemodynamic, respiratory, and oxygen transport variables during active and passive mobilization	To minimize undue stress on oxygen transport; avoid oxygen demands that unduly challenge the patient's capacity to deliver oxygen
Passive range-of-motion exercises	To elicit associated cardiopulmonary responses
Upper extremity	
Trunk	
Lower extremity	

Physical Therapy Diagnosis: Ineffective breathing pattern caused by surgery, anesthesia, posterolateral thoracotomy, chest tubes, pain, decreased lung compliance, increased airflow resistance, recumbency, inability to spontaneously change positions, and restricted mobility

Signs and Symptoms: Depressed respiratory effort, left thoracotomy incision and dressings over incision, pain, radiographic evidence of infiltrates and right upper lobe and left lower lobe atelectasis, increased lung surface tension, decreased functional residual capacity, and increased airway closure

INTERVENTIONS	RATIONALE
Monitor breathing pattern parameters, chest x-rays, breathing symmetry, airway resistance, lung compliance, chest wall retraction, and thoracoabdominal motion	To provide a baseline, ongoing assessment and measure of treatment outcome
Define outcome criteria: reversal or mitigation of the signs and symptoms	To provide a basis for defining treatment goals and criteria for discontinuing treatment

Continued.

INTERVENTIONS	RATIONALE

Body positioning prescription:
  Prone abdomen free
  ¾ prone
  Variants supine, head of bed up and down at various
    angles
  Erect, high Fowler's position (unslumped)
360 degrees positional rotation schedule
Change from one extreme position to another
Frequent body position changes (at least every 1-2 hr)
	Compared with supine, prone has several significant benefits in the neonate (e.g., increased Pao_2, increased lung compliance, increased tidal volume, decreased chest wall asymmetry, decreased number of apneic episodes, increased $TcPo_2$, decreased respiratory rate, less chest wall retraction, improved sleep quality, less crying, less motor activity, more regular respiratory rates, and decreased heart rate)
	
	Prone abdomen free; patient is supported beneath upper chest and pelvis to allow displacement of viscera and to accommodate the umbilical catheter
	¾ prone accommodates umbilical catheter, orotracheal tube, and other lines
	Upright positions maximize lung volumes and capacities and expiratory flow rates, minimize chest wall compression, and displace the viscera caudally, which enhances diaphragmatic descent and excursion

Monitor hemodynamic and respiratory status during and after positioning Observe those positions that optimize oxygen transport and increase time in and frequency of these positions Avoid excessive time (greater than 1-2 hr) in any single position, even one that is beneficial	To avoid deleterious body positions that compromise ABGs and increase respiratory distress To avoid complications in the dependent lung fields

---

Physical Therapy Diagnosis: Physical and psychological stress, pain

Signs and Symptoms: Discomfort, respiratory distress and agitation, crying efforts, increased metabolic cost associated with routine care and handling, breathing, agitation, being startled, temperature regulation, suctioning, tests, assessments, procedures

---

INTERVENTIONS	RATIONALE
Monitor physical and psychological stress and pain	To provide a baseline, ongoing assessment and measure of treatment response
Define outcome criteria: reversal or mitigation of the signs and symptoms	To provide a basis for defining treatment goals and criteria for discontinuing treatment
Maximize comfort	To reduce physiological arousal
Coordinate interventions with analgesia	To reduce oxygen demands and respiratory distress
Reduce agitation	
Handle carefully; not suddenly	
Warm hands before handling	
Warm stethoscope head	
Maximize a quiet, warm environment	
Speak quietly to the child	
Leave patient bundled when appropriate	
Keep area darkened when appropriate	
Minimize disturbances	
Minimize distress and crying efforts	
Double up assessment and treatment with nursing or other procedures when possible	
Maximize quality of rest and sleep	To optimize balance between treatments, physiological work demands, and sleep and rest
Reduce discomfort/pain from the surgical incision by supporting the incision, positioning with care, doubling up with nursing procedures when possible, and not disturbing the patient unnecessarily	The neonate has sufficient neurological function to experience discomfort and pain; minimizing discomfort/pain is a priority to reduce arousal, oxygen demand, and suffering

Physical Therapy Diagnosis: Threats to oxygen transport and gas exchange: prematurity, postsurgical status, intubation, mechanical ventilation, oxygen therapy, and bronchopulmonary dysplasia; risk of prolonged weaning from mechanical ventilation due to respiratory muscle weakness and fatigue and of postextubation complications (predeliction for the right lung > left lung; right upper lobe)

Signs and Symptoms: Decreased airway diameter, low lung surface area, poor surfactant production and distribution, decreased airway stability, increased airway closure, impaired thermoregulation, immunoinsufficiency, recumbency, restricted mobility, thromboemboli, invasive lines, monitoring equipment (e.g., ECG, $TcPo_2$, umbilical arterial catheter), risks of intubation and mechanical ventilation, suctioning, infection, respiratory muscle atrophy, oxygen toxicity, increased secretions, decreased mobility and positioning, trauma to pharynx and airway, decreased cardiac output and venous return, preferential ventilation to upper airways, ventilation and perfusion mismatch, pneumothorax, bronchopulmonary dysplasia, arterial desaturation caused by suctioning, impaired renal perfusion and oliguria, and altered intracerebral pressure; risks associated with limited collateral ventilation, small airway diameters, inefficient respiratory mechanics, susceptibility to postextubation atelectasis (within 24 hours), particularly involving the right upper lobe, susceptibility to postextubation pneumonia and risk of adverse effects of physical therapy (adverse effects of handling); risk of developmental delay (i.e., cardiopulmonary, neuromuscular, and musculoskeletal systems and poor swallowing and gastrointestinal development)

INTERVENTIONS	RATIONALE
Monitor ABGs, hemoglobin, ECG, chest x-rays, pulmonary function, mucociliary transport, secretion retention, vital signs, Sao_2	To provide a baseline, ongoing assessment and measure of treatment response
Monitor for signs of infection (e.g., increased temperature and increased white blood cell count)	
Perform clinical cardiopulmonary assessment	
Monitor mucociliary transport and secretion accumulation	Intubation irritates the trachea and stimulates increased mucus production
Monitor supplemental oxygen levels	Oxygen contributes to depressed ciliary action
Monitor patient's cough efforts	Weak cough reflex contributes to retention of secretions in the postextubation period
Define outcome criteria: prevention, reversal, or mitigation of the signs and symptoms	To provide a basis for defining treatment goals and criteria for discontinuing treatment
Perform assessments and treatments in conjunction with nursing or other procedures whenever possible	To maximize treatment effect, minimize excessive handling and disturbance of the patient, and to promote quality sleep and rest periods
Perform suctioning judiciously as indicated	Suctioning irritates tracheobronchial mucosa and contributes to increased mucus production, immediate hypoxemia, apnea, increased respiratory rate, bradycardia, and atelectasis

Physical Therapy Diagnosis: Risk of the negative sequelae of recumbency

Signs and Symptoms: Reduced stimulation of regulating mechanisms of circulating blood volume, increased work of the heart, altered fluid balance in the lung, impaired pulmonary lymphatic drainage, decreased lung volumes and capacities, decreased functional residual capacity, increased closing volume, and decreased Pao_2 and Sao_2

INTERVENTIONS	RATIONALE
Monitor the negative sequelae of recumbency	To provide a baseline, ongoing assessment and measure of treatment response
Define outcome criteria: prevention, reversal, or mitigation of the signs and symptoms	To provide a basis for defining treatment goals and criteria for discontinuing treatment
Upright body positions	The upright position is essential to shift fluid volume from central to peripheral circulation and maintain fluid volume regulating mechanisms and circulating blood volume

Continued.

INTERVENTIONS	RATIONALE
	The upright position maximizes lung volumes and capacities and functional residual capacity
	The upright position maximizes expiratory flow rate and cough effectiveness
	The upright position optimizes the length-tension relationship of the respiratory muscles and abdominal muscles and maximizes cough effectiveness
	The upright position coupled with mobilization maximizes alveolar ventilation, mucociliary transport, ventilation and perfusion matching, and pulmonary lymphatic drainage

Physical Therapy Diagnosis: Risk of the negative sequelae of restricted mobility

Signs and Symptoms: Reduced spontaneous movement, reduced movement tolerance, muscle atrophy, reduced muscle strength, decreased oxygen transport efficiency, increased heart rate, blood pressure, and minute ventilation at submaximal work rates, reduced respiratory muscle strength and endurance, circulatory stasis, thromboemboli, pressure areas, skin breakdown and ulceration

INTERVENTIONS	RATIONALE
Monitor the negative sequelae of restricted mobility	To provide a baseline, ongoing assessment and measure of treatment response
Define outcome criteria: prevention, reversal, or mitigation of the signs and symptoms	To provide a basis for defining treatment goals and criteria for discontinuing treatment
Facilitate movement; promote spontaneous movement	Mobilization and exercise optimize circulating blood volume and enhance the efficiency of all steps in the oxygen transport pathway
Monitor hemodynamic, respiratory, and gas exchange variables in response to movement and positional stress and other sources of physical stress	
Base parameters of movement stimuli on patient's ongoing response to oxygen transport (i.e., delivery and consumption); pace treatments accordingly	

Physical Therapy Diagnosis: Knowledge deficit

Signs and Symptoms: Lack of information of caregivers and family about infant respiratory distress syndrome complications and cardiopulmonary physical therapy management

INTERVENTIONS	RATIONALE
Assess knowledge deficits related to the patient's condition and cardiopulmonary physical therapy management	To provide a baseline, ongoing assessment and measure of response to interventions
	To identify specific knowledge deficits and address accordingly
Define outcome criteria: reversal or mitigation of the signs and symptoms	To provide a basis for defining treatment goals and criteria for discontinuing interventions
Promote a caring and supportive patient-therapist relationship	To focus on treating the patient with infant respiratory distress syndrome rather than the syndrome
Stress to caregivers the importance of the upright position and prone position, frequent position changes, and facilitation of spontaneous movement in varied positions	Between-treatment interventions are as important as treatments themselves to provide cumulative treatment effect
Teach, demonstrate, and provide feedback on interventions that can be administered by others	
Reinforce the balance of activity and rest	Optimal balance between activity and rest is essential to exploit short-term, long-term, and preventive effects of body positioning and mobilization

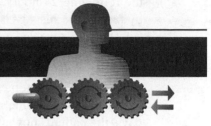

CHAPTER 23

Cardiopulmonary Failure

PATHOPHYSIOLOGY

Cardiopulmonary failure refers to the inability of the cardiopulmonary unit to pump and oxygenate sufficient blood to meet the body's metabolic demands. Such failure can result from heart disease, lung disease, or conditions such as neuromuscular dysfunction and trauma. Cardiopulmonary failure is frequently initiated by left ventricular failure leading to cardiogenic pulmonary edema and subsequent right ventricular failure. Left ventricular stroke volume decreases. The right ventricle continues to pump blood into the pulmonary circulation as left ventricular volume and pressure rise. Rising pressures soon occur in the left atrium and pulmonary circulation, causing dyspnea. Pulmonary capillary oncotic pressure increases, and fluid extravasates into the interstitial spaces, leading to pulmonary edema, which is clinically manifested by cough and sputum production. Continued high pressures cause fluid to move into the alveoli, resulting in frank pulmonary edema. Elevated pressures eventually occur in the right ventricle, causing right ventricular failure. Right atrial pressure rises, which results in systemic venous congestion and the presence of edema. As this process develops and cardiac output falls, the following compensatory mechanisms may be activated: increased sympathetic stimulation, increased peripheral vascular resistance, fluid retention, increased contractility, and ventricular hypertrophy. Compensatory mechanisms provide beneficial effects as long as they remain within normal physiological limits. However, once left ventricular end-diastolic volume and stretch exceed these limits, the muscle fibers can no longer shorten adequately during systole. Contractility decreases, cardiac output decreases, and the typical cycle of heart failure ensues.

Case Study

The patient is a 72-year-old man. He is a retired accountant but continues to do private work. He lives in a retirement community with his wife. Their lifestyle is sedentary. He is about 20 pounds (9 kg) overweight. He has smoked 1½ packs of cigarettes per day for 50 years. His medical history includes a myocardial infarction 15 years ago and adult-onset diabetes. He developed sudden onset of fever, chills, and cough productive of thick, reddish-brown sputum. He reported a sharp, nonradiating pain in his left lateral chest that was aggravated with inspiration. Coarse crackles and harsh rhonchi were audible over the left lung fields with a pleural friction rub. His vital signs were heart rate 120 beats per minute, respiratory rate 26 breaths per minute, blood pressure 155/90 mm Hg, and temperature 102.2°F (39°C). On room air, his arterial blood gases (ABGs) were pH 7.49, arterial oxygen pressure (Pao_2) 70 mm Hg, arterial carbon dioxide pressure ($Paco_2$) 33 mm Hg, bicarbonate (HCO_3) 27, and arterial oxygen saturation (Sao₂) 91%. His white blood cell count was elevated. The patient was put on oxygen by nasal prongs at 3 L/minute and fluids were administered by an intravenous line. Over the following 24 hours, the patient's condition deteriorated significantly. On 50% oxygen delivered by face mask, his ABGs were pH 7.49, Pao₂ 50 mm Hg, Paco₂ 32 mm Hg, HCO₃ 26, and Sao₂ 87%. Chest x-ray revealed complete whiteout on the left side; adventitious lung sounds were audible throughout the left lung. His temperature was now 104°F (40°C) heart rate 146 beats per minute, and blood pressure 175/96 mm Hg. Respiratory rate was 40 to 60 breaths per minute, and respirations were labored. He was intubated and mechanically ventilated on assist control; tidal volume 1100 ml, rate 12 breaths per minute, and fractional inspired oxygen concentration (Fio₂) of 0.50. Over the next 2 days, the patient showed signs of hepatic and gastrointestinal dysfunction. The patient was diagnosed with bacteremia, sepsis, and multiorgan system failure secondary to overwhelming pneumonia.

Oxygen Transport Deficits: Observed and Potential

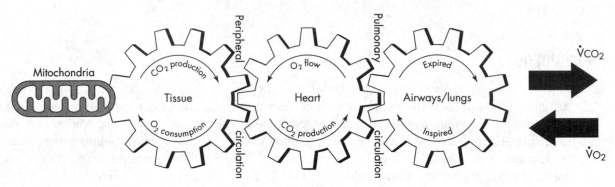

Hypoxia	Ventricular dilatation	Dyspnea
Metabolite accumulation	Impaired myocardial	Respiratory muscle
↑ Oxygen demand	contractility	weakness
	Ineffective pumping	Respiratory muscle fatigue
	action	Pulmonary congestion
	Left ventricular	↓ Compliance
	dysfunction	Discoordinated
	↑ Left heart work	thoracoabdominal motion
	↑ Right heart work	Intercostal retraction
	Cardiac distention	Use of accessory muscles
	Cardiomegaly	Atelectasis
	Dysrhythmias	Ventilation and perfusion
		mismatch
		↓ Surfactant production
		↓ Surfactant distribution
		Impaired diaphragmatic
		descent (due to
		hepatomegaly)
		↓ Mucociliary transport
		↑ Secretion retention
		Bronchospasm

Abnormal vasomotion tone
Systemic hypertension

Hypoxic vasoconstriction
↑ Pulmonary vascular resistance
Shunt
↓ Lymph motion
↓ Lymphatic fluid

Blood: Hypoxemia
    Hypercapnia
    ↓ pH
    Respiratory acidosis
    ↓ Circulatory velocity
    Microemboli
    Polycythemia

↑ Increase
↓ Decrease

PHYSICAL THERAPY DIAGNOSES AND TREATMENT PRESCRIPTION

Physical Therapy Diagnosis: Decreased cardiac output caused by myocardial dysfunction

Signs and Symptoms: $Pao_2 < 104.2 - 0.27$ age (± 7) mm Hg on room air; $Sao_2 < 98\%$, arrhythmias, cardiomegaly, increased work of the heart, changes in blood pressure, abnormal intracardiac pressures, decreased capillary filling, cold and clammy skin, decreased level of consciousness, decreased urinary output, pulmonary congestion, and pulmonary hypoxic vasoconstriction

INTERVENTIONS	RATIONALE
Monitor vital signs, hemodynamic variables, ABGs, electrocardiogram (ECG), fluid balance, and urinary output	To provide a baseline, ongoing assessment and measure of treatment response
Monitor changes in ventilatory support and parameters and supplemental oxygen	To determine the degree to which these factors augment oxygenation versus cardiopulmonary physical therapy interventions
To assess oxygen delivery (Do_2) with changes in the patient's management, such as changes in positive end-expiratory pressure (PEEP): $Do_2 =$ cardiac output (CO) $\times$ arterial O_2 content (Cao_2) $\times 10$, where $Cao_2 = $ (hemoglobin $\times 1.39 \times Sao_2) + (0.003 \times Pao_2)$	To determine the effect of interventions on Do_2; Do_2 was reduced at PEEP of 15 mm Hg compared with 10 mm Hg; normally PEEP is set to maintain $Pao_2 > 60$ mm Hg, $Sao_2 > 90\%$ at an $Fio_2 < 0.60$, but the effect on Do_2 must also be considered
	PEEP reduced cardiac output, which significantly reduced Do_2
To assess oxygen consumption (Vo_2): $Vo_2 = CO \times (Cao_2 - Cvo_2) \times 10$, where $Cvo_2 = $ (hemoglobin $\times 1.39 \times Svo_2) + (0.003 \times Pvo_2)$	The oxygen extraction ratio (i.e., the ratio of oxygen consumption to oxygen delivery) is increased in critically ill patients because oxygen demands increase and oxygen delivery decreases (normal $Vo_2/Do_2 = 23\%$)
Define outcome criteria: reversal or mitigation of the signs and symptoms	To provide a basis for defining treatment goals and criteria for discontinuing treatment
Body positioning:	To reduce the work of the heart and hemodynamic stress
Semirecumbent position (i.e., head up 10-30 degrees) when resting	To stimulate pressure and fluid volume regulating mechanisms to maintain circulating blood volume by eliciting gravitational stress
Reverse-Trendelenburg position (head up and feet down)	
Place in high or semi-Fowler's position as indicated	To decrease work of the heart, work of breathing, and associated oxygen demands
Dangle and progress to chair sitting with an active-assisted transfer	To optimize gas exchange
Monitor vital signs and ECG; check for chest pain during position changes	To detect myocardial ischemia, damage, and cardiac compromise
Assess orthostatic intolerance	To detect orthostatism and prevent syncope associated with orthostatic intolerance

Physical Therapy Diagnosis: Impaired gas exchange caused by alveolar hypoventilation and shunt effect

Signs and Symptoms: Increased work of breathing, reduced arousal, increased (A − a) oxygen gradient; hypoxemia, atelectasis, decreased lung compliance, decreased vital capacity, decreased functional residual capacity, decreased tidal volume, increased respiratory rate, decreased breath sounds, dry crackles, decreased fremitus, dull percussion note, radiographic evidence of alveolar collapse and atelectasis, alveolar consolidation and pneumonia, excessive secretions, hepatomegaly, cardiomegaly, pulmonary congestion, diffusion defect, reduced arousal

INTERVENTIONS	RATIONALE
Monitor respiratory and gas exchange variables, ECG, ABGs, pulmonary function, and chest x-ray	To provide a baseline, ongoing assessment and measure of treatment response
	To assess lung compliance; derive index of the work of breathing and patient's ability to sustain spontaneous ventilation
	To maintain $Pao_2 > 70$ mm Hg to minimize hypoxic pulmonary vasoconstriction and shunting
Assess level of arousal and effect of narcotics on arousal	To help reduce the need for narcotics and increase arousal

Continued.

INTERVENTIONS	RATIONALE
Define outcome criteria: reversal or mitigation of the signs and symptoms	To provide a basis for defining treatment goals and criteria for discontinuing treatment
Coordinate interventions with bronchodilator medications	To maximize treatment effects
Suction judiciously; hyperventilate and hyperoxygenate	To minimize the adverse effects of suctioning

Body positioning:
  Relaxation positions
  360 degrees positional rotating
  High or semi-Fowler's positions
  Reverse-Trendelenburg position (head up and feet down)
  Side lying to either side; modify for left side if untoward hemodynamic effects
  ½ side lying to either side
  ¾ prone; abdomen free
Frequent body position changes; at least every 1-2 hr change from one position to an extreme position
	To maximize period of time (maximum 1-2 hr) in position associated with the least oxygen demands and work of breathing
	To promote physiological "stir-up"
	To exploit the gravitational effects of changes in body positioning (i.e., changes in alveolar volume, distributions of alveolar ventilation, perfusion, and ventilation to perfusion matching, mucuciliary transport, reduced secretion accumulation, increased surfactant production and distribution, increased lymph flow, lymphatic drainage, diaphragmatic descent, decreased intraabdominal pressure, increased functional residual capacity, and reduced airway closure)

Mobilization:
  Indications—patient can tolerate upright positioning, reverse-Trendelenburg with acceptable hemodynamic parameters
  Type—dangling over the edge of bed, transfers to chair, and chair sitting
  Intensity—heart rate increase < 20 beats per minute; blood pressure increase < 30 mm Hg, Sao_2 > 94%
  Duration—5-30 minutes
  Frequency—several to 2 times a day
  Course and progression—as indicated; commensurate with hemodynamic stability
	To exploit the *acute* effects of mobilization (i.e., increase alveolar ventilation, optimize the distribution of ventilation and ventilation and perfusion matching, optimize lung volumes and capacities, expiratory flow rates, lymph flow, lymphatic drainage, increase functional residual capacity, reduce closing volume, reduce the work of breathing and of the heart)

Promote standing and walking preextubation	Mechanical ventilation does not necessarily preclude standing and ambulation; these activities facilitate weaning and potentially reduce morbidity and intensive care unit (ICU) stay

Range-of-motion exercises
  Upper extremities
  Trunk
  Lower extremities
Intensity—low; active assist, increase < 20 beats per minute, blood pressure increase < 30 mm Hg; Sao_2 > 94%
Duration—5-20 minutes
Frequency—several to 2 times a day
Course and progression—as indicated; commensurate with hemodynamic stability
	To exploit the cardiopulmonary effects of range-of-motion exercises (i.e., ventilatory and cardiovascular effects)

Physical Therapy Diagnosis: Ineffective breathing pattern caused by decreased compliance secondary to interstitial pulmonary edema, leading to decreased surfactant, increased alveolar closure

Signs and Symptoms: Chest x-ray shows atelectasis, increased work of breathing, increased respiratory rate, decreased tidal volume, decreased minute ventilation, decreased vital capacity, use of accessory muscles, exertional dyspnea, decreased mobilization/exercise tolerance, hypoxemia, hypoxia, crackles, decreased bibasilar breath sounds, and decreased chest wall movement

INTERVENTIONS	RATIONALE
Monitor breathing pattern (i.e., tidal volume, respiratory rate, chest wall symmetry, and excursion)	To provide a baseline, ongoing assessment and measure of treatment response
Define outcome criteria: reversal or mitigation of the signs and symptoms	To provide a basis for defining treatment goals and criteria for discontinuing treatment
Maintain Fio_2 < 50% with Sao_2 > 90 mm Hg	Increase in Fio_2 > 50% may lead to oxygen toxicity with fibrotic lung change
Observe for signs of ventilatory muscle fatigue	Fatigued respiratory muscles require rest rather than strengthening
Mobilization:	To optimize a more normal breathing pattern in the upright body positions
Dangling; erect, relaxed, sitting over edge of bed transfer to chair	
Chair sitting	
Range-of-motion exercises:	To exploit the ventilatory and cardiovascular effects of range-of-motion exercises
Upper extremities	
Trunk	
Lower extremities	
Monitor hemodynamic responses to physical stressors	To ensure that oxygen demands do not exceed supply

Physical Therapy Diagnosis: Anxiety

Signs and Symptoms: Agitation, distraction, restlessness, fighting the ventilator, sleep disturbance

INTERVENTIONS	RATIONALE
Monitor anxiety and its effect on hemodynamics and gas exchange	To provide a baseline, ongoing assessment and response to treatment
Define outcome criteria: reversal or mitigation of the signs and symptoms	To provide a basis for defining treatment goals and criteria for discontinuing treatment
Interact with patient reassuringly	To exploit nonpharmacological means of reducing anxiety
Reduce metabolic demands	To help reduce the need for narcotic medication
Pace treatments	
Discuss feasibility of alternate medications to narcotics	Narcotics depress the drive to breathe and the patient's ability to cooperate with treatment

Physical Therapy Diagnosis: Decreased activity and exercise tolerance

Signs and Symptoms: Dyspnea, exaggerated increase in heart rate and blood pressure on exertion

INTERVENTIONS	RATIONALE
Monitor hemodynamic, respiratory, and gas exchange effects of exercise	To provide a baseline, ongoing assessment and measure of treatment response
Define outcome criteria: reversal or mitigation of the signs and symptoms	To provide a basis for defining treatment goals and criteria for discontinuing treatment
Mobilization:	To exploit the *long-term* effects of activity and mobilization
Active and active-assisted body position changes every 1-2 hr when recumbent	Patients with extremely impaired oxygen transport are capable of only minimal mobilization stimuli; thus mobilization is prescribed on an interval schedule, low intensity, low duration, and high frequency of sessions; commensurate with patient's hemodynamic status
Dangling over edge of bed	
Transfer to chair	
Standing	
Walking	

Continued.

INTERVENTIONS	RATIONALE
Intensity—commensurate with recovery	
Frequency—several to 2-3 times a day	
Course and progression—as indicated	
Check blood pressure with patient in supine, sitting, and standing positions	To monitor orthostatic hypotension
Monitor heart rate and blood pressure with activity increases	To maintain heart rate increase < 20 beats per minute and blood pressure increase < 20 mm Hg; decreased heart rate and blood pressure suggest a decrease in cardiac output
Prescribe frequent rest periods within and between treatments	To minimize undue oxygen demands and fatigue, thereby increasing work capacity
Strengthening exercises	To optimize functional work capacity
Intensity—low	
Duration—5-20 minutes	
Frequency—daily	
Course and progression—as indicated	

Physical Therapy Diagnosis: Threats to oxygen transport and gas exchange, impaired mucociliary transport, retained secretions, atelectasis, effusion, bronchospasm, inadequate Fio_2; inadequate tidal volume, decreased cardiac output, increased pulmonary vascular resistance, altered cardiopulmonary, cerebral, renal, and peripheral tissue perfusion

Signs and Symptoms: Abnormal ABGs, Pao_2 < 80 mm Hg, $Paco_2$ < 35 or > 45 mm Hg, Sao_2 < 98%, cyanosis, radiographic evidence of atelectasis, effusion, pneumothorax, copious secretions, increased respiratory rate, wheezes, asymmetrical chest wall expansion, change in mental status, and fluid overload; signs of altered cerebral perfusion: mental confusion, dizziness, syncope, convulsions, seizures, transient ischemic attacks, yawning; signs of altered cardiopulmonary perfusion: angina and ischemic changes; signs of altered renal perfusion: oliguria and anuria; signs of altered peripheral perfusion: hypotension, peripheral ischemia, increased temperature and white blood cell count, skin breakdown

INTERVENTIONS	RATIONALE
Assess threats to oxygen transport and gas exchange	To provide a baseline, ongoing assessment and measure of treatment response
Monitor for signs of cerebral perfusion	Modify or discontinue treatment as indicated
Monitor for ECG changes and chest pain	To prevent ischemia and ischemic cardiac damage
Check urinary output	To determine renal function
Monitor peripheral tissue perfusion	To ensure that peripheral perfusion is maintained
Define outcome criteria: prevention, reversal, or mitigation of the signs and symptoms	To provide a basis for defining treatment goals and criteria for discontinuing treatment
360 degrees positional rotation	To promote physiological "stir-up"
Body positioning	
Range-of-motion exercises	
Mobilization	To exploit the *preventive* effects (i.e., increase mucocilary transport, mobilize secretions centrally, open closed alveoli, decrease shunt, and increase oxygen transport efficiency)

Physical Therapy Diagnosis: Knowledge deficit

Signs and Symptoms: Lack of knowledge about cardiopulmonary failure, its precipitating factors, complications, and cardiopulmonary physical therapy management

INTERVENTIONS	RATIONALE
Assess specific knowledge deficits related to cardiopulmonary failure and cardiopulmonary physical therapy management	To provide a baseline, ongoing assessment and measure of response to intervention
Define outcome criteria: reversal or mitigation of the signs and symptoms	To provide a basis for defining treatment goals and criteria for discontinuing treatment
Promote a caring and supportive patient-therapist relationship	To focus on treating the patient with cardiopulmonary failure rather than the cardiopulmonary failure
Consider every patient interaction an opportunity for education commensurate with the patient's level of arousal, alertness, and cognitive capacity	To promote self-responsibility for recovery, wellness, and health promotion
Commensurate with recovery, instruct regarding avoidance of respiratory tract infections, nutrition, hydration, fluid balance, exercise, stress management, and quality sleep	To promote cooperation and active participation in treatment
Reinforce medications, their purposes, and medication schedule	
Reinforce knowledge provided by other team members	
Teach, demonstrate, and provide feedback on interventions that can be self-administered	Between-treatment interventions are as important as treatments themselves to maximize cumulative treatment effect
Teach patient to balance activity and rest	Optimal balance between activity and rest is essential to exploit acute, long-term, and preventive effects of mobilization and exercise

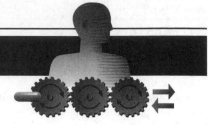

CHAPTER 24

Multiple Trauma

PATHOPHYSIOLOGY

Multiple trauma most frequently results from motor vehicle accidents, industrial accidents, high falls, and assaults with or without weapons. Cardiopulmonary dysfunction and threat to oxygen transport result from injury to the head, central nervous system, thoracic cavity, abdomen, or some combination. External trauma includes fractures, amputations, and contusions and lacerations of the chest wall and extremities. Internal trauma includes contusions, lacerations, and rupture of internal structures and organs. Even in the absence of head injury, trauma to the thorax and abdomen can threaten oxygen transport by its effects on the chest wall, great vessels to and from the heart, lungs, peripheral circulation, and plasma volume and on the local and neural control mechanisms of these organs and structures. Severe injuries are often associated with loss of consciousness, airway obstruction, loss of airway protection, blood loss, internal bleeding, third spacing, open wounds that provide portals for fluid loss and increased risk of infection, recumbency, and restricted mobility. In addition, nutrition and hydration are disrupted. Associated morbidity, complications, and prognosis are significantly influenced by the patient's age, weight, nutritional status, fluid and electrolyte balance, conditioning level, underlying cardiopulmonary or neuromuscular dysfunction, immune status, diabetes, smoking history, and substance abuse. Surgery may be indicated to reduce fractures, debride wounds, investigate the extent of internal injuries, and drain fluid from internal sites of injury. Surgery is itself traumatic and poses a threat to oxygen transport in that it requires anesthesia and sedation commensurate with the type and duration of surgery, prolonged ventilatory support, and prolonged static body positioning. Multiple surgeries may be indicated. Although pharmacological agents such as oxygen and narcotics are indicated in the management of critically ill patients, oxygen has well-known side effects that impair oxygen transport (e.g., contributes to denitrogen atelectasis and ciliary dyskinesia). Narcotic analgesia depresses respiratory drive and significantly reduces arousal and the patient's ability to cooperate with and derive the full benefit of cardiopulmonary physical therapy.

Case Study

The patient is a 59-year-old woman. She is East Indian and speaks little English. She lives with her extended family. She is a lifelong nonsmoker. She is moderately obese; her body mass index is 29. She was a passenger in the front seat of a car involved in a head-on collision with a combined speed

212

of 80 mph. She was not wearing a seat belt. She was thrown forward and hit the windshield. It was unclear whether there was any loss of consciousness. Her vital signs were stable at the scene. She was immobilized on a spine board. An intravenous (IV) line was started and oxygen administered. She was transferred to hospital. She was alert and through an interpreter was oriented to year, month, location, and situation. She had considerable tenderness over her left anterior chest wall, maximally around the eighth to eleventh ribs and shoulder. Her heart sounds were normal. There was no jugular venous distension and no crepitations. There was good air entry bilaterally. The abdomen was tender in the left upper quadrant. The pelvis was tender on the left side. She had lacerations to her face, head, and right elbow. She had several loose teeth. The rectal examination was negative for blood. X-rays confirmed fractures on the left side of the jaw, ribs 8 to 11, ankle, radius, and acetabulum. A chest tube was inserted for a left hemothorax and approximately 500 cc of blood drained. A nasogastric tube and Foley catheter were positioned. Two peripheral IV lines were also placed. Urinary analysis and an IV pylogram suggested a left-sided renal contusion. The patient was intubated and mechanically ventilated on assist control; tidal volume was 700 ml and rate was 18 breaths per minute with a fractional inspired oxygen concentration (Fio_2) of 0.30. Under general anesthesia she underwent closed reduction and splinting of the wrist and ankle fractures. The acetabular fracture was untreated. In addition, she underwent a diagnostic peritoneal lavage, which showed significant intraabdominal contusion. Computed tomography (CT) scan showed a mediastinal hemorrhage and shifting, periaortic hemorrhage and shifting, periaortic hematoma, and cardiac contusion. Aortogram corroborated a rupture of the thoracic aorta, which was surgically repaired. A pulmonary artery catheter was inserted. After surgery, her platelet count and hemoglobin were signficantly low. Chest x-ray showed low lung volumes, left lower lobe atelectasis, and a left pleural effusion extending to the apex. Heart rate was 112 beats per minute and blood pressure 139/69 mm Hg. She had occasional runs of ventricular tachycardia; otherwise she remained in sinus rhythm. She remained hemodynamically stable and values were within acceptable limits. On an Fio_2 of 0.30, arterial blood gas (ABG) analysis was pH 7.45, oxygen pressure (Po_2) 104 mm Hg, carbon dioxide pressure (Pco_2) 33 mm Hg, bicarbonate (HCO_3) 22, arterial oxygen saturation (Sao_2) 92%, and alveolar-arterial oxygen pressure difference ($P[A - a]o_2$) 69 mm Hg. Medications included narcotics, sedatives, and bronchodilators administered as needed. Scheduled medications included stress ulceration prophylaxis and antibiotics.

Oxygen Transport Deficits: Observed and Potential

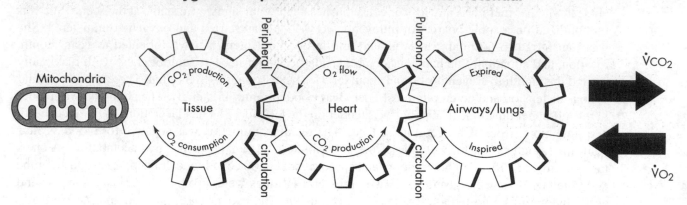

Stress-induced blood
    sugar abnormality
Impaired tissue healing
↑ Oxygen demand

Heart contusion
↑ Work of the heart
Repair of ruptured aorta
Pericardial effusion

↓ Mucociliary transport
↑ Secretion retention
Bronchospasm
↑ Airway resistance
Airway closure
Facial lacerations
Jaw fracture
Loose teeth
↓ Saliva control
↓ Cough reflex
Lung contusion
Rib fractures
Unstable chest wall
↓ Chest wall motion
Asymmetric chest wall
    movement
↑ Abdominal fluid
Third spacing
Encroachment of viscera
    on underside of
    diaphragm; secondary
    to obese abdomen
Ventilation and perfusion
    mismatch
Atelectasis
↓ Functional residual
    capacity
Monotonous tidal
    ventilation
↓ Alveolar volume
↓ Lung volumes and
    capacities
↑ Closing volumes
↓ Forced expiratory flow
    rates
Pleural effusions

↑ Systemic blood pressure

↑ Pulmonary vascular
    resistance
↑ Shunt
Fluid imbalance
↓ Lymph flow
↓ Lymphatic drainage

Blood: Hypoxemia
    Anemia
    Arterial desaturation

↑ Increase
↓ Decrease

PHYSICAL THERAPY DIAGNOSES AND TREATMENT PRESCRIPTION

Physical Therapy Diagnosis: Language and communication problem

Signs and Symptoms: Patient speaks Hindi and does not speak or understand English; fear, apprehension, and anxiety particularly because she is intubated and mechanically ventilated and cannot speak or communicate even with gestures effectively

INTERVENTIONS	RATIONALE
Monitor communication deficit	To provide a baseline and ongoing assessment
Identify means of communicating (e.g., interpreter, family member); prepare a list of key Hindi words at bedside	To reduce fear and arousal
	To promote understanding
	To promote cooperation
	Use her preferred name frequently
Communicate by speaking to the patient using a calm, reassuring voice even when an interpreter is not present	
Communicate by touching and smiling	To rely primarily on nonverbal communication

Physical Therapy Diagnosis: Pain

Signs and Symptoms: Grimacing, guarding, splinting, moaning, reluctance to move and reposition herself, and expressions of discomfort and pain when moving or being repositioned

INTERVENTIONS	RATIONALE
Monitor pain behavior and need for medication	To provide a baseline, ongoing assessment and measure of treatment response
Define outcome criteria: reversal or mitigation of the signs and symptoms	To provide a basis for defining treatment goals and criteria for discontinuing treatment
Ensure that patient is adequately medicated before treatments	To minimize patient's discomfort, pain, and suffering
	To reduce physiological arousal, increased energy and oxygen demands
Have an interpreter explain treatment and what patient is to do initially	Reduce patient's anxiety and apprehension by having treatment and procedures explained
Reduce anxiety	Increased anxiety and arousal lowers pain threshold
Promote pain control	Use voice and nonverbal communication to reassure and calm patient
Pace treatment	
Body positioning for comfort	When positioning the patient provide optimal limb support; request assistance when necessary; optimize body alignment
Transcutaneous electrical nerve stimulation (TENS) for shoulder	A trial of TENS to relieve shoulder pain and to increase comfort during positioning; TENS must be used selectively in the intensive care unit (ICU) because it interferes with the electrocardiogram (ECG) tracing
Promote relaxation	Exploit nonpharmacological pain control interventions to reduce or eliminate the need for medication, particularly narcotic analgesia

Physical Therapy Diagnosis: Abnormal hemodynamic status and increased metabolic demands

Signs and Symptoms: $Pao_2 < 104.2 - 0.27$ age (± 7) mm Hg, $Pao_2 < 75$ mm Hg on room air, $Sao_2 < 90\%$, repaired ruptured aorta, cardiac contusion, periaortic hematoma, reduced cardiac output, thoracotomy, exploratory laparotomy, mechanical ventilation, and decreased hemoglobin

INTERVENTIONS	RATIONALE
Monitor vital signs, ABGs, ECG, hemodynamics, cerebral perfusion, peripheral perfusion, urinary output	To provide a baseline, ongoing assessment and measure of treatment response
Define outcome criteria: reversal or mitigation of the signs and symptoms	To provide a basis for defining treatment goals and criteria for discontinuing treatment

Continued.

INTERVENTIONS	RATIONALE
Body positioning: in upright positions, head of bed up > 30 degrees; right side lying	To reduce hemodynamic stress and work of the heart To maintain systemic blood pressure < 130 mm Hg initially; to relieve stress on aortic repair

Physical Therapy Diagnosis: Alveolar hypoventilation and shunt caused by left hemothorax, left pleural effusion, lung contusion, heart contusion, pain over left upper quadrant, left kidney region, left hip, and from facial lacerations and jaw fracture, moderate obesity, intraabdominal contusion, anesthesia and sedation, surgery, low postoperative hemoglobin, left lower lobe atelectasis, and left pleural effusion; runs of ventricular tachycardia

Signs and Symptoms: $Pao_2 < 104.2 - 0.27$ age (± 7) mm Hg, $Pao_2 < 75$ mm Hg on room air, $Sao_2 < 90\%$, fractured ribs 8 to 11; chest wall contusion; mediastinal hemorrhage and shifting; periaortic hematoma, fluid shifts, third spacing; hypovolemia, increased work of breathing; increased minute ventilation and energy cost of breathing caused by increased respiratory rate and tidal volume; increased myocardial work: cardiac contusion, reduced cardiac output, decreased urinary output, sequelae of orthopedic surgery (closed reduction of ankle and wrist fractures), left thoracotomy for repair of lacerated aorta; exploratory laparotomy surgery: type of surgery, duration, anesthesia and sedation, reduced functional residual capacity and airway closure, narcotic analgesia; chest x-ray: low lung volume, left lower lobe atelectasis, and a left pleural effusion extending to the apex, decreased urinary output, decreased cardiac output, decreased venous return, and circulatory stasis

INTERVENTIONS	RATIONALE
Serial monitoring of vital signs, ABGs, blood work, ECG, Sao_2, Pao_2, Pao_2/Fio_2, Svo_2, heart rate, blood pressure, red and white blood cell counts, chest x-rays, and vital signs	To provide a baseline, ongoing assessment and measure of treatment response
Monitor oxygen transport variables, i.e., delivery, uptake, and extraction	
Cardiopulmonary clinical assessments	
Monitor pulmonary secretions; type, volume, consistency, color	
Define outcome criteria: reversal or mitigation of the signs and symptoms	To provide a basis for defining treatment goals and criteria for discontinuing treatment
Suctioning as indicated, particularly before, during, and after positioning and mobilization	Clear tracheal, bronchial, and oral secretions to maintain clear airways and decrease risk of aspiration
Monitor minute ventilation; respiratory rate and tidal volume; hemodynamics, oxygen, and ventilatory support; mechanical ventilation mode and parameters	To assess oxygen demand and oxygen delivery, which support the need for supplemental oxygen and ventilatory support
	To distinguish changes in gas exchange caused by changes in ventilatory support from cardiopulmonary physical therapy
	To monitor during treatment to minimize work of the heart and maintain systolic blood pressure below 130 mm Hg because of aortic repair
Body position prescription (patient cleared of head injury and spinal cord lesions)	To minimize pain and undue arousal
Ensure that patient is well supported in all positions	
Place in high and semi-Fowler's position	To enhance alveolar volume and the distribution of ventilation; promote mucociliary clearance, airway clearance of accumulated secretions
Place in reverse-Trendelenburg position (head up with feet down)	To elicit fluid shifts by providing a gravitational stimulus; reduce pulmonary blood volume and encroachment of abdominal viscera on the underside of the diaphragm; reduce the work of the heart

INTERVENTIONS	RATIONALE
In the horizontal plane, positional rotation includes ¾ supine to either side, supine, side lying to either side, ¾ prone to right side	To promote three-dimensional chest wall excursion, including bucket handle and pump handle motions
Duration—up to 1-2 hr, provided either beneficial or no change is observed	To minimize chest wall compression and compression of underlying dependent lung fields during static body positioning
Frequency—change body position every 1-2 hr	To simulate frequent changes in gravitational stress on the cardiopulmonary system to effect normal cardiopulmonary function and gas exchange
	To optimize lung movement, lung fluid balance, lymphatic drainage, and chest tube drainage
	To avoid excessive time supine; short durations in supine with head of bed > 10 degrees; longer periods permissible corresponding to increases in head of bed

Positions for the left lower lobe:
  Anterior segment—supine, head of bed down
  Lateral segment—right side lying, head of bed down
  Posterior segment—prone (modified ¾ prone right side), head of bed down
Upper lobe:
  Lingula—¾ supine in right side lying
  Apical segment—high Fowler's
  Anterior segment—semi-Fowler's
Posterior segment—¾ prone in right side lying, head of bed up
	Body positioning to maximize alveolar ventilation to the left lower lobe and upper lobe, enhance mucociliary transport, reduce secretion accumulation, and promote reabsorption of the left pleural effusion
	¾ prone positions on the right displaces protruding abdomen anteriorly, augmenting diaphragmatic descent

Frequent changes in body position	To stimulate physiological "stir-up"
Reposition in extreme positions from previous position	Use of successive extreme positions to place lowermost lung fields uppermost, thereby relieving compressed atelectatic-dependent lung fields, enhancing alveolar ventilation and mucociliary transport, and mobilizing any accumulation of pulmonary secretions
Restrict duration on any given position to 1 to 2 hr	Even beneficial positions become deleterious over time because of dependency and associated compression forces

Mobilization and exercise prescription (with patient appropriately premedicated; preferably nonnarcotic analgesia)
Type—active-assisted range-of-motion exercises, upper and lower extremities, and modified movement of chest wall
  In upright, high and semi-Fowler's positions
  In positions in the horizontal plane
Frequency—3 times a day
Duration—15-20 minutes
Course and progression—increase active participation of patient; as peak allowable systolic blood pressure is increased, low resistance is added to the range-of-motion exercises in extremities without fractures
	To exploit the *acute* effects of active mobilization and exercise on cardiopulmonary function, oxygen transport, and gas exchange (i.e., increase alveolar ventilation, optimize distribution of ventilation, perfusion, and ventilation and perfusion matching, decrease dead space and shunt, facilitate mucociliary transport, clearance of accumulated secretions, lymphatic drainage, lung and chest wall motion, maximize lung volumes and capacities, increase functional residual capacity and decrease airway closure, and optimize chest tube drainage)
	To minimize discomfort, pain, and suffering and maximize patient's ability to cooperate with treatment

Relaxation body positions	To reduce the work of breathing and overall oxygen demands
Continuous use of compression stockings	To optimize the mechanical function of the heart, augment venous return, and reduce circulatory stasis Ensure that compression stockings are applied over the full length of the legs, are of optimal tightness, are not bunched, wrinkled, or twisted, and are reapplied several times daily with 10-15 minutes between reapplications

Continued.

INTERVENTIONS	RATIONALE
Suction judiciously as indicated; prehyperoxygenate	To minimize the adverse effects of airway clearance with suctioning (e.g., arterial disaturation, atelectasis, and arrhythmias)

Physical Therapy Diagnosis: Inefficient breathing pattern: chest wall trauma, intraabdominal trauma, and pain over chest wall (ribs 8 to 11), head and neck, left shoulder, hip, radius, and ankle

Signs and Symptoms: Impaired chest wall motion; loss of three-dimensional motion and bucket handle and pump handle motions; particularly on the left side (ribs 8 to 11), decreased breath sounds, crackles, asymmetry, and pleural effusion of chest wall motion, radiographic evidence of alveolar collapse and atelectasis, reduced lung compliance, increased airway resistance, and obesity

INTERVENTIONS	RATIONALE
Monitor breathing pattern (i.e., tidal ventilation, respiratory rate, chest wall excursion, and symmetry)	To provide a baseline, ongoing assessment and measure of treatment response
Perform serial cardiopulmonary clinical examinations	
Monitor factors that improve and worsen breathing pattern	To assess gas exchange and lung parenchyma, etiology of shunt, and monitor effect of interventions
Monitor ABGs and chest x-rays	To assess gas exchange and left pleural effusion and monitor effect of interventions
Define outcome criteria: reversal or mitigation of the signs and symptoms	To provide a basis for defining treatment goals and criteria for discontinuing treatment
Optimize pain control	To promote more normal respiratory mechanics and breathing pattern
Mobilization	
Body positioning	
360 degrees positional rotation	
Frequent body position changes	

Physical Therapy Diagnosis: Decreased tolerance to physical activity and exercise

Signs and Symptoms: Expressions of pain during physical activity and mobilization, fatigue with minimal exertion, restrictions imposed by musculoskeletal and cardiopulmonary injuries, impaired oxygen transport, intubation and mechanical ventilation, supplemental oxygen, anemia, reduced circulating blood volume, premorbid deconditioning, and obesity

INTERVENTIONS	RATIONALE
Monitor responses to routine procedures and treatment sessions (i.e., ABGs, respiratory, hemodynamic, and gas exchange parameters)	To provide a baseline, ongoing assessment and index of treatment response
Monitor hemoglobin and blood work	
Define outcome criteria: reversal or mitigation of the signs and symptoms	To provide a basis for defining treatment goals and criteria for discontinuing treatment
Mobilization and exercise prescription (cardiopulmonary clinical examination before and after treatment; suction as indicated)	To exploit the *long-term* effects of mobilization and exercise
Type—dangling, transfer to chair, chair sit	Intensity of mobilization is low and sessions are short in duration but frequent while the patient is in the intensive care unit; although she is medically stable, she is still at risk of cardiopulmonary compromise and requires comprehensive ongoing monitoring until she is transferred to the ward
Intensity—low blood pressure restriction	
Duration—10-30 minutes	
Frequency—several times a day	
Course and progression—exercise intensity will be increased significantly when the patient is medically stable, at reduced risk of cardiopulmonary compromise, and transferred to the ward	As patient recovers, upper acceptable limit for blood pressure increased to 150 mm Hg by day 5

INTERVENTIONS	RATIONALE
Body positioning: active-assisted positioning	To encourage active-assisted positioning as much as possible but avoid static contractions and straining
	To avoid undue hemodynamic responses and ECG irregularities
Intersperse rest periods within or between treatments	To maximize the benefits of *acute* mobilization by maximizing treatment duration (hence work output) with interspersed rests
Optimize rest and sleep	
Monitor responses to treatment closely and to rest	To optimize parameters of treatment prescription (i.e., dosage maximally therapeutic with least risk)

Physical Therapy Diagnosis: Threats to oxygen transport, gas exchange, and peripheral tissue perfusion: fluid shifts, cardiac contusion, lung contusion, rib fractures, intraabdominal contusion, pain, medications (e.g., narcotic analgesia), restricted mobility, recumbency, lines, leads, catheters

Signs and Symptoms: Increased work of breathing, increased minute ventilation, increased $P(A - a)o_2$, hypoxemia, anemia, low platelet count, surgery, anesthesia and sedation and related procedures, thoracotomy, laparotomy, closed reduction of extremity fractures, dental surgery, blood transfusions, atelectasis, decreased lung compliance, decreased functional residual capacity, intubation and mechanical ventilation, multiple invasive lines and catheters (including pulmonary artery catheter), anxiety and pain, circulatory stasis, thrombosis formation, thromboemboli, ECG changes, myocardial ischemia, myocardial injury, angina, decreased cardiac output, pulmonary hypoxic vasoconstriction, oliguria, anuria, altered peripheral perfusion, decreased cardiac output, hypotension, impaired capillary filling time, impaired peripheral circulation, peripheral cyanosis, impaired skin nutrition, skin discoloration, skin breakdown, ulceration, impaired peripheral healing

INTERVENTIONS	RATIONALE
Identify threats to oxygen transport, gas exchange, and peripheral tissue perfusion	To provide a baseline, ongoing assessment and index of treatment response
Monitor respiratory, hemodynamic, and gas exchange parameters	
Cardiopulmonary physical therapy assessment	
Monitor signs of altered perfusion of vital organs	
Monitor temperature	
Monitor white blood cell count	
Define outcome criteria: prevention, reversal, or mitigation of the signs and symptoms	To provide a basis for defining treatment goals and criteria for discontinuing treatment
Mobilization and exercise prescription (patient adequately premedicated)	To exploit the *preventive* effects of mobilization and exercise within the limits of the patient's physiological reserve capacity
Type—bed mobility exercises, range-of-motion exercises, transfers	
Intensity—within limits of fatigue caused by anemia, within limits of pain	
Duration—short	
Frequency—frequent	
Course and progression—progress to stand and walk a few steps within patient's hemodynamic status and capacity	
Body positioning prescription:	To exploit the effects of gravity via body positioning and body position changes on cardiopulmonary function and gas exchange
Type—360 degrees positional rotation	
Duration—as per outcomes	
Frequency—1-2 hr	
Course and progression—as indicated	
Communicate through interpreter; verbal and nonverbal communication	Communication will alleviate fears and apprehension and reduce physiological arousal and oxygen demands; the patient will be more cooperative and willing to actively and fully participate in treatments

Continued.

INTERVENTIONS	RATIONALE
Infection control	Meticulous infection control practices are essential in handling and performing procedures on the patient (e.g., hand washing, gown, glove, and mask); avoid coming into contact with any bodily fluids
Minimize risk of pulling out lines and catheters when handling and treating patient	Inadvertent removal and reinsertion of lines and catheters can increase patient's risk of infection

Physical Therapy Diagnosis: Risk of the negative sequelae of recumbency

Signs and Symptoms: Within 6 hours reduced circulating blood volume, decreased blood pressure on sitting and standing compared with supine, light-headedness, dizziness, syncope, increased hematocrit and blood viscosity, increased work of the heart, altered fluid balance in the lung, impaired pulmonary lymphatic drainage, decreased lung volumes and capacities, decreased functional residual capacity, increased closing volume, and decreased Pao_2 and Sao_2

INTERVENTIONS	RATIONALE
Monitor the negative sequelae of recumbency	To provide a baseline, ongoing assessment and measure of treatment response
Define outcome criteria: prevention, reversal, or mitigation of the signs and symptoms	To provide a basis for defining treatment goals and criteria for discontinuing treatment
Sitting upright position, standing and walking	The upright position is essential to shift fluid volume from central to peripheral circulation and maintain fluid volume regulating mechanisms and circulating blood volume
	The upright position maximizes lung volumes and capacities and functional residual capacity
	The upright position maximizes expiratory flow rate and cough effectiveness
	The upright position optimizes the length-tension relationship of the respiratory muscles and abdominal muscles and optimizes cough effectiveness
	The upright position coupled with mobilization maximizes alveolar ventilation, ventilation and perfusion matching, and pulmonary lymphatic drainage; effects are augmented when patient is extubated and can coordinate breathing control and coughing maneuvers with mobilization

Physical Therapy Diagnosis: Risk of negative sequelae of restricted mobility

Signs and Symptoms: Reduced activity and exercise tolerance, muscle atrophy and reduced muscle strength, decreased oxygen transport efficiency, increased heart rate, blood pressure, and minute ventilation at submaximal work rates, reduced respiratory muscle strength, circulatory stasis, thromboemboli (e.g., pulmonary emboli), pressure areas, skin breakdown and ulceration, reduced premorbid fitness, and obesity

INTERVENTIONS	RATIONALE
Monitor the negative sequelae of restricted mobility	To provide a baseline, ongoing assessment and measure of treatment response
Define outcome criteria: prevention, reversal, or mitigation of the signs and symptoms	To provide a basis for defining treatment goals and criteria for discontinuing treatment
Mobilization and exercise prescription	Mobilization and exercise optimize circulating blood volume and enhance the efficiency of all steps in the oxygen transport pathway

Physical Therapy Diagnosis: Knowledge deficit

Signs and Symptoms: Lack of information about the effects of trauma, surgery, complications, and cardio-pulmonary physical therapy management

INTERVENTIONS	RATIONALE
Through an interpreter, determine the specific knowledge deficits related to injury, surgery, and cardiopulmonary physical therapy management	To address specific knowledge deficits in a simplified manner through an interpreter
Define outcome criteria: reversal or mitigation of the signs and symptoms	To provide a basis for defining treatment goals and criteria for discontinuing treatment
Promote a caring and supportive patient-therapist relationship	To focus on treating the patient with multiple trauma rather than the trauma
Consider every patient interaction an opportunity for education	To promote patient's sense of responsibility for recovery, wellness, and health promotion; even within limits of communication barrier, gestures of positive reinforcement and encouragement are understood
Through an interpreter, teach, demonstrate, and provide feedback on interventions that can be self-administered	Between-treatment interventions are as important as treatments themselves to provide cumulative treatment effect
Through an interpreter, teach patient to balance activity and rest	Optimal balance between activity and rest is essential to exploit short-term, long-term, and preventive effects of mobilization and exercise

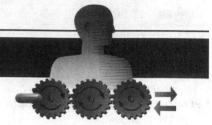

CHAPTER 25

Head Injury

PATHOPHYSIOLOGY

Head injuries are commonly associated with multiple trauma resulting from motor vehicle accidents, industrial accidents, high falls, and assaults with or without weapons. Injuries to the head are always a medical priority in that contusion to the brain results in increased blood flow, swelling, and cerebral compression. The adult cranial vault is noncompliant; therefore increased blood flow (increased pressure) threatens cerebral perfusion. The three main categories of head injuries are focal brain injuries, diffuse head injuries, and skull fractures. Severe head injuries involve a combination of these types of injuries. Cardiopulmonary dysfunction and threat to oxygen transport results from primary injury to the vital centers of the brain and from injuries to the thoracic and abdominal cavities. Severe head injuries are complicated by unconsciousness, obstructed airway, loss of airway protection, fluid loss, internal bleeding, spinal injuries, chest wall injuries, limb complications, burns, open wounds (which provide portals for continued fluid loss and increased risk of infection), recumbency, and restricted mobility. In addition, nutrition and hydration are compromised. Associated morbidity, complications, and prognosis are significantly influenced by the patient's age, weight, nutritional status, fluid and electrolyte balance, conditioning level, underlying cardiopulmonary or neuromuscular dysfunction, immune status, diabetes, smoking history, and substance abuse. Surgery may be indicated to reduce cerebral pressure and to insert a subarachnoid screw for intracranial pressure monitoring. Surgery is itself traumatic and poses further threat to oxygen transport in that it requires anesthesia and sedation commensurate with the type and duration of surgery, prolonged ventilatory support, and prolonged static body positioning. In addition, pharmacological agents such as oxygen and narcotics are indicated. Although essential in the management of critically ill patients, oxygen has well-known side effects that impair oxygen transport (e.g., contributes to denitrogen atelectasis and ciliary dyskinesia). Narcotic analgesia depresses respiratory drive and significantly reduces arousal and the patient's ability to cooperate with and derive the full benefit of cardiopulmonary physical therapy. In addition, coma or neuromuscular blockade may be indicated to minimize metabolic demands.

Case Study

The patient is a 37-year-old man. He is a rancher who lives with his wife and 6-year-old daughter. He was thrown from his horse, fell down an embankment, and hit his head on a rock. At the site of the accident, he was confused and disoriented. Ranch workers reported that he lost consciousness for several minutes. On arrival at the hospital, his vital signs were heart rate 60 beats per minute, blood pressure 165/90 mm Hg, and respiratory rate 15 breaths per minute and regular. His pupils were equal and reactive to light but were sluggish. His breathing became increasingly labored. The patient became progressively obtunded and was responding to pain with incomprehensible sounds. The Glasgow Coma scale rating was 8 (eye response rated 2, verbal response rated 3, and motor response rated 3). The patient was placed on mechanical ventilatory support to provide hyperventilation, that is, tidal volume 1200 ml, respiratory rate 10 breaths per minute, and a fractional inspired oxygen concentration (Fio_2) of 0.50. Arterial blood gases (ABGs) were pH 7.51, arterial oxygen pressure (Pao_2) 225 mm Hg, and arterial carbon dioxide pressure ($Paco_2$) 28 mm Hg. Heart rate was 72 beats per minute and blood pressure was 140/74 mm Hg. There was no evidence of spinal cord involvement or significant other injuries other than bruising and superficial lacerations of the chest wall and arms. The patient went to the operating room for removal of a bone flap on the left side to reduce cerebral pressure and insertion of a subarachnoid screw for intracranial pressure (ICP) monitoring. The ICP rose to 30 to 35 mm Hg despite hyperventilation and sedation. A pulmonary artery catheter was inserted to monitor the patient's hemodynamic status during the fluid and inotropic therapy and the institution and maintenance of barbiturate coma with pentobarbital. Muscle relaxants were also administered. After stabilization, hemodynamic profile was blood pressure 105/65 mm Hg, central venous pressure 7 mm Hg, pulmonary artery capillary wedge pressure 8 mm Hg, cardiac index 3.0, intracranial pressure 18 mm Hg, and cerebral perfusion pressure 60 mm Hg.

Oxygen Transport Deficits: Observed and Potential

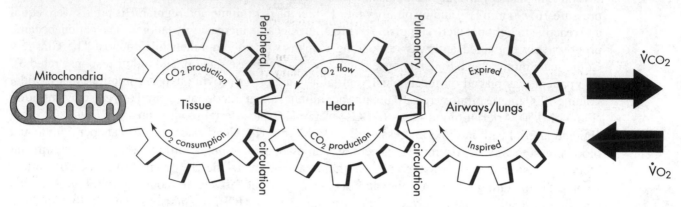

↑ Intracranial pressure
↓ Cerebral perfusion
↑ Systemic metabolic
   demands
↓ Oxygen uptake

↑ Work of the heart

↓ Gag reflex
↓ Cough reflex
↓ Upper airway tone
↓ Mucociliary transport
↓ Secretion clearance
Aspiration
↑ Airflow resistance
Monotonous tidal
   ventilation
Atelectasis
↓ Compliance
↓ Lung volumes and
   capacities
↓ Functional residual
   capacity
↑ Closing volumes
Acute lung injury

Circulatory stasis
Thrombus formation

Fluid imbalance
Neurogenic pulmonary
   edema
Alveolar capillary
   membrane leak
↓ Lymph flow
↓ Lymph drainage

Blood: ↓ Blood volume
        ↓ Hemoglobin

↑ Increase
↓ Decrease

PHYSICAL THERAPY DIAGNOSES AND TREATMENT PRESCRIPTION

Physical Therapy Diagnosis: Decreased cerebral perfusion pressure related to increased ICP, cerebral edema, and hypertension

Signs and Symptoms: ICP > 20 mm Hg, $Paco_2$ > 25 and < 35 mm Hg, spiking of ICP with handling of patient, suctioning, and noxious stimulation; decreased pupillary response, motor dysfunction, sensory dysfunction, altered level of consciousness, altered vital signs, cognitive impairment, seizure activity, confusion, impaired sleep, and restlessness

INTERVENTIONS	RATIONALE
Serial monitoring of ICP	To provide a baseline, ongoing assessment and measure of treatment response
	Patients with increased ICP are mechanically hyperventilated to maintain low $Paco_2$; CO_2 is a cerebral vasodilator that increases cerebral volume and pressure and reduces cerebral perfusion
	Extremely low $Paco_2$ levels can impair perfusion because of excessive vasoconstriction
Serial monitoring of mechanical ventilator parameters, especially positive end-expiratory pressure (PEEP) and the effect on ICP	PEEP increases intrathoracic pressure, which decreases cardiac output; it increases ICP in patients with poor cerebral compliance
Define outcome criteria: reversal or mitigation of the signs and symptoms	To provide a basis for defining treatment goals and criteria for discontinuing treatment
Maintain head of bed > 30 degrees	To minimize obstruction of venous drainage and reduce ICP
Position patient in high or semi-Fowler's position Monitor ICP in response to upright positions	Erect upright positions may compromise cerebral perfusion pressure (CPP), an indirect measure of cerebral blood flow; CPP = MAP (mean arterial pressure) − ICP
	Hypertensive therapy may need to be instituted to maintain cerebral blood flow in upright positions
Maintain head, neck, and upper body in a neutral position with sandbags and rolled blankets	Turning and flexion of the head may obstruct venous drainage and increase ICP
Minimize flexion, extension, and rotation of the head and neck	
Monitor responses to head-turned positions	Right head turning may increase ICP more than left head turning; the right internal jugular vein is usually larger than the left
Monitor responses to turning to either side	Some patients do not tolerate turning to either side
Turn patient with assistance; one person maintains the head and neck in a neutral position	Extreme caution is used to change patient's body position to ensure that ICP is not increased
Allow for stabilization period if ICP spikes during treatment	Intracranial pressure increases should not exceed 40 mm Hg for prolonged periods and should only spike to higher pressures and not be sustained
	Persistently increased ICP is indicative of impaired cerebral compliance, reduced cerebral perfusion, and potential cerebral injury and damage
	To minimize MAP and ICP
Ensure that patient is well supported	Patient is on muscle relaxants and is less able to support himself in a given position
Range-of-motion exercises are performed such that mean arterial pressure does not significantly increase	All physical therapy interventions can increase ICP; these must be performed within acceptable limits and with appropriate rests between
Coordinate treatments with nursing and other interventions	
Pace treatments	
Optimize sleep and rest periods	To minimize excessive physical demands on the patient
Suction judiciously; preoxygenate and limit suction catheter pass time < 10-15 seconds with rest periods between	Suctioning significantly increases ICP because of induced hypoxemia and tracheal irritation

Continued.

INTERVENTIONS	RATIONALE
When patient is no longer under an induced coma, promote relaxation during and between treatments	To exploit nonpharmacological means of optimizing ICP
Avoid breath holding, static posturing, and the Valsalva maneuver	Breath holding and the Valsalva maneuver increase intra-thoracic and intraabdominal pressures which increases mean arterial pressure and ICP
Avoid activities requiring excessive postural stabilization and isometric muscle contraction	Static muscle contractions are associated with increased hemodynamic stress and increased intraabdominal pressure, which increases mean arterial pressure and ICP

Physical Therapy Diagnosis: Alveolar hypoventilation and shunt

Signs and Symptoms: ABGs on Fio_2 0.50, Pao_2 225 mm Hg, $Paco_2$ 28 mm Hg, pH 7.51, Sao_2 92%, anesthesia, sedation, induced paralysis, increased pulmonary secretions, atelectasis, increased respiratory rate, decreased air entry, decreased chest wall excursion, and closure of dependent airways

INTERVENTIONS	RATIONALE
Serial monitoring of ABGs, ECG, hemodynamics, chest x-rays, and fluid balance	To provide a baseline, ongoing assessment and measure of treatment response
Monitor oxygen transport variables, i.e., delivery, uptake, and extraction	Patients with increased ICP are mechanically hyperventilated to maintain low $Paco_2$; CO_2 is a vasodilator of cerebral blood vessels that increases cerebral blood volume and pressure and reduces cerebral perfusion; extremely low $Paco_2$ levels, however, also impair cerebral blood flow and perfusion because of excessive vasoconstriction
Continuous monitoring of ICP and CPP during treatments to guide their prescription parameters	To establish an index of cerebral compliance
	To determine what interventions and physical perturbations increase ICP, decrease ICP, or have no effect
	To use ICP changes as a guide to modifying treatment
Define outcome criteria: reversal or mitigation of the signs and symptoms	To provide a basis for defining treatment goals and criteria for discontinuing treatment
Body positioning prescription: ECG, hemodynamic, respiratory, Sao_2, and ICP responses are monitored before, during, and after treatment	Monitoring untoward hemodynamic and ICP responses is essential to avoid cerebral ischemia and injury
Body support during handling and positioning	Induced paralysis increases patient's susceptibility to musculoskeletal and neuromuscular trauma and skin breakdown
Type — place in upright positions with the head, neck, upper body, and trunk in neutral alignment Right side lying Modified side lying ¾ prone	Erect upright positions decrease hydrostatic pressure, hence ICP Erect, upright positions elicit a gravity stimulus, which maximizes lung volumes and capacities, functional residual capacity, expiratory flow rates, minimizes closing volumes, optimizes the position of the respiratory muscles on their length-tension curves, reduces the work of breathing, reduces thoracic blood volume, increases lung compliance and alveolar volume, and reduces the work of the heart
Intensity — within therapeutic limits of oxygen transport variables and hemodynamic and ICP values	
Duration — as long as beneficial effects occur	
Frequency — 1-2 hr	Positioning the head to the left in left side lying is contraindicated in this patient because of the left bone flap removal
Course and progression — as indicated	Patient is turned into each position gradually to reduce physical stress of body position change
	Positions < 30 degrees and prone are not tolerated well by patients with poor cerebral compliance

INTERVENTIONS	RATIONALE
Monitor CPP and ICP responses during positioning, particularly head up > 30 degrees and side lying	CPP may decrease in upright positions because of decreased hydrostatic pressure ICP may increase in side lying if neck position is not controlled
Frequent body position changes	Frequent body position changes are indicated to minimize deleterious effects in the dependent lung fields; attempt to reposition from one position to an extreme position within limits of acceptable ICP levels
Range-of-motion exercises (passive): hemodynamic, respiratory, ICP, and Sao_2 responses monitored before, during, and after treatment Upper extremity Lower extremity, including hip and knee and foot and ankle exercises Intensity — minimal hemodynamic response, minimal to moderate respiratory and hemodynamic responses, ICP response within acceptable levels Duration — as required to complete range of motion of limbs Frequency — 2-3 times a day Course and progression — include chest wall mobility exercises as the induced coma is discontinued and increased ICP resolves and patient can be dangled over edge of bed and transferred to chair	Range-of-motion exercises elicit important cardiopulmonary reflexes and significant cardiopulmonary effects (i.e., stimulate increased tidal volume and breathing frequency and respiratory muscle recruitment) Range-of-motion exercises augment circulatory flow rates and tissue perfusion Modify range-of-motion exercises from passive to active-assist based on hemodynamic, respiratory, and ICP responses

Physical Therapy Diagnosis: Ineffective breathing pattern caused by location and severity of head injury and cerebral edema, associated trauma, discomfort and pain, intubation, and mechanical ventilation

Signs and Symptoms: Abnormal chest wall symmetry, abnormal chest wall movement, abnormal coordination of thoracic and abdominal movement, radiographic evidence of atelectasis

INTERVENTIONS	RATIONALE
Serial monitoring of breathing pattern; tidal volume, respiratory rate, and chest wall excursion and symmetry Serial monitoring of ABGs Monitor changes in the absence or presence of breath sounds and adventitious sounds Monitor symmetry of chest wall motion Monitor chest wall motion in three planes Monitor thoracoabdominal motion Monitor respiratory muscle accessory activity Monitor cardiorespiratory distress	To provide a baseline, ongoing assessment and measure of treatment response
Define outcome criteria: reversal or mitigation of the signs and symptoms	To provide a basis for defining treatment goals and criteria for discontinuing treatment
Body position prescription: Identify those body positions that promote a relaxed, efficient breathing pattern Place patient in relaxation positions (i.e., optimize ABGs and decrease the work of breathing)	Breathing pattern reflects the most mechanically and metabolically efficient pattern of breathing for the patient; body positioning alters breathing pattern by manipulating airway resistance, lung compliance, intraabdominal pressure, thoracoabdominal motion, and thoracic blood volume, which influence breathing pattern
Place in high and semi-Fowler's positions; monitor CPP and ICP in head-up positions > 30 degrees	To optimize breathing pattern and minimize the work of breathing

Continued.

Physical Therapy Diagnosis: Impaired mucociliary transport

Signs and Symptoms: Abnormal breath sounds, adventitious sounds (i.e., crackles and wheezes), increased airway resistance, increased system pressure on mechanical ventilator, increased secretions, increased work of breathing, respiratory distress, arterial desaturation, and radiographic evidence of atelectasis

INTERVENTIONS	RATIONALE
Serial monitoring of mucociliary transport Serial monitoring of secretions: quantity and quality Serial monitoring of ABGs	To provide a baseline, ongoing assessment and measure of treatment response
Monitor neck veins for jugular venous distention	To assess changes in central venous pressure
Define outcome criteria: reversal or mitigation of the signs and symptoms	To provide a basis for defining treatment goals and criteria for discontinuing treatment
Suction as indicated	Prolonged or excessive suctioning causes hypoxemia, altered breathing pattern, and agitation
Hyperoxygenate and hyperventilate with 100% oxygen before and after suctioning	To minimize hypoxemia and hypercapnea, which precipitate cerebral vasodilation
Suction pass < 15 seconds	
Body positioning prescription for postural drainage: Modified side lying positions	To facilitate mucociliary transport and drain pulmonary secretions
Coordinate modified postural drainage positions with manual chest wall vibration if indicated	Postural drainage positions are restricted to head of bed at 30 degrees (i.e., no head down)
Duration—based on airway clearance and avoidance of adverse responses	Manual vibration is performed continuously and modified according to respiratory, hemodynamic, and ICP responses
Frequency—as indicated	
Course and progression—as indicated; positioning challenge to assess cerebral compliance and whether horizontal or head down position can be tolerated	As patient improves and cerebral edema resolves, cerebral compliance improves; the patient will be able to tolerate a modified head of bed < 30 degrees and eventually head down position
	A position challenge provides an index of cerebral compliance; the degree to which ICP drops after being increased (poor compliance if ICP fails to drop after an ICP challenge such as head of bed < 30 degrees or head down)

Physical Therapy Diagnosis: Agitation and restlessness after discontinuation of induced coma

Signs and Symptoms: Excessive activity, impaired rest and sleep periods, inadequate rest and sleep, increased hemodynamic and ICP responses, and increased energy and oxygen demand

INTERVENTIONS	RATIONALE
Serial monitoring of agitation and restlessness	To provide a baseline, ongoing assessment and measure of treatment response
Monitor effect of medications	To identify interventions and factors that increase, decrease, and do not affect agitation and restlessness, hence ICP
Coordinate treatments with medications to control agitation	To determine the relationship between agitation/restlessness and ICP and CPP
Define outcome criteria: reversal or mitigation of the signs and symptoms	To provide a basis for defining treatment goals and criteria for discontinuing treatment
Relaxation procedures: Talk calmly to patient	To minimize physiological arousal and psychological distress
Use touch and reassuring voice to calm patient	
Prepare patient for position changes, suctioning, and mobilization	
Provide adequate support and assist to handle and move patient	
Suction pass < 15 seconds in duration	
Play tapes of patient's favorite music	

INTERVENTIONS	RATIONALE

Pain control strategies:
  Coordinate treatments with pain medications
  Provide support to injury sites when treating
  Minimize excessive time in any given position
  Frequent position changes
  Minimize undue arousal associated with treatments
	To minimize discomfort/pain to reduce suffering and maximize cooperation with treatment and treatment response

Physical Therapy Diagnosis: Altered orthostatic tolerance

Signs and Symptoms: Hypotension, dizziness and light-headedness, decreased heart rate with the upright position, syncope, and fatigue

INTERVENTIONS	RATIONALE
Monitor blood pressure and hemodynamic responses to approximating the upright position	To provide a baseline, ongoing assessment and measure of treatment response To introduce a gravitational stimulus gradually (i.e., the upper body erect, followed by dependency of the legs)
Define outcome criteria: reversal or mitigation of the signs and symptoms	To provide a basis for defining treatment goals and criteria for discontinuing treatment
Body position prescription: place in upright positions with the head, neck, upper body, and trunk in neutral position with the legs dependent in the supported reverse-Trendelenburg position (i.e., head of bed up and foot of bed down)	In addition to the benefits of upright position on cardiopulmonary function and gas exchange, dependency of the legs prime the fluid volume regulating mechanisms that help maintain a normovolemic state Compared with the high Fowler's position, the reverse-Trendelenburg position decreases hip flexion and intra-abdominal pressure, which can increase ICP
Monitor ICP in head-up positions > 30 degrees or head down < 30 degrees	To ensure that CPP is not compromised or ICP unduly increased

Physical Therapy Diagnosis: Reduced activity and exercise capacity

Signs and Symptoms: Induced paralysis and sedation

INTERVENTIONS	RATIONALE
Monitor degree of induced muscle relaxation	To provide a baseline, ongoing assessment and measure of treatment response
Monitor effect of muscle relaxation on CPP and ICP	To select mobilization prescription parameters based on CPP, ICP, muscle relaxants, and hemodynamic responses
Monitor effect of muscle relaxants on oxygen transport, including delivery and consumption	Muscle relaxants are used to reduce the metabolic cost and hemodynamic demands of patients with head injuries; as ICP is reduced to normal levels, muscle relaxants are discontinued, and active mobilization can be initiated Induced coma contributes further to muscular and aerobic deconditioning

Range-of-motion exercises:
  Upper extremities
  Trunk
  Lower extremities
	To exploit the *acute* effects of range-of-motion exercises and pulmonary and cardiovascular function

Mobilization as soon as induced coma is discontinued	To exploit the *long-term* effects of mobilization on oxygen transport

Continued.

Physical Therapy Diagnosis: Threats to cardiopulmonary function and oxygen transport from cerebral trauma, increased ICP, decreased CPP, fluid and electrolyte imbalance, infection, pain, stiffness, altered bowel function, skin breakdown, recumbency, and restricted mobility

Signs and Symptoms: Persistently elevated ICP and impaired cerebral perfusion, motor, sensory and cognitive deficits indicative of compression of vital centers in the brain, impaired fluid and electrolyte status, altered hematocrit, altered blood urea nitrogen, creatinine, and serum osmolality, increased temperature, increased white blood cell count, hyperthermia, change in sputum characteristics, altered level of consciousness, verbalization and physical expressions of pain, circulatory stasis, venous thrombosis, and pulmonary emboli

INTERVENTIONS	RATIONALE
Monitor threats to cardiopulmonary function and oxygen transport	To provide a baseline and ongoing assessment
Serial monitoring of signs and symptoms of compromised cardiopulmonary function and oxygen transport	
Serial monitoring of fluid and electrolyte balance and body weight	
Serial monitoring of signs of infection	To distinguish cardiopulmonary infection from other sites
	To monitor risk of cardiopulmonary infection if infection elsewhere
	To modify treatment with respect to oxygen demands
Define outcome criteria: prevention, reversal, or mitigation of the signs and symptoms	To provide a basis for defining treatment goals and criteria for discontinuing treatment
Pain control strategies	To minimize adverse effects of pain on oxygen transport and gas exchange
	To modify treatment accordingly
Range-of-motion exercises	In addition to their cardiopulmonary benefits, perform range-of-motion exercises to preserve joint mobility and muscle structure and lengths, optimize function, and reduce complications
Maximize frequency of body positioning progressing to mobilization as indicated by hemodynamic and respiratory status and ICP	To maximize treatment effects by maintaining safe therapeutic limits of hemodynamic and cardiopulmonary effects, minimizing ICP and optimizing CPP
When induced coma is discontinued, mobilization is instituted with acceptable limits of ICP and CPP	To exploit the *preventive* effects of mobilization and being upright commensurate with the patient's status; mobilization prescribed accordingly

Physical Therapy Diagnosis: Risk of the negative sequelae of recumbency

Signs and Symptoms: Within 6 hours reduced circulating blood volume, decreased blood pressure on sitting and standing compared with supine, light-headedness, dizziness, syncope, increased hematocrit and blood viscosity, increased work of the heart, altered fluid balance in the lung, impaired pulmonary lymphatic drainage, decreased lung volumes and capacities, decreased functional residual capacity, increased closing volume, and decreased Pao_2 and Sao_2

INTERVENTIONS	RATIONALE
Monitor the negative sequelae of recumbency	To provide a baseline and ongoing assessment
Define outcome criteria: prevention, reversal, or mitigation of the signs and symptoms	To provide a basis for defining treatment goals and criteria for discontinuing treatment
Place in upright positions	To optimize gravitational stimulation on hemodynamics and minimize the negative sequelae of recumbency
Place in reverse-Trendelenburg position (head up and feet down)	

INTERVENTIONS	RATIONALE
Dangling over bed, chair sit, standing and walking when induced coma discontinued and within acceptable limits of ICP	The upright position is essential to shift fluid volume from central to peripheral circulation and maintain fluid volume regulating mechanisms and circulating blood volume The upright position maximizes lung volumes and capacities and functional residual capacity The upright position maximizes expiratory flow rate and cough effectiveness The upright position optimizes the length-tension relationship of the respiratory muscles and abdominal muscles and optimizes cough effectiveness The upright position coupled with mobilization and breathing control and coughing maneuvers maximizes alveolar ventilation, ventilation and perfusion matching, mucociliary transport, mucociliary clearance, and pulmonary lymphatic drainage

Physical Therapy Diagnosis: Risk of negative sequelae of restricted mobility

Signs and Symptoms: Reduced activity and exercise tolerance, muscle atrophy and reduced muscle strength, decreased oxygen transport efficiency, increased heart rate, blood pressure, and minute ventilation at submaximal work rates, reduced respiratory muscle strength, circulatory stasis, thromboemboli (e.g., pulmonary emboli), pressure areas, skin redness, skin breakdown and ulceration

INTERVENTIONS	RATIONALE
Monitor the negative sequelae of restricted mobility Define outcome criteria: prevention, reversal, or mitigation of the signs and symptoms Mobilization and exercise prescription: passive range of motion and body positioning initially, followed by active mobilization as ICP is less of a threat and induced coma discontinued	To provide a baseline and ongoing assessment To provide a basis for defining treatment goals and criteria for discontinuing treatment Mobilization and exercise optimize circulating blood volume and enhance the efficiency of all steps in the oxygen transport pathway

Physical Therapy Diagnosis: Knowledge deficit

Signs and Symptoms: Lack of information about injury, complications, and prognosis

INTERVENTIONS	RATIONALE
Assess patient's specific knowledge deficits related to injury and cardiopulmonary physical therapy management Define outcome criteria: reversal or mitigation of the signs and symptoms Promote a caring and supportive patient-therapist relationship Consider every patient interaction an opportunity for education when induced coma discontinued Teach, demonstrate, and provide feedback on interventions that can be administered by staff (e.g., positioning schedule) Reinforce patient's need for rest and sleep to optimize therapeutic response to treatment and recovery	To provide a baseline and ongoing assessment To address specific knowledge deficits To provide a basis for defining treatment goals and criteria for discontinuing treatment To focus on treating the patient with a head injury rather than the head injury To promote patient's sense of responsibility for recovery, wellness, and health promotion Between-treatment interventions are as important as treatments themselves to provide cumulative treatment effect Optimal balance between activity and rest is essential to exploit short-term, long-term, and preventive effects of mobilization and exercise

Bibliography

Adams, M. A., & Chandler, L. S. (1974). Effects of physical therapy program on vital capacity of patients with muscular dystrophy. *Physical Therapy, 54,* 494–496.

Albert, R. K., Leasa, D., Snaderson, M., Robertson, H. T., & Hlastala, M. P. (1987). The prone position improves arterial oxygenation and reduces shunt in oleic-acid induced acute lung injury. *American Review of Respiratory Diseases, 135,* 626–633.

Alexander, J. K. (1985). The cardiomyopathy of obesity. *Progress in Cardiovascular Diseases, 28,* 325–334.

Alexander, J. L., Spence, A. A., Parikh, R. K., & Stuart, B. (1973). The role of airway closure in postoperative hypoxaemia. *British Journal of Anaesthesiology, 59,* 1070–1079.

American College of Sports Medicine. (1991). *Guidelines for exercise testing and prescription* (4th ed.). Philadelphia: Lea & Febiger.

Andreoli, K. G., Fowkes, V. K., Zipes, D. P., & Wallace, A. G. (Eds.). (1991). *Comprehensive cardiac care* (7th ed.). St. Louis: Mosby.

Arita, K. I., Nishida, O., & Hiramoto, T. (1981). Physical exercise in 'pulmonary fibrosis'. *Hiroshima Journal of Medical Science, 30,* 149–159.

Astrand, P. O., & Grumby, G. (Eds.), (1986). Physical activity in health and disease. *Acta Medica Scandinavica,* Suppl. 711, 1–249.

Austin, G. L., & Greenfield, L. J. (1980). Respiratory care in cardiac failure and pulmonary edema. *Surgical Clinics in North America, 60,* 1565–1575.

Bach, J. R. (1992). Pulmonary rehabilitation considerations for Duchenne muscular dystrophy: The prolongation of life by respiratory muscle aids. *Critical Reviews in Physical and Rehabilitation Medicine, 3,* 239–269.

Bach, J. R. (1993). Mechanical insufflation-exsufflation. Comparison of peak expiratory flows with manually assisted and unassisted coughing techniques. *Chest, 104,* 1553–1562.

Bach, J. R., Alba, A. S., Bodofsky, E., Curran, F. J., & Schultheiss, M. (1987). Glossopharyngeal breathing and noninvasive aids in the management of post-polio respiratory insufficiency. *Birth Defects, 23,* 99–113.

Bach, J. R., Alba, A. S., & Shin, D. (1989). Management alternatives for post-polio respiratory insufficiency. Assisted ventilation by nasal or oro-nasal interface. *American Journal of Physical Medicine and Rehabilitation, 68,* 264–271.

Bach, J. R., O'Brien, J., Krotenberg, R., & Alba, A. S. (1987). Management of end stage respiratory failure in Duchenne muscular dystrophy. *Muscle and Nerve, 10,* 177–182.

Bach, J. R., Smith, W. H., Michaels, J., Saporito, L., Alba, A. S., Dayal, R., & Pan, J. (1993). Airway secretion clearance by mechanical exsufflation for post-poliomyelitis ventilator-assisted individuals. *Archives of Physical Medicine and Rehabilitation, 74,* 170–174.

Bain, J., Bishop, J., & Olinsky, A. (1988). Evaluation of directed coughing in cystic fibrosis. *British Journal of Diseases of the Chest, 82,* 138–148.

Bake, B., Dempsey, J., & Grimby, G. (1976). Effects of shape changes of the chest wall on distribution of inspired gas. *American Review of Respiratory Diseases, 114,* 1113–1120.

Bannister, R. (1988). *Autonomic failure* (2nd ed.). Oxford: Oxford Medical Publications.

Barrach, A. L. (1974). Chronic obstructive lung disease: Postural relief of dyspnea. *Archives of Physical Medicine and Rehabilitation, 55,* 494–504.

Barrach, A. L., & Beck, G. J. (1954). Ventilatory effects of head-down position in pulmonary emphysema. *American Journal of Medicine, 16,* 55–60.

Barrach, A. L., Beck, G. J., Bickerman, H. A., & Seanor, J. H. (1952). Physical methods of stimulating cough mechanisms. Use in poliomyelitis, bronchial asthma, and bronchiectasis. *Journal of the American Medical Association, 50,* 1380–1385.

Bartlett, R. H., Gassaniga, A. B., & Geraphty, T. R. (1973). Respiratory maneuvers to prevent postoperative pulmonary complications. A critical review. *Journal of the American Medical Association, 224,* 1017–1021.

Bartlett, J. G., & Gorbach, S. L. (1976). The triple threat of pneumonia. *Chest, 68,* 4–10.

Baskin, M. W. (1996). Respiratory care practice review. In D. L. Frownfelter & E. Dean (Eds.), *Principles and practice of cardiopulmonary physical therapy* (3rd ed.). St Louis: Mosby.

Bates, D. V. (1989). *Respiratory function in disease* (3rd ed.). Philadelphia: W. B. Saunders.

Behrakis, P. K., Baydur, A., Jaeger, M. J., & Milic-Emili, J. (1983). Lung mechanics in sitting and horizontal body positions. *Chest, 83,* 643–646.

Belman, M. J., & Kendregan, B. A. (1981). Exercise training fails to increase skeletal muscle enzymes in patients with chronic obstructive pulmonary disease. *American Review of Respiratory Diseases, 123,* 256–261.

Belman, M. J., & Wasserman, K. (1981). Exercise training and testing in patients with chronic obstructive pulmonary disease. *Basics of Respiratory Diseases, 10,* 1–6.

Bennett, W. D., Foster, W. M., & Chapman, W. F. (1990). Cough-enhanced mucus clearance in the normal lung. *Journal of Applied Physiology, 69,* 1670–1675.

Berry, J., Covey, M., & Shekleton, M. (1996). Respiratory muscle fatigue and training. In D. L. Frownfelter & E. Dean (Eds.), *Principles and practice of cardiopulmonary physical therapy* (3rd ed.). St. Louis: Mosby.

Bishop, M. H., Shoemaker, W. C., Appel, P. L., Wo, C-J., Zwick, C., Kram, H. B., Meade, P., Kennedy, F., & Fleming, A. W. (1993). Relationship between supranormal circulatory values, time dealsy, and outcome in severely traumatized patients. *Critical Care Medicine, 21,* 56–63.

Bjore, D. (1972). Post myocardial infarctions: A program of graduated exercises. *Physiotherapy Canada, 24,* 22–25.

Black, L. F., & Hyatt, R. E. (1971). Maximal static respiratory pressures in generalized neuromuscular disease. *American Review of Respiratory Diseases, 103,* 641–650.

Blair, S. N., Painter, P., Pate, R. R., Smith, L. K., & Taylor, C. B. (1988). *Resource manual for guidelines for exercise testing and prescription.* Philadelphia: Lea & Febiger.

Blomqvist, C. G., & Stone, H. L. (1983). Cardiovascular adjustments to gravitational stress. *Handbook of physiology* (Vol. 2). Washington, DC: American Physiological Society.

Boggs, R. L., & Wooldridge-King, M. (1993). *AACN procedure manual for critical care* (3rd ed.). Philadelphia: W. B. Saunders.

Borozyny, M. L. (1987). Intracranial hypertension: Implications for the physiotherapist. *Physiotherapy Canada, 39,* 360–366.

Bourn, J., & Jenkins, S. (1992). Post-operative respiratory physiotherapy. Indications for treatment. *Physiotherapy, 78,* 80–85.

Braun, N. M. T., Arora, N. S., & Rochester, D. F. (1983). Respiratory muscle and pulmonary function in polymyositis and other proximal myopathies. *Thorax, 38,* 616–623.

Brooks, G. (1996). Clinical assessment of the cardiopulmonary systems. In D. L. Frownfelter & E. Dean (Eds.), *Principles and practice of cardiopulmonary physical therapy* (3rd ed.). St Louis: Mosby.

Brunner, J. X., & Wolff, G. (1988). *Pulmonary function indices in critical care patients.* New York: Springer-Verlag.

Bulton, S. (1996). Clinical assessment of the cardiopulmonary system. In D. L. Frownfelter & E. Dean (Eds.), *Principles and practice of cardiopulmonary physical therapy* (3rd ed.). St Louis: Mosby.

Burke, C. M., Glanville, A. R., Theodore, J., & Robin, E. D. (1987). Lung immunogenicity, rejection, and obliterative bronchiolitis. *Chest, 92,* 547–549.

Burns, J. R., & Jones, F. L. (1975). Early ambulation of patients requiring ventilatory assistance. *Chest, 68,* 608.

Calabrese, L. H. (1991). Exercise, immunity, cancer, and infection. In C. Bouchard, R. J. Shephard, T. Stephens, J. R. Sutton, B. C. McPherson (Eds.), *Exercise, fitness, and health, A consensus of current knowledge.* Champaign, IL: Human Kinetics Books.

Campbell, J., & Ball, J. (1978). Energetics of walking in cerebral palsy. *Orthopedic Clinics of North America, 9,* 374–377.

Cane, R. D., Shapiro, B. A., & Davison, R. (1990). *Case studies in critical care medicine* (2nd ed.). Chicago: Year Book Medical Publishers.

Carrico, C. J., Meakins, J. L., & Marshall, J. C. (1993). Multiple organ failure syndrome. The gastrointestinal tract: The motor of MOF. *Archives of Surgery, 121,* 197–208.

Casciari, R. J., Fairshter, R. D., Harrison, A., Morrison, J. T., Blackburn, C., & Wilson, A. F. (1981). Effects of breathing retraining in patients with chronic obstructive pulmonary disease. *Chest, 79,* 393–398.

Chatham, K., Berrow, S., Beeson, C., Griffiths, L., Brough, D., & Musa, I. (1994). Inspiratory pressures in adult cystic fibrosis. *Physiotherapy, 80,* 748–752.

Chung, F., & Dean, E. (1989). Pathophysiology and cardiorespiratory consequences of interstitial lung disease — review and clinical implications. *Physical Therapy, 69,* 956–966.

Civetta, J. M., Taylor, R. W., & Kirby, R. R. (1988). *Critical Care.* Philadelphia: J. B. Lippincott.

Clanton, T. L., & Diaz, P. T. (1995). Clinical assessment of the respiratory muscles. *Physical Therapy, 75,* 983–995.

Clauss, R. H., Scalabrini, B. Y., Ray, R. F., & Reed, G. E. (1968). Effects of changing body position upon improved ventilation-perfusion relationships. *Circulation, 37* (Suppl. 4), 214–217.

Cotton, D. J., Graham, B. L., Mink, J. T., & Habbick, B. F. (1985). Reduction of the single breath diffusing capacity in cystic fibrosis. *European Journal of Respiratory Diseases, 66,* 173–180.

Curran, F. J. (1981). Night ventilation to body respirators for patients in chronic respiratory failure due to late stage muscular dystrophy. *Archives of Physical Medicine and Rehabilitation, 62,* 270–274.

Curran, F. J., & Colbert, A. P. (1989). Ventilator management in Duchenne muscular dystrophy and postpoliomyelitis syndrome: Twelve years' experience. *Archives of Physical Medicine and Rehabilitation, 70,* 180–185.

Dantzker, D. R. (1983). The influence of cardiovascular function on gas exchange. *Clinics in Chest Medicine, 4,* 149–159.

Dantzker, D. R. (1985). Effect of body position upon improved ventilation-perfusion relationships. *Circulation, 37* (Suppl. 4), 214–217.

Dantzker, D. R. (1988). Oxygen transport and utilization. *Respiratory Care, 33,* 874–880.

Dantzker, D. R. (1991). *Cardiopulmonary critical care* (2nd ed.). Philadelphia: W. B. Saunders.

Dantzker, D. R. (1993). Adequacy of tissue oxygenation. *Critical Care Medicine, 21,* S40–S43.

Dean, E. (1985). Effect of body position on pulmonary function. *Physical Therapy, 65,* 613–618.

Dean, E. (1987). Assessment of the peripheral circulation: An update for practitioners. *The Australian Journal of Physiotherapy, 33,* 164–172.

Dean, E. (1991). Clinical decision making in the management of the late sequelae of poliomyelitis. *Physical Therapy, 71,* 752–761.

Dean, E. (1993). Advances in rehabilitation for older persons with cardiopulmonary dysfunction. In P. R. Katz, R. L. Kane, & M. D. Mezey (Eds.), *Advances in long-term care* (Vol. 2) New York: Springer Publishing

Dean, E. (1994). Cardiopulmonary development. In B. R. Bonder, & M. B. Wagner, (Eds.), *Functional performance in older adults.* Philadelphia: F. A. Davis.

Dean, F (1994). Physiotherapy skills: Positioning and mobilization of the patient. In B. A. Webber, & J. A. Pryor, (Eds.), *Physiotherapy for respiratory and cardiac problems.* Edinburgh: Churchill Livingstone.

Dean, E. (1994). Invited commentary on 'Are incentive spirometry, intermittent positive pressure breathing, and deep breathing exercises effective in the prevention of postoperative pulmonary complications after upper abdominal surgery? A systematic overview and meta-analysis.' *Physical Therapy, 74,* 10–15.

Dean, E. (1996). Acute surgical conditions. In D. L. Frownfelter & E. Dean (Eds.), *Principles and practice of cardiopulmonary physical therapy* (3rd ed.). St Louis: Mosby.

Dean, E. (1996). Cardiopulmonary manifestations of systemic conditions. In D. L. Frownfelter & E. Dean (Eds.), *Principles and practice of cardiopulmonary physical therapy* (3rd ed.). St Louis: Mosby.

Dean, E. (1996). Monitoring systems in the intensive care unit. In D. L. Frownfelter & E. Dean (Eds.), *Principles and practice of cardiopulmonary physical therapy* (3rd ed.). St Louis: Mosby.

Dean, E. (1996). Optimizing treatment prescription: relating treatment to the underlying pathophysiology. In D. L. Frownfelter & E. Dean (Eds.), *Principles and practice of cardiopulmonary physical therapy* (3rd ed.). St Louis: Mosby.

Dean, E. (1996). Mobilization and exercise. In D. L. Frownfelter & E. Dean (Eds.), *Principles and practice of cardiopulmonary physical therapy* (3rd ed.). St Louis: Mosby.

Dean, E. (1996). Body positioning. In D. L. Frownfelter & E. Dean (Eds.), *Principles and practice of cardiopulmonary physical therapy* (3rd ed.). St Louis: Mosby.

Dean, E., Hammon, B. E., & Hobson, L. (1996). Acute medical conditions. In D. L. Frownfelter & E. Dean (Eds.), *Principles and practice of cardiopulmonary physical therapy* (3rd ed.). St Louis: Mosby.

Dean, E., & Frownfelter, D. L. (1996). Primary cardiopulmonary pathophysiology. In D. L. Frownfelter & E. Dean (Eds.), *Principles and practice of cardiopulmonary physical therapy* (3rd ed.). St Louis: Mosby.

Dean, E., & Frownfelter, D. L. (1996). Secondary cardiopulmonary pathophysiology. In D. L. Frownfelter & E. Dean (Eds.), *Principles and practice of cardiopulmonary physical therapy* (3rd ed.). St Louis: Mosby.

Dean, E. (1996). Comprehensive patient management in the intensive care unit. In D. L. Frownfelter & E. Dean (Eds.), *Principles and practice of cardiopulmonary physical therapy* (3rd ed.). St Louis: Mosby.

Dean, E. (1996). ICU management of primary cardiopulmonary dysfunction. In D. L. Frownfelter & E. Dean (Eds.), *Principles and practice of cardiopulmonary physical therapy* (3rd ed.). St Louis: Mosby.

Dean, E. (1996). ICU management of secondary cardiopulmonary dysfunction. In D. L. Frownfelter & E. Dean (Eds.), *Principles and practice of cardiopulmonary physical therapy* (3rd ed.). St Louis: Mosby.

Dean, E. (1996). Complications, adult respiratory distress syndrome, sepsis and multiorgan system failure. In D. L. Frownfelter & E. Dean (Eds.), *Principles and practice of cardiopulmonary physical therapy* (3rd ed.). St Louis: Mosby.

Dean, E., Murphy, S., Parrent, L., & Rousseau, M. (1995). Metabolic consequences of physical therapy in critically-ill patients. *Proceedings of the world confederation of physical therapy congress*, Washington, DC: World Confederation of Physical Therapy.

Dean, E., & Ross, J. (1989). Integrating current literature in the management of cystic fibrosis: a rejoinder. *Physiotherapy Canada, 41*, 46–47.

Dean, E., & Ross, J. (1991). Effect of modified aerobic training on movement energetics in polio survivors. *Orthopedics, 14*, 1243–1246.

Dean, E., & Ross, J. (1992). Mobilization and exercise conditioning. In C. C. Zadai (Ed.), *Pulmonary management in physical therapy.* New York: Churchill Livingstone.

Dean, E., & Ross, J. (1992). Discordance between cardiopulmonary physiology and physical therapy. *Chest, 101*, 1694–1698.

Dean, E., & Ross, J. (1992). Oxygen treatment. The basis for contemporary cardiopulmonary physical therapy and its optimization with body positioning and mobilization. *Physical Therapy Practice, 1*, 34–44.

Dean, E., & Ross, J. (1993). Movement energetics of individuals with a history of poliomyelities. *Archives of Physical Medicine and Rehabilitation, 74*, 478–483.

Dean, E., & Ross, J., & MacIntyre, D. (1989). A rejoinder to 'Exercise programs for patients with post-polio syndrome: a case report.' *Physical Therapy, 69*, 695–698.

Dean, E., Ross, J., Road, J. D., Courtenay, L., & Madill, K. (1991). Pulmonary function in individuals with a history of poliomyelitis. *Chest, 100*, 118–123.

Demling, R. H. (1980). The pathogenesis of respiratory failure after trauma and sepsis. *Surgical Clinics of North America, 60*, 1373–1390.

Dickey, B. F., & Myers, A. R. (1988). Pulmonary manifestations of collagen-vascular diseases. In A. P. Fishman (Ed.), *Pulmonary diseases and disorders.* New York: McGraw-Hill.

Don, H. F., Craig, D. B., Wahba, W. M., & Couture, J. G. (1971). The measurement of gas trapped in the lungs at functional residual capacity and the effects of posture. *Anesthesiology, 35*, 582–590.

Douglas, W. W., Rehder, K., Beynen, F. M., Sessler, A., D., & Marsh, H. M. (1977). Improved oxygenation in patients with acute respiratory failure: The prone position. *American Review of Respiratory Disease, 115*, 559–566.

Downs, A. (1996). Physiological basis for airway clearance techniques. In D. L. Frownfelter & E. Dean (Eds.), *Principles and practice of cardiopulmonary physical therapy* (3rd ed.). St Louis: Mosby.

Downs, A., & Frownfelter, D. L. (1996). Clinical application of airway clearance techniques. In D. L. Frownfelter & E. Dean (Eds.), *Principles and practice of cardiopulmonary physical therapy* (3rd ed.). St Louis: Mosby.

Dresen, M. H. W., de Groot, J. R., & Bouman, L. N. (1985). Aerobic energy expenditure of handicapped children after training. *Archives of Physical Medicine and Rehabilitation, 66*, 302–306.

Dripps, R. D., & Waters, R. M. (1941). Nursing care of the surgical patient. 1. The 'stir-up.' *American Journal of Nursing, 41*, 53–34.

Druz, W. S., & Sharp, J. T. (1982). Electrical and mechanical activity of the diaphragm accompanying body position in severe chronic obstructive pulmonary disease. *American Review of Respiratory Diseases, 125*, 275–280.

Dull, J. L., & Dull, W. L. (1983). Are maximal inspiratory breathing exercises or incentive spirometry better than early mobilization after cardiopulmonary bypass surgery? *Physical Therapy, 63*, 655–659.

Dureuil, B., Viires, N., & Cantineau, J. P. (1986). Diaphragmatic contractility after upper abdominal surgery. *Journal of Applied Physiology, 61*, 1775–1780.

Ekblom, B., & Nordemar, R. (1987). Rheumatoid arthritis. In J. S. Skinner (Ed.), *Exercise testing and training for special cases.* Philadelphia: Lea & Febiger.

Epidemiology Standardization Project. American Thoracic Society. (1989). *American Review of Respiratory Diseases, 118*, 1–120.

Epstein, C. D., & Henning, R. J. (1993). Oxygen transport variables in the identification and treatment of tissue hypoxia. *Heart and Lung, 22*, 328–348.

Estenne, M., & Gorino, M. (1992). Action of the diaphragm during cough in tetraplegic subjects. *Journal of Applied Physiology, 72*, 1074–1080.

Ewing, D. J., & Clarke, B. F. (1986). Autonomic neuropathy: its diagnosis and prognosis. In P. J. Watkins (Ed.), *Clinics in endocrinology and metabolism.* London: W. B. Saunders.

Fell, T., & Cheney, F. W. (1971). Prevention of hypoxia during endotracheal suction. *Annals of Surgery, 174*, 24–28.

Fenwick, J. C., Dodek, P. M., Ronco, J. J., Phang, P. T., Wiggs, B., & Russell, J. A. (1990). Increased concentrations of plasma lactate predict pathologic dependence of oxygen consumption on oxygen delivery in patients with adult respiratory distress syndrome. *Journal of Critical Care, 5*, 81–86.

Ferris, B. G., & Pollard, D. S. (1960). Effect of deep and quiet breathing on pulmonary compliance in man. *Journal of Clinical Investigations, 39*, 143–149.

Fluck, D. C. (1966). Chest movements in hemiplegia. *Clinical Science, 31,* 382–388.

Ford, G. T., & Guenter, C. A. (1984). Toward prevention of postoperative complications. *American Review of Respiratory Diseases, 130,* 4–5.

Froelicher, V. F. (1987). *Exercise and the heart. Clinical concepts* (2nd ed.). St. Louis: Year Book Medical Publishers.

Froese, A. B., & Bryan, A. C. (1974). Effects of anesthesia and paralysis on diaphragmatic mechanics in man. *Anesthesiology, 41,* 242–255.

Frownfelter, D. L. (1996). Pulmonary function tests. In D. L. Frownfelter & E. Dean (Eds.), *Principles and practice of cardiopulmonary physical therapy* (3rd ed.). St Louis: Mosby.

Frownfelter, D. L. (1996). Arterial blood gases. In D. L. Frownfelter & E. Dean (Eds.), *Principles and practice of cardiopulmonary physical therapy* (3rd ed.). St Louis: Mosby.

Frownfelter, D. L. (1996). The patient in the community. In D. L. Frownfelter & E. Dean (Eds.), *Principles and practice of cardiopulmonary physical therapy* (3rd ed.). St Louis: Mosby.

Frownfelter, D. L., & Dean, E. (Eds.). (1996). *Principles and practice of cardiopulmonary physical therapy* (3rd ed.). St Louis: Mosby.

Frownfelter, D. L., & Massery, M. (1996). Clinical application of airway clearance techniques. In D. L. Frownfelter & E. Dean (Eds.), *Principles and practice of cardiopulmonary physical therapy* (3rd ed.). St Louis: Mosby.

Frownfelter, D. L., & Massery, M. (1996). Facilitating ventilatory patterns and breathing strategy. In D. L. Frownfelter & E. Dean (Eds.), *Principles and practice of cardiopulmonary physical therapy* (3rd ed.). St Louis: Mosby.

Fugl-Meyer, A. R., & Grimby, G. (1984). Respiration in tetraplegia and in hemiplegia: A review. *International Rehabilitation Medicine, 6,* 186–190.

Gallagher, T. J., & Civetta, J. M. (1980). Goal-directed therapy of acute respiratory failure. *Anesthesia & Analgesia, 59* (11), 831–834.

Gaskell, D. V., & Webber, B. A. (1988). *The Brompton hospital guide to chest physiotherapy* (5th ed.). Oxford: Blackwell Scientific Publications.

Gattinoni, L., Bombino, M., Pelosi, P., Lissoni, A., Pensenti, A., Fumagalli, R., & Tagliabue, M. (1989). Lung structure and function in different stages of severe adult respiratory distress syndrome. *Journal of the American Medical Association, 271,* 1772–1779.

Geddes, D. M. (1984). Chronic airflow obstruction. *Postgraduate Medicine, 60,* 194–200.

Gentilello, L., Thompson, D. A., Tonnesen, A. S., Hernandez, D., Kapadia, A. S., Allen, S. J., Houtchens, B. A., & Miner, M. E. (1988). Effect of a rotating bed on the incidence of pulmonary complications in critically ill patients. *Critical Care Medicine, 16,* 783–786.

Gibson, G. J., Pride, N. B., Davis, J. N., & Loh, L. C. (1977). Pulmonary mechanics in patients with respiratory muscle weakness. *American Review of Respiratory Diseases, 115,* 389–395.

Gilman, A. G., Goodman, L. S., & Gilman, A. (1990). *Goodman and Gilman's the pharmacological basis of therapeutics* (8th ed.). New York: Macmillan Publishing.

Glaister, D. H. (1967). The effect of posture on the distribution of ventilation and blood flow in the normal lung. *Clinical Science, 33,* 391–398.

Goldberger, E. (1990). *Essentials of clinical cardiology.* Philadelphia: J. B. Lippincott.

Gordon, S. (1994). Inside the patient-driven system. *Critical Care Nurse,* Suppl., 1–28.

Gray, I. R., (1989). Cardiovascular manifestations of collagen vascular diseases. In D. G. Julian, A. J. Camm, K. M. Fox, R. J. C. Hall, & P. A. Poole-Wilson (Eds.), *Diseases of the heart.* Philadelphia: Bailliere Tindall.

Griggs, R. C., & Donohoe, K. M. (1982). Recognition and management of respiratory insufficiency in neuromuscular disease. *Journal of Chronic Diseases, 35,* 497–500.

Grimby, G. (1974). Aspects of lung expansion in relation to pulmonary physiotherapy. *American Review of Respiratory Diseases, 110,* 145–153.

Gross, D. (1980). The effect of training on strength and endurance on the diaphragm in quadriplegia. *American Journal of Medicine, 68,* 27–35.

Gutierrez, G. (1991). Cellular energy metabolism during hypoxia. *Critical Care Medicine, 19,* 619–626.

Guyton, A. C. (1991). *Textbook of medical physiology* (8th ed.). Philadelphia: W. B. Saunders.

Hammon, W. E. (1987). Pathophysiology of chronic pulmonary disease. In D. L. Frownfelter (Ed.), *Chest physical therapy and pulmonary rehabilitation* (2nd ed.). Chicago: Year Book Medical Publishers.

Hanson, P., & Nagle, F. (1987). Isometric exercise: Cardiovascular responses in normal and cardiac populations. In Hansen, P. (Ed.), *Exercise and the heart.* Philadelphia: W. B. Saunders.

Hapke, E. J., Meek, J. C., & Jacobs, J. (1972). Pulmonary function in progressive muscular dystrophy. *Chest, 61,* 41–47.

Harkcom, T. M., Lampman, R. M., Branwell, B. F., & Castor, C. W. (1985). Therapeutic value of graded aerobic exercise training in rheumatoid arthritis. *Arthritis and Rheumatism, 28,* 32–39.

Hasani, A., Pavia, D., Agnew, J. E., & Clarke, S. W. (1991). The effect of unproductive coughing/PET on regional mucus movement in the human lungs. *Respiratory Medicine, 85,* 23–26.

Hayes, M. A., Yau, E. H. S., Timmins, A. C., Hinds, C. J., & Watson, D. (1993). Response of critically-ill patients to treatment aimed at achieving supranormal oxygen delivery and consumption. *Chest, 103,* 886–895.

Hedenstierna, G., Standberg, A., Brismar, B., Lundquist, H., Svenson, L., & Tokics, L. (1985). Functional residual capacity, thoracoabdominal dimensions and central blood volume during general anesthesia with muscle paralysis and mechanical ventilation. *Anesthesiology, 62,* 247–254.

Hedenstierna, G., Tokics, L., Strandberg, A., Lundquist, H., & Brismar, B. (1986). Correlation of gas exchange impairment to development of atelectasis during anaesthesia and muscle paralysis. *Acta Anaesthesiologica Scandinavica, 30,* 183–191.

Hietpas, B. G., Roth, R. D., & Jensen, W. M. (1979). Huff coughing and airway patency. *Respiratory Care, 24,* 710.

Hillegass, E. A., & Sadowsky, H. S. (Eds.), (1994). *Essentials of cardiopulmonary physical therapy.* Philadelphia: W. B. Saunders.

Hoeppner, V. H., Cockcroft, D. W., Dosman, J. A., & Cotton, D. J. (1984). Nighttime ventilation improves respiratory failure in secondary kyphoscoliosis. *American Review of Respiratory Diseases, 129,* 240–243.

Holten, K. (1972). Training effect in patients with severe ventilary failure. *Scandinavian Journal of Respiratory Diseases, 53,* 65–76.

Howard, R. S., Wiles, C. M., & Spencer, G. T. (1988). The late sequelae of poliomyelitis. *Quarterly Journal of Medicine, 66,* 219–232.

Hunt, B., & Geddes, D. M. (1985). Newly diagnosed cystic fibrosis in middle and later life. *Thorax, 40,* 23–26.

Imle, P. C. & Klemic, N. (1989). Changes with immobility and methods of mobilization. In C. F. Mackenzie, P. C. Imle, & N. Ciesla (Eds.), *Chest physiotherapy in the intensive care unit,* (2nd ed.). Baltimore: Williams & Wilkins.

Inkley, S. R., Alderberg, F. C., & Vignos, P. C. (1974). Pulmonary function in Duchenne muscular dystrophy related to stage of disease. *American Journal of Medicine, 56,* 297–306.

Irwin, S., & Teeklin, J. S. (Eds.), (1995). *Cardiopulmonary physical therapy* (3rd ed.). St Louis: Mosby.

Jardin, F., Farcot, J. C., Boisante, L., Curien, N., Margairaz, A., & Bourdarias, J. P. (1981). Influence of positive end-expiratory pressure on left ventricular performance. *New England Journal of Medicine, 304,* 387–392.

Jernudd-Wilhelmsson, Y., Hornblad, Y., & Hedenstierna, G. (1986). Ventilation perfusion relationships in interstitial lung disease. *European Journal of Respiratory Disease, 68,* 39–49.

Juergens, J. L., Spittell, J. A., & Fairbairn, J. F. (1980). *Peripheral vascular diseases* (5th ed.). Philadelphia: W. B. Saunders.

Kaneko, K., Milic-Emili, J., Dolovich, M. B., Dawson, A., & Bates, D. V. (1966). Regional distribution of ventilation and perfusion as a function of body position. *Journal of Applied Physiology, 21,* 767–777.

Kariman, K., & Burns, S. R. (1985). Regulation of tissue oxygen extraction is disturbed in adult respiratory distress syndrome. *American Review of Respiratory Diseases, 132,* 109–114.

Keens, T. G., Krastins, I. R. B., Wannamaker, E. M., Levison, H., Crozier, D. N., & Bryan, A. C. (1977). Ventilatory muscle endurance training in normal subjects and patients with cystic fibrosis. *American Review of Respiratory Diseases, 116,* 853–860.

Kilborn, K. H., Eagan, J. T., Sieker, H. O., & Heyman, A. (1959). Cardiopulmonary insufficiency in myotonic and progressive muscular dystrophy. *New England Journal of Medicine, 261,* 1089–1096.

Kirilloff, L. H., Owens, G. R., Rogers, R. M., & Mazzocco, M. C. (1985). Does chest physical therapy work? *Chest, 88,* 436–444.

Kollberg, H. (1988). Cystic fibrosis and physical activity. *International Journal of Sports Medicine, 9* (Suppl. 1), 1–64.

Krug, P. (1996). Exercise testing and training: Secondary cardiopulmonary dysfunction. In D. L. Frownfelter & E. Dean (Eds.), *Principles and practice of cardiopulmonary physical therapy* (3rd ed.). St Louis: Mosby.

Kumar, A., Pontoppiaan, H., Falke, K. J., Wilson, R. S., & Laver, M. B. (1973). Pulmonary barotrauma during mechanical ventilation. *Critical Care Medicine, 1,* 181–186.

Landau, L. I., & Phelan, P. D. (1973). The spectrum of cystic fibrosis. *American Review of Respiratory Diseases, 108,* 593–602.

Lane, D. J., Hazleman, B., & Nichols, P. J. R. (1974). Late onset respiratory failure in patients with previous poliomyelitis. *Quarterly Journal of Medicine, 43,* 551–568.

Lange, R. A., Katz, J., McBridge, W., Moore, D. M., & Hillis, L. D. (1988). Effects of supine and lateral positions on cardiac output and intracardiac pressures. *American Journal of Cardiology, 62,* 330–333.

Langer, M., Mascheroni, D., Marcolin, R., & Gattinoni, L. (1988). The prone position in ARDS patients. A clinical study. *Chest, 94,* 103–107.

Langou, R. A., Wolfson, S., Olson, E. G., & Cohen, L. S. (1977). Effects of orthostatic postural changes on myocardial oxygen demands. *American Journal of Cardiology, 39,* 418–421.

Leaver, H., Conway, J. H., & Holgate, S. T. (1994). The incidence of post-operative hypoxaemia following lobectomy and pneumonectomy: A pilot study. *Physiotherapy, 80,* 521–527.

Leblanc, P., Ruff, F., & Milic-Emili, J. (1970). Effects of age and body position on 'airway closure' in man. *Journal of Applied Physiology, 28,* 448–451.

Leon, A. S. (1987). Diabetes. In J. S. Skinner (Ed.), *Exercise testing and exercise prescription for special cases. Theoretical basis and clinical application.* Philadelphia: Lea & Febiger.

Levine, R. D. (1984). *Anesthesiology. A manual for medical students.* Philadelphia: J. B. Lippincott.

Levine, S. A., & Lown, B. (1952). 'Armchair' treatment of acute coronary thrombosis. *Journal of the American Medical Association, 148,* 1365–1369.

Lewis, F. R. (1980). Management of atelectasis and pneumonia. *Surgical Clinics of North America, 60,* 1391–1401.

Lipman, R. L. (1972). Glucose tolerance during decreased physical activity in man. *Diabetes, 21,* 101–105.

Lisboa, C., Moreno, R., Fava, M., Ferreti, R., & Cruz, E. (1985). Inspiratory muscle function in patients with severe kyphoscoliosis. *American Review of Respiratory Diseases, 132,* 48–52.

Ludwick, S. (1996). Exercise testing and training: Primary cardiopulmonary dysfunction. In D. L. Frownfelter & E. Dean (Eds.), *Principles and practice of cardiopulmonary physical therapy* (3rd ed.). St Louis: Mosby.

Mackenzie, C. F., Shin, B., Hadi, F., & Imle, P. C. (1980). Changes in total lung/thorax compliance following chest physiotherapy. *Anesthesia & Analgesia, 59,* 207–210.

Mackenzie, C. F., Imle, P. C., & Ciesla, N. (1989). *Chest physiotherapy in the intensive care unit* (2nd ed.). Baltimore: Williams & Wilkins.

Macklem, P. T., & Roussos, C. S. (1977). Respiratory muscle fatigue: A cause of respiratory failure? *Clinical Science & Molecular Medicine, 53,* 419–422.

Make, B. (1983). Medical management of emphysema. *Clinics in Chest Medicine, 4,* 465–482.

Malamed, S. F. (1989). *Sedation. A guide to patient management* (2nd ed.). St. Louis: Mosby.

Malouin, F., Potvin, M., Prevost, J., Richards, C. L., & Wood-Dauphinee, S. (1992). Use of an intensive task-oriented gait training program in a series of patients with acute cerebrovascular accidents. *Physical Therapy, 72,* 781–793.

Mansell, A., Dubrawsky, C., Levison, H., Bryan, A. C., & Crozier, D. N. (1974). Lung elastic recoil in cystic fibrosis. *American Review of Respiratory Diseases, 109,* 190–197.

Marini, J. J. (1984). Postoperative atelectasis: Pathophysiology, clinical importance, and principles of management. *Respiratory Care, 29,* 516–528.

Marini, J. J., & Wheeler, A. P. (1989). *Critical Care Medicine—The Essentials.* Baltimore: Williams & Wilkins.

Matthay, R. A., Bromberg, S. I., & Putman, A. M. (1980). Pulmonary-renal syndromes—a review. *Yale Journal of Biology and Medicine, 53,* 497–523.

Matthay, M. A. (Ed.). (1985). Pathophysiology of pulmonary edema. *Clinics in Chest Medicine, 6,* 301–314.

McArdle, W. D., Katch, F. I., & Katch, V. L. (1991). *Exercise physiology. Energy, nutrition, and performance* (3rd ed.). Philadelphia: Lea & Febiger.

McAslan, T. C., & Cowley, R. A. (1979). The preventive use of PEEP in major trauma. *American Surgeon, 45,* 159–167.

McCook, F. D., & Tzelepis, G. E. (1995). Inspiratory muscle training in the patient with neuromuscular diseases. *Physical Therapy, 75,* 1006–1114.

Mendelson, L. S. (1996). Care of the patient with an artificial airway. In: D. L. Frownfelter & E. Dean (Eds.), *Principles and practice of cardiopulmonary physical therapy* (3rd ed.). St Louis: Mosby.

Moerchen, V. A., & Crane, L. (1996). Cardiopulmonary physical therapy for neonatal and pediatric patients. In D. L. Frownfelter & E. Dean (Eds.), *Principles and practice of cardiopulmonary physical therapy* (3rd ed.). St Louis: Mosby.

Moerchen, V. A., & Crane, L. D. (1996). The neonatal and pediatric patient. In D. L. Frownfelter & E. Dean (Eds.), *Principles and practice of cardiopulmonary physical therapy* (3rd ed.). St Louis: Mosby.

Moorman, J. R., Coleman, E., Packer, D. L., Kisslo, J. A., Bell, J., Hettlemna, B. C., Stajich, Mossberg, K. A., Linton, K. A. J., & Roses, A. D. (1985). Cardiac involvement in myotonic muscular dystrophy. *Medicine, 64,* 371–387.

Mossberg, K. A., Linton, K. A., Friske, K. (1990). Ankle-foot orthoses: Effect of energy expenditure of aids in spastic diplegia children. *Archives of Physical Medicine and Rehabilitation, 71,* 490–494.

Moylan, J. A. (Ed.). (1988). *Trauma Survey.* Philadelphia: J. B. Lippincott.

Muller, N., Volgyesi, G., Becker, L., Bryan, M. H., & Bryan, A. C. (1979). Diaphragmatic muscle tone. *Journal of Applied Physiology, 47,* 279–284.

Muller, R. E., Petty, T. L., & Filley, G. F. (1970). Ventilation and arterial blood gas changes induced by pursed-lip breathing. *Journal of Applied Physiology, 28,* 784–789.

Murray, E. (1993). Anyone for pulmonary rehabilitation? *Physiotherapy, 79,* 705–710.

Murray, J. E., & Nadel, J. A. (1988). *Textbook of respiratory medicine, Part 1.* Philadelphia: W. B. Saunders.

Murray, J. E., & Nadel, J. A. (1988). *Textbook of respiratory medicine, Part 2.* Philadelphia: W. B. Saunders.

Murray, J. F. (1979). The ketchup-bottle method. *New England Journal of Medicine, 300,* 1155–1157.

Nakano, K. K., Bass, H., Tyler, H. R., & Carmel, R. J. (1976). Amyotrophic lateral sclerosis: A study of pulmonary function. *Diseases of the nervous system, 37,* 32–35.

Neiderman, M. S., Clemente, P. H., Fein, A. M., Feinsilver, S. H., Robinson, D. A., Howite, J. S., & Bernstein, M. G. (1991). Benefits of a multidisciplinary pulmonary rehabilitation program: Improvements are independent of lung function. *Chest, 99,* 798–804.

Nightingale, P. (1993). Optimization of oxygen transport to the tissues. *Acta Anaesthesiologica Scandinavica, 98,* 32–36.

Nunn, J. F. (1989). The influence of anesthesia on the respiratory system. In K. Reinhart & K. Eyrich (Eds.), *Clinical aspect of O_2 transport and tissue oxygenation.* New York: Springer-Verlag.

Nunn, J. F., Coleman, A. J., Sachithanandan, T., Bergman, N. A., & Laws, J. W. (1965). Hypoxaemia and atelectasis produced by forced expiration. *British Journal of Anesthesia, 37,* 3–12.

Oldenburg, F. A., Dolovich, M. B., Montgomery, J. M., & Newhouse, M. T. (1979). Effects of postural drainage, exercise, and cough on mucus clearance in chronic bronchitis. *American Review of Respiratory Diseases, 120,* 739–745.

Orlava, O. E. (1959). Therapeutic physical culture in the complex treatment of pneumonia. *Physical Therapy Review, 39,* 153–160.

Painter, P. L., Nelson-Worel, J. N., Hill, M. M., Thornbery, D. R., Shelp, W. R., Harrington, A. R., & Winstein, A. B. (1986). Effects of exercise training during hemodialysis. *Nephron, 43,* 87–92.

Pallares, L. C. M., & Evans, T. W. (1992). Oxygen transport in the critically ill. *Respiratory Medicine, 86,* 289–295.

Pape, H. C., Regel, G., Borgman, W., Sturm, J. A., & Tacherne, H. (1994). The effect of kinetic positioning on lung function and pulmonary haemodynamics in posttraumatic ARDS: A clinical study. *International Journal of the Care of the Injured, 25,* 51–57.

Pardy, R. L., & Leith, D. E. (1984). Ventilatory muscle training. *Respiratory Care, 29,* 278–284.

Perez-Padilla, R., West, P., & Lertzman, M. (1985). Breathing during sleep in patients with interstitial lung disease. *American Review of Respiratory Diseases, 132,* 224–229.

Perloff, J. K., de Leon, A. C., & O'Doherty, D. (1966). The cardiomyopathy of progressive muscular dystrophy. *Circulation, 33,* 625–648.

Petty, T. L. (1982). *Intensive and rehabilitative respiratory care* (3rd ed.). Philadelphia: Lea & Febiger.

Petty, T. L. (1985). *Chronic obstructive pulmonary disease* (2nd ed.). New York: Marcel Dekker.

Phang, P. T., & Russell, J. A. (1993). When does Vo_2 depend on Do_2? *Respiratory Care, 38,* 618–630.

Piehl, M. A., & Brown, R. S. (1976). Use of extreme position changes in acute respiratory failure. *Critical Care Medicine, 4,* 13–14.

Poelaert, J., Lannoy, B., Volegaers, D., Evaert, J., Decruyenaere, J., Capiau, P., & Colardyn, F. (1991). Influence of chest physiotherapy on arterial oxygen saturation. *Acta Anaesthesiologica Belgica, 42,* 165–170.

Prakash, R., Parmley, W. W., Dikshit, K., Forrester, J., & Swan, H. J. (1973). Hemodynamic effects of postural changes in patients with acute myocardial infarction. *Chest, 64,* 7–9.

Protas, B. (1996). The aging patient. In D. L. Frownfelter & E. Dean (Eds.), *Principles and practice of cardiopulmonary physical therapy* (3rd ed.). St Louis: Mosby.

Pryor, J. A. (1991). Respiratory care. Edinburgh: Churchill Livingstone.

Pyne, D. B. (1994). Regulation of neutrophil function during exercise. *Sports Medicine, 17,* 245–258.

Rankin, J. A., & Matthay, R. R. (1982). Pulmonary renal syndromes. II. Etiology and pathogenesis. *Yale Journal of Biology and Medicine, 55,* 11–26.

Ray, J. F., III, Yost, L., Moallem, S., Sanoudos, G. M., Villamena, P., Paredes, R. M., & Clauss, R. H. (1974). Immobility, hypoxemia, and pulmonary arteriovenous shunting. *Archives of Surgery, 109,* 537–541.

Reid, W. D., & Dechman, G. (1995). Considerations when testing and training respiratory muscles. *Physical Therapy, 75,* 971–982.

Reid, W. D., & Samrai, B. (1995). Respiratory muscle training for patients with chronic obstructive lung disease. *Physical Therapy, 75,* 996–1005.

Reid, W. D., & Warren, C. P. W. (1984). Ventilatory muscle strength and endurance training in elderly subjects and patients with chronic airflow limitation: A pilot study. *Physiotherapy Canada, 36,* 305–311.

Ries, A. L., Ellis, B., & Hawkins, R. W. (1988). Upper extremity exercise training in chronic obstructive pulmonary disease. *Chest, 93,* 688–692.

Remolina, C., Khan, A. U., Santiago, T. V., & Edelman, N. H. (1981). Positional hypoxemia in unilateral lung disease. *New England Journal of Medicine, 304,* 523–525.

Rochester, D. F., & Arora, N. S. (1983). Respiratory muscle failure. *Medical Clinics of North America, 67,* 573–597.

Rochester, D. F., & Essau, S. A. (1984). Malnutrition and the respiratory system. *Chest, 85,* 411–415.

Ross, J., Bates, D. V., Dean, E., & Abboud, J. T. (1992). Discordance of airflow limitation and ventilation inhomogeneity in asthma and cystic fibrosis. *Clinical and Investigative Medicine, 15,* 97–102.

Ross, J., & Dean, E. (1989). Integrating physiological principles into the comprehensive management of cardiopulmonary dysfunction. *Physical Therapy, 69,* 255–259.

Ross, J., & Dean, E. (1992). Body positioning. In C. C. Zadai (Ed.), *Pulmonary management in physical therapy.* New York: Churchill Livingstone.

Ross, J., Dean, E., & Abboud, R. T. (1992). The effects of postural drainage positioning on ventilation homogeneity in healthy subjects. *Physical Therapy, 72,* 794–799.

Roukonen, E., Takala, J., & Kari, A. (1991). Septic shock and multiple organ failure. *Critical Care Medicine, 19,* 1146–1151.

Roussos, C. S., Fixley, M., Geriest, J., Cosio, M., Kelly, S., Martin, R. R., & Engel, L. A. (1977). Voluntary factors influencing the distribution of inspired gas. *American Review of Respiratory Diseases, 116,* 457–467.

Sannerstedt, R. (1987). Hypertension. In J. S. Skinner (Ed.), *Exercise testing and exercise prescription for special cases. Theoretical basis and clinical application.* Philadelphia: Lea & Febiger.

Scharf, S. M., & Cassidy, S. S. (Eds.). (1989). *Heart-lung interactions in health and disease.* New York: Marcel Dekker.

Sciaky, A. (1996). Patient education. In D. L. Frownfelter & E. Dean (Eds.), *Principles and practice of cardiopulmonary physical therapy* (3rd ed.). St Louis: Mosby.

Sciaky, A. (1996). Principles and practice of cardiopulmonary patient education. In D. L. Frownfelter & E. Dean (Eds.), *Principles and practice of cardiopulmonary physical therapy* (3rd ed.). St Louis: Mosby.

Scott, T. E., Wise, R. A., Hochberg, M. C., & Wigley, F. M. (1987). HLA-DR4 and pulmonary dysfunction in rheumatoid arthritis. *The American Journal of Medicine, 82,* 765–771.

Seaton, D., Lapp, N. I., & Morgan, W. K. C. (1979). Effect of body position on gas exchange after thoracotomy. *Thorax, 34,* 518–522.

Segal, A. M., Calabrese, L. H., Ahmad, M., Tubbs, R. R., & White, C. S. (1985). The pulmonary manifestations of systemic lupus erythematosus. *Seminars in Arthritis and Rheumatism, 14,* 202–224.

Shephard, R. J., Verde, T. J., Thomas, S. G., & Shek, P. (1991). Physical activity and the immune system. *Canadian Journal of Sports Science, 16,* 163–185.

Shoemaker, W. C. (Ed.). (1984). *Critical care: State of the art.* Fullerton, CA: Society of Critical Care Medicine.

Shoemaker, W. C., Thompson, W. L., & Holbrook, P. R. (Eds.). (1984). *Textbook of critical care.* Philadelphia: W. B. Saunders.

Sinha, R., & Bergofsky, E. H. (1972). Prolonged alteration of lung mechanics in kyphoscoliosis by positive pressure hyperinflation. *American Review of Respiratory Diseases, 106,* 47–57.

Smith, P. E. M., Calverley, P. M. A., Edwards, R. H. T., Evans, G. A., & Campbell, E. J. M. (1987). Practical problems in the respiratory care of patients with muscular dystrophy. *New England Journal of Medicine, 316,* 1197–1205.

Smith, P. E. M., Edwards, R. H. T., & Calverley, P. M. A. (1989). Oxygen treatment of sleep hypoxaemia in Duchenne muscular dystrophy. *Thorax, 44,* 997–1001.

Smith, E. L., Smith, K. A., & Gilligan, C. (1991). Exercise, fitness, osteoarthritis, and osteoporosis. In C. Bouchard, R. J. Shephard, J. R. Sutton, & B. C. McPherson (Eds.), *Exercise, fitness, and health. A consensus of current knowledge.* Champaign, IL: Human Kinetics Books.

Sokolow, M., McIlroy, M. B., & Cheitlin, M. D. (1990). *Clinical cardiology* (5th ed.). Norwalk: Appleton & Lange.

Sonnenblick, E. H., Ross, J., Jr., & Brauwald, E. (1968). Oxygen consumption of the heart. Newer concepts of its multifactorial determination. *American Journal of Cardiology, 22,* 328–336.

Stillwell, S. (1992). *Critical care nursing reference.* St Louis: Mosby.

Stokes, D. C., Wohl, M. E. B., Khaw, K. T., & Strieder, D. J. (1985). Postural hypoxemia in cystic fibrosis. *Chest, 87,* 785–789.

Sutton, P. P., Pavia, D., Bateman, J. R. M., & Clarke, S. W. (1982). Chest physiotherapy—a review. *European Journal of Respiratory Disease, 63,* 188–201.

Underhill, S. L., Woods, S. L., Froelicher, E. S. S., & Halpenny, C. J. (1989). *Cardiac nursing* (2nd ed.). Philadelphia: J. B. Lippincott.

Veis, S. L., & Logemann, J. A. (1985). Swallowing disorders in persons with cardiovascular accident. *Archives of Physical Medicine and Rehabilitation, 66,* 372–375.

Vignos, P. J., & Watkins, M. P. (1966). The effects of exercise in muscular dystrophy. *Journal of the American Medical Association, 197,* 843–848.

Vincent, J. L., & Suter, P. M. (1987). *Cardiopulmonary interactions in acute respiratory failure.* New York: Springer-Verlag.

Vincent, J. L. (1991). Advances in the concepts of intensive care. *American Heart Journal, 121,* 1859–1865.

Vincent, J. L. (1993). Oxygen transport in severe sepsis. *Acta Anaesthesiology Scandinavica, 37* (Suppl. 98), 29–31.

Walsh, J. M., Vanderwarf, C., Hoscheit, D., & Fahey, P. J. (1989). Unsuspected hemodynamic alterations during endotracheal suctioning. *Chest, 95,* 162–165.

Wasserman, K. L., & Whipp, B. J. (1975). Exercise physiology in health and disease. *American Review of Respiratory Diseases, 112,* 219–249.

Watchie, J. (1995). *Cardiopulmonary physical therapy. A clinical manual.* Philadelphia: W.B. Saunders.

Waxman, K., & Shoemaker, W. C. (1980). Management of postoperative and posttraumatic respiratory failure in the intensive care unit. *Surgical Clinics of North America, 60,* 1413–1428.

Webber, B.A., & Pryor, J. A. (1994). *Physiotherapy for respiratory and cardiac problems.* Edinburgh: Churchill Livingstone.

Weber, K. T., Janicki, J. S., Shroff, S. C., & Likoff, M. J. (1983). The cardiopulmonary unit: The body's gas exchange system. *Clinics in Chest Medicine, 4,* 101–110.

Weinstein, M. E., & Skillman, J. J. (1980). Management of severe respiratory failure. *Surgical Clinics of North America, 60,* 1403–1412.

Weissman, C., & Kemper, M. (1993). Stressing the critically ill patient: The cardiopulmonary and metabolic responses to an acute increase in oxygen consumption. *Journal of Critical Care, 8,* 100–108.

Weissman, C., Kemper, M., Damask, M. C., Askanazi, J., Hyman, A. I., & Kinney, J. M. (1984). Effect of routine intensive care interactions on metabolic rate. *Chest, 86,* 815–818.

Weissman, C., Kemper, M., Elwyn, D. H., Askanzi, J., Hyman, A. I., & Kinney, J. M. (1989). The energy expenditure of the mechanically ventilated critically ill patient. *Chest, 2,* 254–259.

West, J. B. (1995). *Respiratory physiology—The essentials* (5th ed.). Baltimore: Williams & Wilkins.

West, J. B. (1987). *Pulmonary pathophysiology.* Baltimore: Williams & Wilkins.

Whipp, B. J., & Ward, S. A. (1982). Cardiopulmonary coupling during exercise. *Journal of Experimental Biology, 100,* 175–193.

Wilson, J. D., Braunwald, E., Isselbacher, K. J., Martin, J. B., Fauci, A. S., & Root, R. K. (Eds.). *Harrison's principles of internal medicine* (12th ed.). St. Louis: McGraw-Hill.

Wilson, R. F. (1992). *Critical care manual* (2nd ed.). Philadelphia: F. A. Davis.

Wolff, R. K., Dolovich, M. B., Obminski, G., & Newhouse, M. T. (1977). Effects of exercise and eucapnic hyperventilation on bronchial clearance in man. *Journal of Applied Physiology, 43,* 46–50.

Wood, R. E., Wanner, A., Hirsch, J., & Farrell, P. M. (1975). Tracheal mucociliary transport in patients with cystic fibrosis and its stimulation by terbutlaine. *American Review of Respiratory Diseases, 111,* 733–738.

Wright, P. C. (1984). Fundamentals of acute burn care and physical therapy management. *Physical Therapy, 64,* 1217–1231.

Wysocki, M., Besbes, M., Roupie, E., & Brun-buisson, C. (1992). Modification of oxygen extraction ratio by change in oxygen transport in septic shock. *Chest, 102,* 221–226.

Yu, M., Levy, M. M., Smith, P., Takiguchi, S. A., Miyasaki, A., & Myers, S. A. (1993). Effect of maximizing oxygen delivery on morbidity and mortality rates in critically ill patients: A prospective, randomized, controlled study. *Critical Care Medicine, 21,* 830–838.

Zach, M., Oberwaldner, B., & Hausler, F. (1982). Cystic fibrosis: Physical exercise versus chest physiotherapy. *Archives of Diseases in Children, 57,* 587–589.

Zack, M. B., Pontoppidan, H., & Kazemi, H. (1974). The effect of lateral positions on gas exchange in pulmonary disease. *American Review of Respiratory Diseases, 110,* 149–153.

Zadai, C. C. (Ed.), (1992). *Clinics in physical therapy. Pulmonary management in physical therapy.* New York: Churchill Livingstone.

Zinman, R. (1984). Cough versus chest physiotherapy. *American Review of Respiratory Diseases, 129,* 182–184.

ZuWallack, R. L., Patel, K., Reardon, J. Z., Clark, B. A., & Normandin, E. A. (1991). Predictors of improvement in the 12-minute walking distance following a six-week outpatient pulmonary rehabilitation program. *Chest, 99,* 805–808.